Dr Agarwals' Textbook on
CORNEAL TOPOGRAPHY

Dr Agarwals' Textbook on
CORNEAL
TOPOGRAPHY

Editors

Sunita Agarwal
Athiya Agarwal
Amar Agarwal

Associate Editors
Soosan Jacob
Nilesh Kanjani
Neera Kanjani

Dr Agarwal's Group of Eye Hospitals and
Eye Research Centre
Chennai, Bangalore, Jaipur, Trichy, Salem (India)

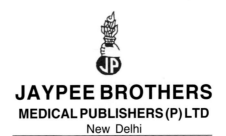

JAYPEE BROTHERS
MEDICAL PUBLISHERS (P) LTD
New Delhi

Published by

Jitendar P Vij

Jaypee Brothers Medical Publishers (P) Ltd

EMCA House, 23/23B Ansari Road, Daryaganj

New Delhi 110 002, India

Phones: +91-11-23272143, +91-11-23272703, +91-11-23282021, +91-11-23245672

Fax: +91-11-23276490, +91-11-23245683   e-mail: jaypee@jaypeebrothers.com

Visit our website: www.jaypeebrothers.com

Branches

- 202 Batavia Chambers, 8 Kumara Krupa Road, Kumara Park East,
  Bangalore 560 001, Phones: +91-80-22285971, +91-80-22382956, +91-80-30614073
  Tele Fax: +91-80-22281761   e-mail: jaypeebc@bgl.vsnl.net.in
- 282 IIIrd Floor, Khaleel Shirazi Estate, Fountain Plaza
  Pantheon Road, **Chennai** 600 008, Phones: +91-44-28262665, +91-44-28269897
  Fax: +91-44-28262331   e-mail: jpchen@eth.net
- 4-2-1067/1-3, Ist Floor, Balaji Building, Ramkote
  Cross Road, **Hyderabad** 500 095, Phones: +91-40-55610020, +91-40-24758498
  Fax: +91-40-24758499   e-mail: jpmedpub@rediffmail.com
- 1A Indian Mirror Street, Wellington Square, **Kolkata** 700 013,
  Phones: +91-33-22456075, +91-33-22451926 Fax: +91-33-22456075
  e-mail: jpbcal@cal.vsnl.net.in
- 106 Amit Industrial Estate, 61 Dr SS Rao Road, Near MGM Hospital
  Parel, **Mumbai** 400 012, Phones: +91-22-24124863, +91-22-24104532, +91-22-30926896
  Fax: +91-22-24160828   e-mail: jpmedpub@bom7.vsnl.net.in
  e-mail: jpmedpub@bom7.vsnl.net.in
- Kamalpushpa, 38 Reshimbag, Opp. Mohota Science College, Umred Road
  Nagpur 440 009, Phone: +91-0712-3945220

Dr Agarwals' Textbook on Corneal Topography

This book has been published in good faith that the material provided by contributors is original. Every effort is made to ensure accuracy of material, but the publisher, printer and editors will not be held responsible for any inadvertent error(s). In case of any dispute, all legal matters to be settled under Delhi jurisdiction only.

First Edition: **2006**

ISBN   81-8061-630-4

Typeset at   JPBMP typesetting unit
Printed at   Gopsons Papers Ltd., Noida.

This book is dedicated to

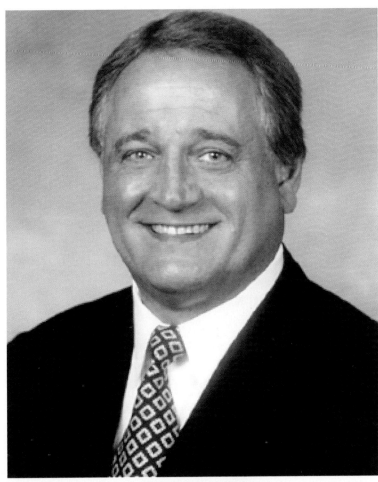

JACK HOLLADAY

for being a great friend and an even greater human being

Contributors

Guillermo L Simón
Chief Anterior Segment Surgeon
Refractive Surgery Unit
Simon Eye Clinic
Barcelona, Spain

Dra Sarabel Simón
Simon Eye Clinic
Barcelona, Spain

José Ma Simón
Chairman
Simon Eye Clinic
Barcelona, Spain

Dra Cristina Simón
Simon Eye Clinic
Barcelona, Spain

J Agarwal, FORCE DO FICS
Dr Agarwal's Group of Eye Hospitals & Eye Research Centre
Chennai, Bangalore, Jaipur, Trichy, Salem
19 Cathedral road, Chennai-600 086, India

Amar Agarwal, MS FRCS FRCOphth
Dr Agarwal's Group of Eye Hospitals & Eye Research Centre
Chennai, Bangalore, Jaipur, Trichy, Salem
19 Cathedral road, Chennai-600 086, India

Athiya Agarwal, MD FRSH DO
Dr Agarwal's Group of Eye Hospitals & Eye Research Centre
Chennai, Bangalore, Jaipur, Trichy, Salem
19 Cathedral road, Chennai-600 086, India

Sunita Agarwal, MS FSVH DO
Dr Agarwal's Group of Eye Hospitals & Eye Research Centre
Chennai, Bangalore, Jaipur, Trichy, Salem
19 Cathedral road, Chennai-600 086, India

Gregg Feinerman, MD FACS
Feinerman Vision Center
320 Superior Avenue, Suite #350
Newport Beach, California 92663, USA
(949) 631-4780 Phone
(949) 631-7854 Fax
www.FeinermanVision.com

N Timothy Peters, MD FACS
Clear Advantage Vision Correction Center
30 Borthwick Ave Suite 306
Portsmouth, New Hampshire 03801, USA

Kim Nguyen
USA

Sheila Scott
USA

Francisco Sánchez León, MD
Instituto NovaVision
Medical Director
Cornea, Refractive and Anterior Segment Clinic
Cd de México, Acapulco, Mexico
pacornea@yahoo.com

Tracy Schroeder Swartz, OD MS
Wang Vision Institute
Adjunct Faculty
Indiana University School of Optometry
Bloomington, IN, USA

Ming Wang, MD PhD
Clinical Associate Professor of Ophthalmology
University of Tennessee
Staff physician
Thomas Hospital
Director, Wang Vision Institute, USA

Arun C Gulani, MD MS
Director,
Gulani Vision Institute
4500 Salisbury Rd. Suite 160
Jacksonville, Florida, USA

Soosan Jacob, MS FRCS DNB MNAMS
Dr Agarwal's Group of Eye Hospitals & Eye Research Centre
Chennai, Bangalore, Jaipur, Trichy, Salem (India)
19 Cathedral road, Chennai-600 086, India

Nilesh Kanjani, DO DNB FERC
Dr Agarwal's Group of Eye Hospitals & Eye Research Centre
Chennai, Bangalore, Jaipur, Trichy, Salem (India)
19 Cathedral road, Chennai-600 086, India

Jorge L Alió, MD, PhD
Instituto Oftalmologico De Alicante
Alicante, Spain

José I Belda Sanchis, MD PhD
Instituto Oftalmologico De Alicante
Alicante, Spain

Ahmad MM Shalaby, MD
Instituto Oftalmologico De Alicante
Alicante, Spain

Erik L Mertens, MD FEBO
Medical Director
Antwerp Eye Center
Kapelstraat 8, B-2660 Antwerp
Belgium

Paul Karpecki, OD
Director of Research
Moyes Eye Center
Kansas City, USA

Guillermo Avalos, MD
Guadalajara, Mexico

Noel A Alpins, FRACO FRCOphth FACS
Australia

Gemma Walsh B Optom
Australia

Masanao Fujieda, MA
Nidek Ltd., Co., Japan

Mukesh Jain, PhD
Nidek Ltd., Co., Japan

Peter Keller, PhD
Department of Optometry & Vision Sciences
University of Melbourne, Australia

Roberto Pinelli, MD
Scientific Director
Instituto Laser Microchirurgia Oculare
Crystal Palace
Via Cefalonia 70
25124 Brescia, Italy
Ph. +39 030 2428343
Fax. +39 030 2428248
www.ilmo.it

Terry E Burris, MD
Northwest Corneal Services
6950 SW Hampton, Suite 150
Portland, OR 97223, USA
Phone: (503) 624-4814
Fax: (503) 624-4904

Debby Holmes-Higgin, MS
Northwest Corneal Services
6950 SW Hampton, Suite 150
Portland, OR 97223, USA
Phone: (503) 624-4814
Fax: 6(503) 624-4904

T Agarwal, FORCE DO FICS
Dr Agarwal's Group of Eye Hospitals & Eye Research Centre
Chennai, Bangalore, Jaipur, Trichy, Salem (India)
19 Cathedral road, Chennai-600 086, India

Mrcus Solorzano
USA

Foreword

Computer-assisted corneal topography represents indispensable technology in today's practice of cataract and refractive surgery. Building on the foundation of keratometry and keratoscopy laid earlier by Helmholtz, Placido and Gullstrand, the quantitative analysis performed by Rowsey and especially the image enhancement and color-coded maps introduced by Klyce led to rapid adoption of corneal topography among refractive surgeons.[1] Corneal topography quickly enabled a new understanding of corneal degenerations such as keratoconus and pellucid marginal, as well as of the effects of contact lens wear and incisional keratorefractive surgery. The standard of care for all types of corneal refractive surgery has evolved to include preoperative corneal topography. More recently, the calculation of intraocular lens power in the setting or prior keratorefractive surgery has come to rely on data from corneal topography as well.[2]

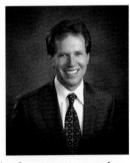

As a diagnostic and research tool corneal topography provides an essential complement to wavefront aberrometry.[3] Our ability to adapt corneal refractive procedures to minimize total postoperative aberrations, and conversely to customize intraocular lens design to complement inherent corneal aberrations both rely upon topography and aberrometry data. Additional imaging modalities such as Scheimpflug photography and anterior segment optical coherence tomography can also complement corneal topography and wavefront analysis to allow further enhancement of our understanding of diagnostic challenges.[4]

In this text, Amar Agarwal and his co-editors have assembled a wealth of knowledge and talent in the fields of cataract and refractive surgery to provide a thorough review of the state-of-the art of corneal topography and its applications. This information and experience represents a critical foundation for clinical practice. The development and commercial availability of new technology always poses a dilemma to the practising surgeon: the question of when and whether to make a potentially large financial investment and perhaps an even greater clinical commitment. This text will allow the clinicians to view the field with an experienced eye and make the best possible decision.

Mark Packer MD, FACS
Clinical Assistant Professor
Department of Ophthalmology
Oregon Health and Science University
Drs Fine, Hoffman & Packer
Eugene, OR

References

1. Wilson SE, Klyce SD. Advances in the Analysis of Corneal Topography. Surv Ophthalmol 35; 1991, 269-77.
2. Hamilton DR, Hardten DR. Cataract surgery in patients with prior refractive surgery. Curr Opin Ophthalmol 2003 Feb;14(1):44-53.
3. Marcos S, Barbero S, Jiménez-Alfaro I. Optical quality and depth-of-field of eyes implanted with spherical and aspheric intraocular lenses. J Refract Surg 2005 May-Jun;21(3):223-35.
4. Cazal J, Lavin-Dapena C, Marín J, Vergés C. Accommodative intraocular lens tilting. Am J Ophthalmol 2005 Aug;140(2):341-4.

Preface

Medical frontiers are never ending, there can be no end to division, the more you go deeper and deeper into any subject, the more we understand how little we know of it. "Multiplication ruins everything", says Lao-Tsu the author of Tao Te Ching.

However we still need to understand the lakes, mountains and valleys of the corneal surface, for us to be able to understand how to modify the surface to suit the patients refractive needs. Just as we understand the geography of the land by seeing from far its topography, so to the corneal surface.

Today we not only use the topographical analysis for our Lasik cases, with our knowledge on relaxing incisions we have stretched the doors to include cataract cases where incisions can be made to decrease the preoperative astigmatism. Wavefront technology heralds yet another dimension when the topography is fed into the Lasik machine to give us a customized ablation.

Aberrations have long played havoc with vision, and doctors world over have only now really understood where the problem really lies. The understanding has brought in better modalities of its treatment, we not only have Lasik treating aberrations, we have customized intraocular lenses taking the aberrations into consideration.

The same concept is also being used for the making of lens power to be fitted to spectacles where not only the spherical and cylindrical diopters are fed into lens power cutting machines, they are surface modified to fit the aberration as well, thus we come into an era of customized fittings of eye glass power.

Authors from all over the world give you a taste of their facts and figures with their cohesive findings for topographical documentation and assessment. To grasp a meaning into this world of multicolored charts we bring this textbook on corneal topography to keep on your desk, to enable you to read a picture effortlessly.

Sunita Agarwal
Athiya Agarwal
Amar Agarwal

Contents

Section III
Other Refractive Procedures

Section IV
Cataract

Section

I

Introduction to Corneal Topography

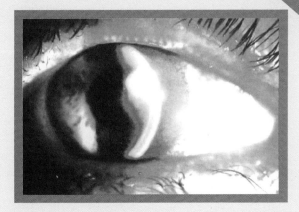

Chapter

1

Fundamentals on Corneal Topography

Guillermo L Simón Castellvi
Sarabel Simón
José Mª Simón
Cristina Simón

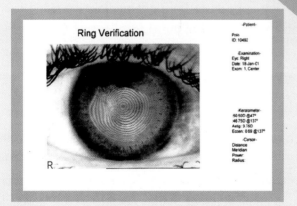

INTRODUCTION: HUMAN OPTICS AND THE NORMAL CORNEA

The cornea is the highest diopter of human eye, accounting alone for about **43-44 diopters** at corneal apex (about two thirds of the total dioptric power of the eye). It has an average **radius of curvature of 7-8 mm**. A healthy cornea is not absolutely transparent: it scatters almost 10 percent of the incident light, primarily due to the scattering at the stroma.

The corneal geography can be divided into **four geographical zones** from apex to limbus, which can be easily differentiated in color corneal videokeratoscopy:

1. The **central zone (4 central millimeters)**: it overlies the pupil and is responsible for the high definition vision. The central part is almost spherical and called **apex**.
2. The **paracentral zone**: where the cornea begins to flatten.
3. The **peripheral zone.**
4. The **limbal zone.**

Refractive surgery refers to a surgical or laser procedure performed on the cornea, to alter its refractive power. The major refractive component of the cornea being its front surface, it is not difficult to understand that most refractive techniques have involved this frontal surface (PRK, radial keratotomies, …). Nevertheless, posterior surface of the cornea also accounts, and that is the reason why a "posterior surface corneal topographer" like the Orbscan™-Bausch & Lomb® was developed by Orbtek®, in the race for a more precise refractive surgery.

The cornea of an eagle is almost as transparent as glass: there is almost no scattering of incident light. That alone explains the resolution of an eagle's eye being much better than ours. As we are never satisfied, we are now developing new tools and extremely promising laser surgical techniques that have proven to increase the human being's visual acuity by reducing corneal aberrations: we reduce diopters and also improve visual acuity. The new dream is "super-vision". Topographic and aberrometer-linked LASIK are on the way to achieve this goal of better-than-normal vision. Bausch & Lomb®'s *Zywave*™ combines topography and wavefront measurements to achieve customized computer-controlled flying spot excimer laser ablation, which appears to be fundamental in treating irregular astigmatisms or retreating unsatisfied LASIK patients to regularize the corneal shape. Regularizing the corneal shape has the theoretical advantage of improving the quality of vision by means of reduction of halos, glare and any other optical aberrations. We are on the way to achieve an aberration-free visual system, though the influence of all other dioptric surfaces (vitreous, lens, …) and interfaces still has to be ascertained.

In this chapter, we will try to introduce the novice to this interesting new world of instruments recently developed due to the advent of refractive corneal surgery. We have tried to show different maps from different systems, trying to make an interesting basic atlas of corneal topography. Corneal maps of rare cases and complications can be found in the different chapters of this book. Please refer to them for better knowledge. There is no perfect system to assess true corneal surface shape, but we still have to rely on the instruments we have, waiting for new instruments and methods being developed for better accuracy. With that goal in mind, BioShape AG® has developed the *EyeShape*™ system, based on a principle called **fringe projection**. Patterns of parallel lines are first imaged onto a reference and then onto the surface to be measured. Detection of the lines with a digital camera under a tilted angle yields distorted line patterns. The deviation of the detected lines from the original lines together with the tilt make it possible to calculate the absolute height at any point on the surface of the cornea (or not).

INSTRUMENTS TO MEASURE THE CORNEAL SURFACE

The normal corneal surface is smooth: a healthy tear film neutralizes corneal irregularities. The cornea, acting as a convex "almost transparent" mirror, reflects part of the incident light. Different instruments have been developed to assess and measure this corneal reflex. These noncontact instruments use a light target (lamp, mires, Placido disks, …) and a microscope or another optic system to measure corneal reflex of these light targets.

Keratometry

A keratometer **quantitatively** measures the radius of curvature of different corneal zones of 3 mm (diameter). The present-day keratometer allows the operator to precisely measure the size of the reflected image, converting the image size to corneal radius using a mathematical relation $r = 2\,a\,Y/y$ where

    r : anterior corneal radius

    a : distance from mire to cornea (75 mm in keratometer)

    Y : image size

    y : mire size (64 mm in keratometer)

    The keratometer can convert from corneal radius r (measured in meters) into refracting power (RP) (in Diopters) using the relationship:

$$RP = 337,5\,/\,r$$

Modern-automated or not-keratometers also known as ophthalmometers directly convert from radius to diopters and inversely. They are mainly used to calculate the power of intraocular lenses (IOLs) through different formulas (Hoffer, SRK-T, SRK-II, Holladay, Enrique del Rio and S. Simón, …). Although the theory of measuring corneal reflex may appear to be simple, it is not, since eye movement, decentration or any tear film deficiency may difficult the measure creating errors. Modern video methods (topographers) can freeze the reflected cornea image, and perform the measurements once the image is captured on the video or computer screen, allowing greater precision. Notice that most traditional keratometers perform measurements of the central 3 mm, while computerized topographers can cover almost the whole corneal surface.

Keratoscopy or Photokeratoscopy

It is a method to evaluate **qualitatively** the reflected light on the corneal surface. The projected light may be a simple flash lamp or a Placido disk target, which is a series of concentric rings (10 or 12 rings) or a tube (cone) with illuminated rings lining the inside surface. When we look at the keratoscope, an elliptical distortion of mires suggest astigmatism, and small, narrow and closely spaced mires suggest corneas that have high power (steep regions or short radius of curvature) (Figure 1.1).

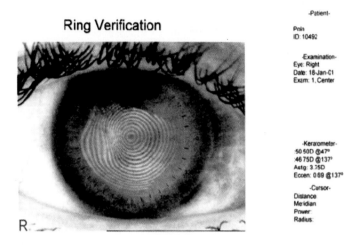

FIGURE 1.1: The "ring verification display" in modern videokeratoscopes is a static picture of what the explorer viewed at the keratoscope. Looking at the keratoscope, the explorer is able to evaluate qualitatively the corneal surface. In this case, notice the huge distortion of the mires on the temporal side of a right eye of a patient who underwent a keratoplasty for a keratoconus, and is wearing a soft plano-T therapeutic contact lens. The distortion of the mires is due to an irregularity at contact lens surface: air is in between the cornea and the lens

The use of keratoscopes is being abandoned in favor of computerized modern topographers which allow qualitative and quantitative measurements of the corneal surface, with higher definition and accuracy (more than 20 rings), and more sensitivity in the peripheral cornea.

Some of the known deficiencies of the Placido method are:
• It requires assumptions about the corneal shape
• It misses data on the central cornea (not all topographers)
• It is only able to acquire limited data points
• It measures slope not height.

Some more subjective complaints include:
• It is difficult to focus and align
• In most topographers, the patient is exposed to high light.

Large **Placido disk** systems work far away from the eye, while small **Placido cones** get much closer to the eye. While Placido disk systems easily create shadows caused by the nose and brow blocking the light of the rings, small cone systems fit under the brow and beside the nose, avoiding shadows, but can get in contact with large noses and make the patient blink and be afraid. Most small cones have a reputation for difficult focusing: some manufacturers—like Optikon 2000®—have worked out worthwhile automatic capture devices for improved accuracy, precision, and repeatability of measurements.

Computerized Videokeratoscopy: Modern Corneal Topographers

Corneal topography has gained wide acceptance as a clinical examination procedure with the advent of modern laser refractive surgery. It has many advantages over traditional keratometers or keratoscopes: they measure a greater area of the cornea with a much higher number of points and produce permanent records that can be used for follow-up (Tables 1.1 to 1.3).

Basically, a projection corneal topographer consists of a Placido disk or cone (large or small) that illuminates the cornea by sending a mire of concentric rings, a video camera that captures the corneal reflex from the tear layer and a computer and software that perform the analysis of the data through different computer algorithms. The computer evaluates the distance between a series of concentric rings of light and darkness in a variable number of points. The shorter the distance, the higher the corneal power, and inversely. Final results can be printed in colors or black-and-white.

The Placido disk (Figure 1.2) consists of a series of concentric dark and light rings in the configuration of a disk or a cone, of different sizes, depending on the number of rings and the manufacturer. Usually, it is better to have a large number of rings, since more corneal radius values can be measured. The mires of most systems exclude the very central cornea and the paralimbal area.

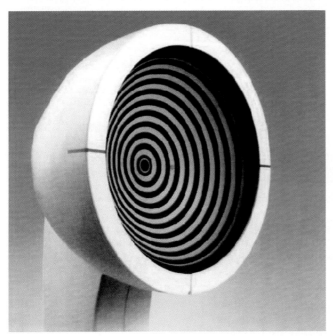

FIGURE 1.2: The Placido cone consists of a series of concentric dark and light rings in the configuration of a cone of different sizes depending on the number of rings and the manufacturer. Usually, it is better to have a large number of rings, since more corneal radius values can be measured: notice that while describing the technical characteristics of videokeratographers some manufactures count both clear and dark rings, while others only count light ones. The mires of most systems exclude the very central cornea (where the video camera or CCD is located) and the paralimbal area. The figure shows a large cone of the Haag-Streit® Keratograph CTK 922™ with 22 rings (dark and light rings) (Published with permission from Haag-Streit® AG International)

The reproducibility of videokeratography measurements is mainly dependent on the accuracy of manual adjustment in the focal plane. Videokeratoscopes having small Placido cones show a considerable amount of error when the required working distance between cornea and keratoscope is not maintained. The advantages of small cones (optimal illumination and the reduction of anatomically caused shadows) are in no proportion to the disadvantage—poor depth of focus, resulting in poor reproducibility. Which one should you choose, a small Placido cone or large Placido disk? Not easy to answer: each family of topographers has advantages and disadvantages. Being no ideal instrument, topographer potential buyers will have to decide upon other important factors, like software ability to exactly reproduce real corneal height, number of rings, price, ...

There are two main groups of corneal topographers: those which use the principle of reflection (most), and those which use the principle of projection.

The image captured by most topographers is produced by the thin tear layer covering the cornea that almost reproduces the shape or contour of the corneal surface. Most instruments perform indirect measurements of the corneal surface (***reflection technique***) and extrapolate to know the height of each point of the cornea. Reflection techniques amplify the corneal topographic distortions (Figure 1.3).

Euclid Systems Corporation® ET-800 uses a completely different method of topography called **Fourier profilometry** using filtered blue light that induces fluorescence of a liquid that has been applied to the tear film before the examination. This ***projection technique*** visualizes the surface directly while a reflection technique amplifies the corneal topographic distortions.

TABLE 1.1: Advantages and disadvantages of projection-based systems over reflection-based ones

Advantages:
 Measurement of direct corneal height
     Ability to measure: irregular corneal surfaces
                          non-reflective surfaces
     Higher resolution (theoretical)
 Uniform accuracy across the whole cornea
 Less operator dependent
 Do not suffer from spherical bias
 	
 Disadvantages:
 Not standard instruments (most are still prototypes):
     complex to use
     need clinical experience validation
     nonstandard presentation maps (more difficult to learn)
 	
 Longer examination time: longer image acquisition time
                                      longer image analysis
 Fluorescein instillation needed (in some, like the Euclid Systems Corporation® ET-800™)

Causes of Artefacts of the Corneal Topography Map

a. Shadows on the cornea from large eye-lashes (Figure 1.4) or trichiasis.

b. Ptosis or non-sufficient eye opening (Figure 1.5).

c. Irregularities of the tear film layer (dry eye, mucinous film, greasy film) (Figure 1.6).

d. Too short working distance of the small Placido disk cone.

e. Incomplete or distorted image (corneal pathology) (Figures 1.7 and 1.8).

TABLE 1.2: Indications and uses of corneal topographers

The use of computerised corneal topography is indicated in the following conditions:
1. Preoperative and postoperative assessment of the refractive patient
2. Preoperative and postoperative assessment of penetrating keratoplasty
3. Irregular astigmatism
4. Corneal dystrophies, bullous keratopathy
5. Keratoconus (diagnostic and follow-up)
6. Follow-up of corneal ulceration or abscess (Figure 1.3)
7. Post-traumatic corneal scarring
8. Contact lens fitting
9. Evaluation of tear film quality
10. Reference instrument for IOL-implants to see the corneal difference before and after surgery
11. To study unexplained low visual acuity after any surgical procedure (trabeculectomy, extracapsular lens extraction, ...)
12. Preoperative and postoperative assessment of Intacs™ corneal rings (intrastromal corneal rings)

TABLE 1.3: Different methods of measuring corneal surface used by modern corneal topographers

- **Placido systems (small cone or large disk)** are the most popular
- Placido cone **with arc-step mapping** (*Keratron™ from Optikon 2000®*)
- Placido disk **with arc-step mapping** (*Zeiss Humphrey® Atlas™*)
- **Slit-lamp topo-pachymetry** (*Orbscan™-Bausch & Lomb®*)
- **Fourier profilometry** (*Euclid Systems Corporation® ET-800™*)
- **Fringe projection** or **Moiré interference fringes** (*EyeShape® from BioShape AG™*)
- **Triangulation ellipsoid topometry** (*Technomed™ color ellipsoid topometer*)
- **Laser interferometry** (experimental method, it records the interference pattern generated on the corneal surface by the interference of two lasers or coherent wave fronts)

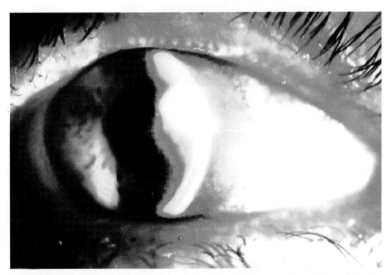

FIGURE 1.3: There are different methods of following the clinical course of a corneal ulceration or corneal abscess. While daily slit-lamp examination and daily photographs are invaluable, corneal topographic maps, being less "explorer dependent", can also be very useful in the follow-up

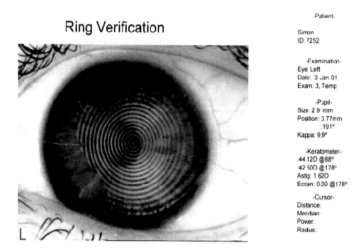

FIGURE 1.4: With large Placido disk topographers, large eyelashes project shadows on the superior cornea: the topographer will be unable to accurately perform the map of that zone. Danger is that extrapolation performed by some systems distorts the true map of the paracentral cornea. Trichiasic cilia projects a shadow that may interfere with the mapping. This situation should be addressed prior to corneal topography

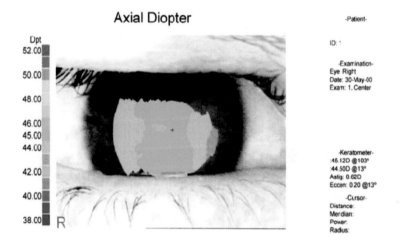

FIGURE 1.5: Ptosis or non-sufficient eye opening because of induced photophobia or patient anxiety limits and distorts the mapping of the cornea. Notice that the map is not round but oval

UNDERSTANDING AND READING CORNEAL TOPOGRAPHY

The meaningful interpretation of topographic maps requires the examiner to have detailed knowledge and clinical experience on the patterns detailed in them. At first, one must understand how to read the color scales. The untrained eye may find some confusion and sometimes misinterpretation in evaluating

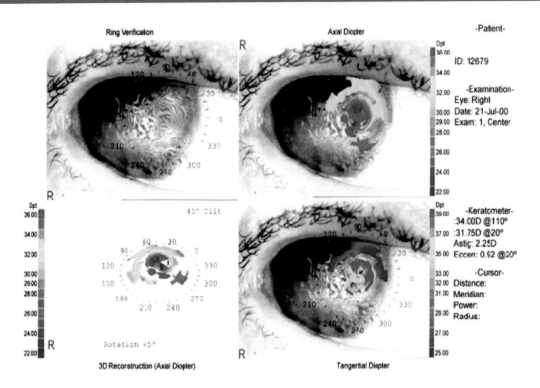

FIGURE 1.6: An advanced corneal herpetic keratopathy produces an irregular completely distorted corneal map in which no regular pattern can be identified. Notice that the low-vision patient is unable fixate to the fixation light

corneal maps. Modern topographers (videokeratographers) use the Louisiana State University Color-Coded Map (See Box) to display corneal superficial powers. The power values (measured in diopters) are preferred by clinicians over the radius values (measured in millimeters), although all topographers can map the corneas using both values.

Projection-based topography systems, adopted a similar color scale to represent their height maps. High areas are depicted by warm colors, while low areas are depicted by cool colors.

The Louisiana State University Color-Coded Map:

colors correspond to the following:

Cool colors (violets and blues): *low powers. They correspond to flat curvatures (low diopter)*

Greens and yellows: colors found in the normal corneas

Warm or hot colors (oranges and reds): higher powers. They correspond to steep curvatures (high diopter).

Facing a corneal topography, care has to be taken to interpret colored maps, since scales (and sometimes color coding) can be modified in most topographers' software. For patient examination, the

11

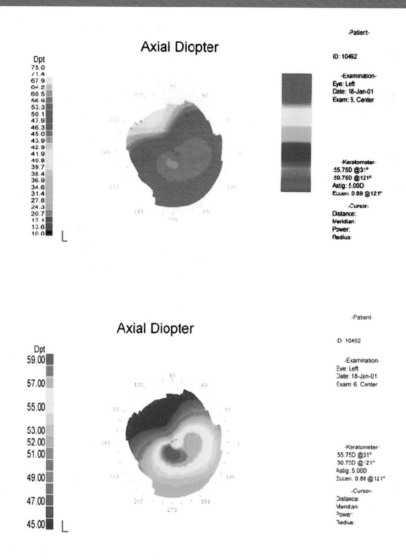

FIGURES 1.7 and 1.8: These two maps may look different but are the same axial diopter map of the left eye of the same patient (**keratoconus**) measured in different scales, absolute on the left and relative on the right. Notice very high diopter values under corneal vertex, where corneal surface is most elevated

manufacturer sets default values which are operator adjustable (diopter interval, radius interval). When the operator adjusts the values to new parameters, color scales are modified.

Rare are the topographers that directly measure the corneal elevation: most act by extrapolation from corneal curvature and power at each measured point. The Optikon 2000® Keratron™ is one of those systems that accurately maps aspheric surfaces by means of its own method of arc-step mapping.

The range of powers found in the normal cornea range from 39 D found at peripheral cornea, close to the limbus, to 48 D found at corneal apex.

The colors do not always represent an elevation map, they correspond to curvature values. Therefore, the cornea is most curved towards the center (green) and flattens out towards the periphery (blue). The nasal side becomes blue more quickly, indicating that the nasal cornea is flatter than the temporal. Some advanced instruments like the Optikon 2000® Keratron™, are able to directly represent a colored elevation map.

Apart from color maps, most topographers also display values of **simulated keratometry**, that should be equivalent to those obtained by a keratometer. Simulated keratometry values are obtained from the radius values at the corneal position (3 central millimeters) where the reflection from the keratometer mires would take place.

Topographic Scales

Two basic scales are commonly used: absolute and relative.

Absolute, Standardized or International Standard Scale

Same scale for every map produced. Good for direct comparisons between different maps, for screening and for gross pathologies. It was designed to make only clinically relevant information obvious, by setting the interval between the contours of the power plot (i.e. in practice, the contours of colors) at 1.5 diopters (which means it has low resolution).

Relative, Normalized or Adaptative Color Scale

Different scale for each map. The computer determines maximum and minimum curvatures for the map and automatically distributes the range of colors. The computer contracts or expands its color range according to the range of colors present in a given cornea. It is best suited for looking at variations for a particular cornea. It has the advantage of offering great topographic detail since incremental steps are smaller (around 0.8 diopters) giving high resolution, but suffers from some inconveniences: the meanings of colors are lost (explorer and clinician have to carefully check the meaning of the colors, according to the new scale), a normal cornea may look abnormal while abnormal corneas may appear closer to normal. With this scale, subtle features are made apparent, being good for detail.

Computer Displays: Presentation of Topographic Information

When confronted to a topography display, either a printed report or on screen, one should study it in a structured way to avoid mistakes in interpretation, and get the most of it.

Proceed as follows:

- Check the name of the patient, date of exam and examined eye
- Check the scale
- Type of measurement (height in microns, curvature in mm, power in diopters)
- Step interval
- Study the map (type of map, form of abnormalities, …)

- Evaluate statistical information (cursor box, statistical indices when given …)
- Compare with topography of the other eye (always perform bilateral exams, when possible)
- Compare with the previous maps first verifying they are in the same scale
- Apply statistical analysis or other needed software application (contact lens fit, surgical modules, 3-D color maps, neural networks, …)
- Explain the exam's results to the patient.

To present a corneal topography, each software application (i.e. each instrument) has a large number of computer displays. Most are produced from data of a single application, and are software dependent. Most instruments are able to show: a ring verification, a numerical display, a large number of corneal maps, a simulated keratometry, a meridional plot, and some can display a 3-D reconstruction of the corneal surface.

Ring Verification (keratoscopic raw image) (Figure 1.1)

Displays a keratoscopic image of the Placido rings reflex on the examined cornea. It is a raw image, that allows qualitative evaluation of the image taken (irregularity of tear film layer, lids aperture, …), helping the examiner to either accept or reject the taken image. It is very useful when there is a question regarding the accuracy of the displayed data.

Numeric Display (Figures 1.9 and 1.10)

Numeric display of a number of corneal power values along several meridians shown in a radial display. Helpful to make the data amenable to statistical methods.

Corneal Maps (Figures 1.11 to 1.13)

Corneal maps details of the most common (axial, tangential, 3-D, …) will be discussed later in this chapter. Each topographer offers different maps or ways of presenting the results. Please refer to your topographer's manual for more details.

Simulated keratometry readings (SimK)

SimK are obtained from the radius values at the corneal position (3 millimeters central zone) where the reflection from the keratometer mires would take place. The major axis is that with the greatest power, and the minor axis is at 90° to it (perpendicular axis). The cylinder is the difference between the major and minor axis. The meridian with the lowest mean power can also be displayed.

Meridional Plot

Meridional plot shows the minimum and the maximum corneal power values, displaying a cross-sectional profile of the cornea along the chosen meridian. It is used to show the general shape of the cornea to the patient, and assessing the toricity for contact lens adaptation. This helps in identifying the ablation zone limits following LASIK or PRK.

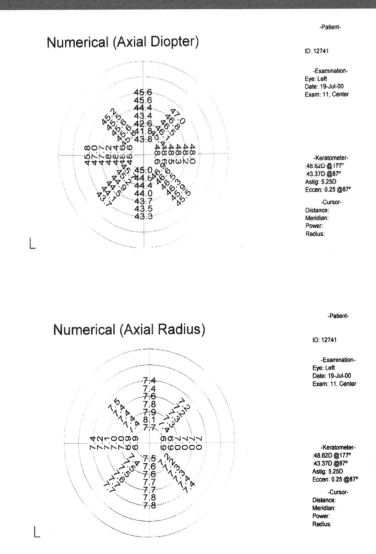

FIGURES 1.9 and 1.10: The numeric display shows a number of corneal power values along several meridians in a radial display. It is a very helpful presentation to make the data amenable to statistical methods. Notice that Figure 1.9 (Axial Diopter) displays corneal powers in diopters and that Figure 1.10 (Axial Radius) shows the same values in millimeters (corneal radius). Most topographers allow you to choose the way you want the results to be shown

COMMON CORNEAL MAPS

Axial Map

The axial map is the original and most commonly used map (Figure 1.14). It provides measurements based on the keratometer formula. It is helpful in evaluating the overall characteristics of the cornea and classify the corneal map (normal or abnormal) (Figures 1.15 to 1.17). It can differentiate between

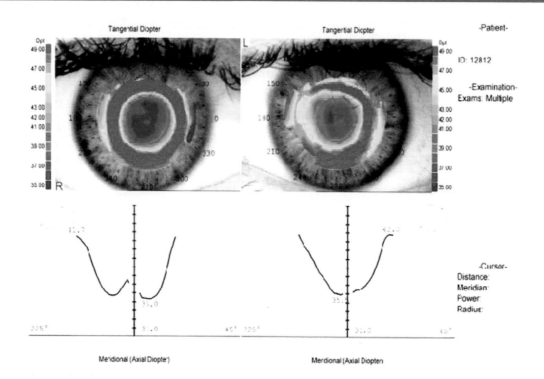

FIGURE 1.11: Shows a "multiple exams" of both eyes of the same patient, a 38 year old man who underwent LASIK in both eyes at a time for high myopia. Corneal map is overlaid upon the keratoscope eye image to aid interpretation. The overlay shows the spatial relationship between the pupil, the ablation zone and the cornea. Notice that immediately after surgery (the day after), ablation zones differ from each other: it is due to the fact that a different excimer laser was used for each eye. Schwind® Keratom™ was used on right eye, while left eye was operated using the Bausch & Lomb® -Chiron Technolas 217™. Although ablation zone seems more perfect and regular on right eye (tangential diopter map), this does not mean that visual result is better. The **meridional plots** shown under tangential diopter maps help the surgeon to evaluate the effectiveness and ablation pattern of the excimer laser he or she uses

spherical, astigmatic or irregular corneas. It is the most stable type of map, but may confuse the explorer when evaluating the peripheral cornea (see Figure 1.18).

Height Map

True height data (in microns) is immediately available from systems using the principle of projection, although a reflection system like the Optikon 2000® Keratron™ does a good job with its own arc-step method of representing corneal height. Very useful in numeric or cross-sectional format to quantify the elevation or the depth of a corneal defect (ulceration, laser ablation zone, keratoconus, …). Some topographers display the spherical height map relative to a reference spherical surface, by comparing to a best fit calculated reference sphere.

Tangential Map (see Figure 1.11)

The tangential map is a very useful display which provides a measurement of corneal power over a large portion of the cornea, based on a mathematical radius formula. It is more accurate than axial map in the corneal periphery, but it is subject to greater variation when comparing several exams that are repeated. It may help detecting mild corneal changes that might not be detected by standard axial map. It is used for locating corneal distances on the map, and to locate a cone or peak position in keratoconus, as well as to locate the ablation diameter and position after laser refractive surgical ablation.

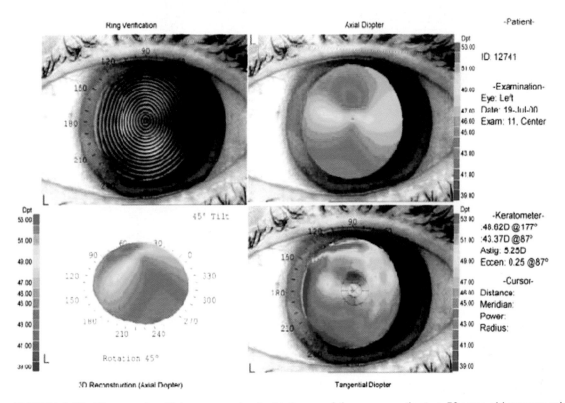

FIGURE 1.12: Shows a "multiple exams view" of left eye of the same patient, a 58-year-old women who underwent (a couple of years before consultation) complicated phacoemulsification converted to extracapsular surgery. In the hurry, the surgeon sutured the cornea too loose, thus creating a peripheral superior corneal wound defect. High **against-the-rule astigmatism** is well represented by the axial diopter display (superior right), and well measured by the keratometer display (5.25 D at 87 °). But only tangential diopter map (down-right) accurately represented the corneal wound **suture defect**: notice the red superior area where the sutures used to be

Refractive Map

The refractive map is based on an axial map, using Snell's law to calculate the refractive power of the cornea. It is mainly used in pre- and post-corneal surgery.

Elliptical Elevation Map

The elliptical elevation map represents the height of the cornea in microns, at different corneal positions, relative to a reference elliptical surface. It is useful to visualize corneal shape. In contrast to the spherical height map—which uses a simple spherical reference—the elliptical elevation map matches better to the inherently elliptical shape of the healthy cornea.

17

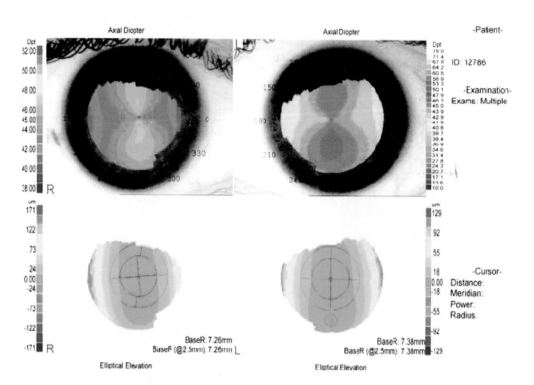

FIGURE 1.13: Shows a "multiple exams view" of both eyes of the same patient, a young man referred for refractive surgery who—to our surprise—was never diagnosed astigmatic. Axial diopter maps are displayed, in normalized (right eye) and absolute scales (left eye). Elliptical elevation with keratometer overlay maps help better assess true corneal shape and direction or axis of astigmatism. Radius of the reference ellipse are displayed and can be modified by operator: BaseR refers to central radius value, and BaseR (2.5 mm) refers to the radius value at 2.5 mm

3-D Reconstruction Map

The 3-D reconstruction map is used to visualize the overall shape of the cornea in a more realistic way. Understandable for the patient, it can be rotated and tilted as desired. Some instruments like OCULUS® Keratograph and Haag-Streit® Keratograph CTK 922 offer excellent comprehensive kinetic three-dimensional (3-D) analysis of corneal topography for simple explanation to the patient.

Irregularity Map

The irregularity map calculates a best sphere/cylinder correction for the cornea, subtracting the correction from either axial or tangential data and presents the remaining irregularities. Used after refractive surgery to detect irregularities that may explain a low visual acuity. It reports an index that measures eccentricity (a measure of asphericity) and the amount of astigmatism that has been subtracted from the original corneal data.

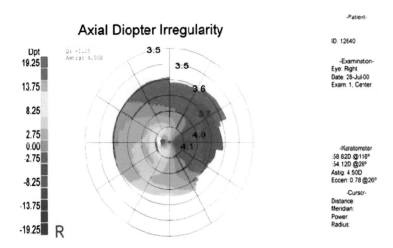

FIGURE 1.14: Shows an **axial irregularity map** in diopters of the right eye of a 55-year-old man suffering from a paracentral progressive corneal ectasia (central **keratoconus**). Notice the Q index with a value of −1.25 (measuring eccentricity) and an astigmatism of 4.5 D, resulting from the subtraction of the original corneal data and the best sphere/cylinder for that cornea. An overlay option adds an irregularity index to the map for increasing circles of 1 mm radius, best visualized thanks to the overlay circular grid option. Normal values would be 0.2 or 0.4, but this exceptional case shows 3.5 and 4.0 zonal indices

TABLE 1.4: Common overlays that can be added to a topography map to help interpretation

- **Pupil margin:** displays the visually important region. Helps evaluating photopic pupillary size, and the centration or refractive surgery
- **Grids square:** helps defining size and location of abnormalities
  - **Circular:** helps defining size and location of abnormalities
  - **Polar:** helps defining axis of abnormalities and the assessment of radial keratotomies
- **Optical zone:** useful in refractive surgery for planning procedures or assessing results
- **Angular scale:** useful in refractive surgery of astigmatism for planning procedures or assessing results. It is similar in use to polar grid
- **Eye image:** more realistic than a simple map, it eases the patient's interpretation of the map
- **Keratoconus:** a peak or keratoconus overlay can be applied by Dicon's CT-200. It is called Bull's Eye target: if one peak area exists with an index of 10 or greater, the system automatically marks it with a target, indicating the location of this elevation to some but not all maps (see Figures 1.12 and 1.15)
- **Keratometer mires:** it is a graphic reference showing a 3 mm circle with both major and minor meridians, representing the calculated keratometry readings, 90 degrees apart (perpendicular). It also shows a 5 mm with the steepest and flattest meridians (see Figure 1.13)

SPECIAL SOFTWARE APPLICATIONS AND DISPLAYS

Each available instrument is sold with standard software package and most offer optional packages at additional price (Table 1.4). The most common are as follows:

19

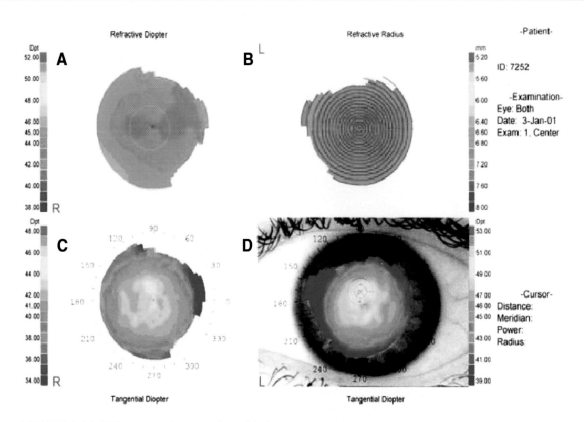

FIGURE 1.15: Different overlays can be added to a topography to help interpretation. The figure shows a quadruple view of an almost normal cornea of a young contact lens user with mild corneal warpage only diagnosed by means of the tangential maps (**C** and **D**). Notice that **B**) is displayed in radius (mm) while the rest of maps are displayed in diopters (see the color scale). Map **A** displays a center overlay (small red cross) that indicates where the true center of the cornea is, and a pupil outline overlay that reproduces pupil margin, the visually important region. Map **B** shows a "verify rings" overlay, to better assess the quality of the taken image. Red and green concentric rings should alternate and not cross. The red rings should be located on the outer edge of the white rings, and the green rings should be located on the outer edge of the black rings. Map **C** shows an angular scale that helps to locate the axis of astigmatism. Map **D** shows "eye image" overlay, the image of the patient's eye is displayed to ease the patient's interpretation of the map. Notice that a paracentral target marks an elevation zone that has to be carefully inspected. Angular scale is also displayed in map **D**

Multiple Display Option

Multiple display option is a customizable multiple display which allows simultaneous screen display for rapid analysis and ease of use. Depending on the software of your topographer, you can simultaneously view either one, two or four maps. Extremely practice in daily use to ease work and interpretation.

Surgical Applications

Surgical applications used to predict the results of refractive surgery, and for postoperative evaluation. Some—but not all—allow refractive surgery simulations and topography-linked laser refractive surgery with special excimer laser brand names.

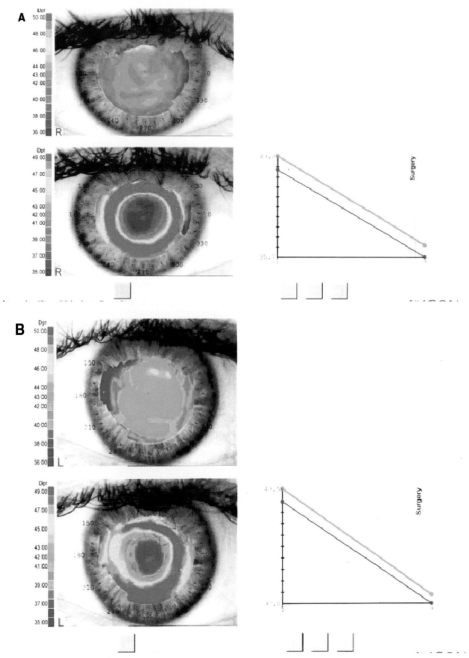

FIGURES 1.16A and B: Dicon's CT200™ **trend analysis** displays a series of exam maps (preoperative exam, first postoperative exam, most recent exam and a choice of a K-trend graph, a pre/postoperative difference map or a post-last difference map. Shown are trend analysis of both eyes of a patient who underwent myopic LASIK with two different excimer lasers. Shown are axial diopter preoperative, tangential diopter immediate postoperative and K-trend graph. Notice that immediately after surgery (the day after), ablation zones differ from each other: it is due to the fact that a different excimer laser was used for each eye. Schwind® Keratom™ was used on right eye, while left eye was operated using the Bausch & Lomb®-Chiron Technolas 217™. K-trend graph shows the major (green) and minor (blue) K values for all exams in the series. The Y axis is power in diopters, and the X axis is the exam's number spaced out over time. The vertical line marks the date of surgery. Trend analysis eases a rapid overview of healing trend over time

Contact Lens Fitting Application

They are used for contact lens fitting, and help choosing the best suggested lens for each case, by simulating the fluorescein pattern and contact lens position of rigid contacts. Not all topographers offer this feature: in some cases, this software module is sold as an option. For instance, Dicon's CT200™ offers as standard the Mandell Contact Lens Module "Easy-Fit™", and as an option the Mandell Contact Lens Module "Advanced-Fit"™ for toric, bi-toric, keratoconic fitting and postsurgical fitting with Labtalk™. Contact your dealer for more precise information.

The simulated fluorescein feature is intended to reduce fitting time by viewing the effect of changing lens parameters on a personalized basis, depending on the patient's corneal exam. Let us notice that the true *"in vivo"* result of any computerized fluorescein test may vary due to differences caused by lid action on the lens (aperture and weight).

Ask the manufacturer of your topographer for special software applications, and for the possibility to link your topographer and your excimer laser for better results.

TOPOGRAPHY MAPS OF THE NORMAL CORNEA

When considering the topography of a normal cornea, we feel the need to remember that there is a **wide spectrum of normality**. No human cornea demonstrates the kind of regularity found in the calibration spheres of a topographer: the eye is not molded glass-made. Normal corneal topography can take on many topographic patterns (Table 1.5).

TABLE 1.5: Normal topographic patterns		
Spherical (Round) (Figure 1.19)		20%
With-the-rule	**(Oval)** (Figure 1.20)	20%
With-the-rule	**(Symmetric bow tie)**	17%
With-the-rule	**(Asymmetric bow tie)**	30%
Against-the-rule		
Displaced apex:	**Inferiorly**	
	Nasally	
Irregular		7%
causes of irregularity:	Dry eye	
	Corneal scar or ulceration	
	Trauma	
	Corneal degeneration	
	Corneal edema	
	Pterygium	
	Contact lens overuse (corneal warpage)	
	Surgery (cataract, keratoplasty, ...)	

Regular astigmatism (**with-the-rule**) gives an oval axial corneal map, being the most common deviation from optically perfect spherical (round) cornea. If the bow tie is vertical (the long axis is near the vertical meridian) in an axial map, it represents a cornea having with-the-rule-astigmatism. If the bow tie is horizontal, it represents an "**against-the-rule**" astigmatism, ninety degrees rotated when compared to a with-the-rule astigmatism.

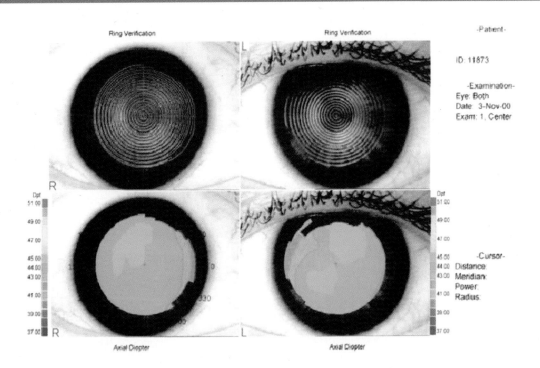

FIGURE 1.17: Shows a "multiple exams view" of left both eyes of the same patient, a 38-year-old woman prior to LASIK surgery. Corneal topography remains a routine exam for preoperative and postoperative assessment of the refractive patient. This report shows **normal, spherical (round), corneas** in both eyes (44 D at vertex, and mostly green color in the map). The color zones are approximately circular in shape. Notice that lid aperture is not the same in both eyes, thus making it more difficult to map superior corneal periphery in left eye.

When the bow tie is diagonal, it represents a cornea having an **oblique** astigmatism. The shape and colors of the bow tie are influenced by the rate of peripheral corneal flattening, and the appearance is influenced by the scale interval chosen by the explorer. The bow tie may be symmetrical or asymmetrical along the perpendicular meridian: one half of the bow tie is significantly larger than the other, the corneal apex being located in the direction of the larger bow half, slightly decentered from the visual axis.

In the normal eye, **nasal cornea is flatter than temporal**. The nasal side of a healthy corneal map becomes blue more quickly, indicating that the nasal cornea is flatter than the temporal. There is a physiological astigmatism of around 0.75 diopter. Physiologically, the axis may not be the same superiorly than inferiorly. In an axial map, the rate of flattening is greater when the color scale interval is larger, and there are many color zones. A focal steepening inferiorly may exist due to the lower tear meniscus.

Generally, **the two eyes of the same subject are very similar, and present a mirror image of each other** (Figures 1.18 and 1.19). This phenomenon is called **enantiomorphism**. The knowledge of this fact is useful to decide whether a cornea is normal or not, by comparing to the map of contralateral eye.

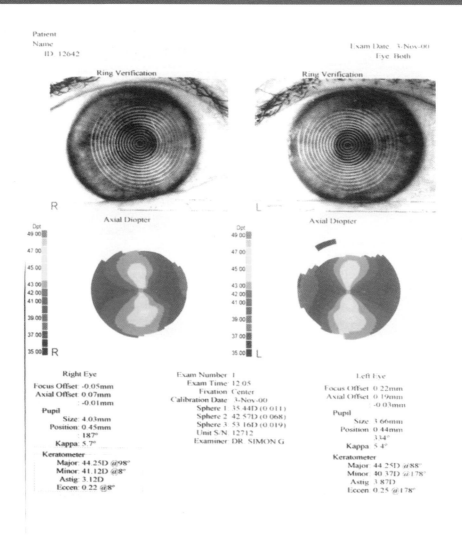

FIGURE 1.18: Axial diopter displays are showed for both right and left eyes. The patient suffered from regular astigmatism (**with-the-rule**), that gives an oval corneal map, being the most common deviation from optically perfect spherical (round) cornea. The long axis is near the vertical meridian. The shape and colors of the bow tie are influenced by the rate of peripheral corneal flattening: notice the nasal peripheral flattening in left eye (purple color). This binocular report from Dicon's CT-200 topographer shows **pupil size** and **simulated keratometry** of both eyes. RE size pupil is 4.03 mm, and astigmatism 3.12 D at 8°. Notice that the two eyes present a mirror image of each other: this phenomenon is called **enantiomorphism**.

Small changes in corneal shape do occur throughout life:
- In **infancy**, the cornea is fairly spherical
- In **childhood** and **adolescence**, probably due to eyelid pressure on a young tissue, cornea becomes slightly astigmatic with-the-rule
- In the **middle age**, cornea tends to recover its sphericity
- Late in life, against-the-rule astigmatism tends to develop.

Short-term fluctuation and diurnal variations are not rare, and usually remain unnoticed by individuals with normal corneas. Some conditions like corneal distrophies, ocular hypotony, radial keratotomies or contact lens use can make them apparent (Table 1.6).

TABLE 1.6: Factors that slightly affect the normal curvature of the cornea
• Lid closure during sleep time • Tear film quallly • Lid pressure on the cornea (weight, exoftalmos) • Intraocular pressure • Menstruation • Pregnancy

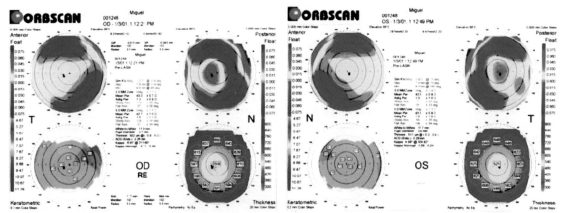

FIGURE 1.19: Enantiomorphism is the phenomenon wherein an individual's topographies are non-superimposable almost mirror images of each other. The knowledge of this fact is useful to decide whether a cornea is normal or not, by comparing to the map of contralateral eye. Notice that even pachymetry maps reflect this phenomenon (corneal thickness was mapped with Bausch & Lomb® Orbscan™ topo-pachymeter)

Comparing Displays

Maps can be compared directly only on the same scale, when taken with the same instrument, and preferably by the same explorer. It is not a good idea to compare maps taken with different instruments: every instrument uses a different measuring algorithm that may confuse you, especially when comparing subtle details.

Most software applications allow the comparison of different maps over time, and even subtract values from two different exams (subtraction or difference maps) (Figures 1.20 to 1.22). They are invaluable to the refractive surgeon (Table 1.7).

TABLE 1.7: Uses of subtraction or difference maps
• Validation of various exams taken in a same session • Ascertain the existence of progressive corneal astigmatism • Comparison of preoperative and postoperative corneal maps (LASIK and PRK) • Follow-up of myopic regression (LASIK and PRK) • Establishing ablation zone centration (LASIK and PRK) • Assessing resolution of corneal warpage in rigid contact lens users • Assessing evolution of a corneal ulcer or abscess

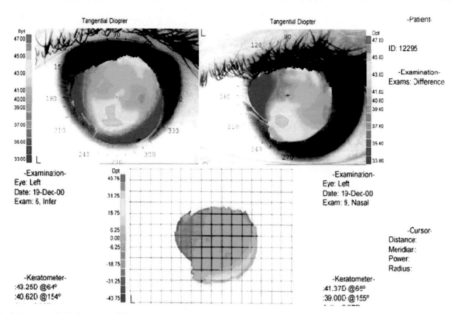

FIGURE 1.20: A tangential diopter difference map of the left eye of a 21-year-old patient is shown. The subtraction has been performed **between two different eye fixations** to determine the existence of any irregularity in the ablation zone. The patient underwent a successful bilateral LASIK surgery to correct a high myopic astigmatism in both eyes a year before

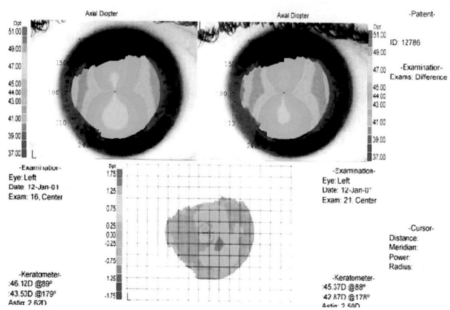

FIGURE 1.21: A diopter difference map is useful to assess the validity of the different exams with the same fixation performed in the same session. Low differences due to tear film irregularities, lid aperture and blinking is acceptable. In case of difference between maps taken at the same moment, they need to be repeated, after a few blinks from the patient. If significant difference persists, try instillating a tear substitute in both eyes and wait for a few minutes. Should differences persist, repeat the exams in a few days. Image shows a left eye with regular (with-the-rule) high astigmatism: both axial diopter maps were taken in the same session: differences exist between the exams. Eye fixation is the same (center): differences are attributable to different lid aperture and from blinking. Axial diopter difference (down, with a square grid overlay) shows that differences are almost nonsignificant (around 0.25-0.50 diopters), but exist. Such differences are physiological: difference maps allow validation of various exams taken in a same session

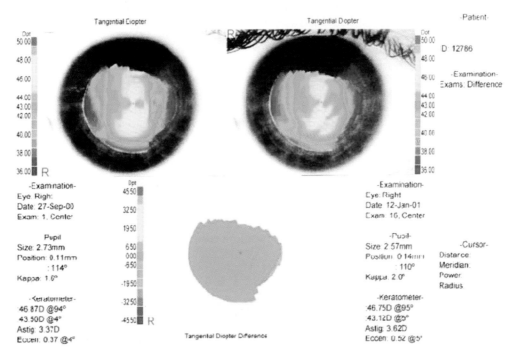

FIGURE 1.22: Difference maps ease the astigmatism progression follow-up . Tangential diopter displays show right eye maps of a 22-year-old myopic patient referred for refractive surgery. To our surprise, neither glasses nor contacts had astigmatism. The existence of astigmatism was ascertained with the keratometer, subjective refraction and skiascopy. Corneal topography was performed and helped the demonstration of its existence. The figure shows a difference map between two exams taken with a 3 months delay (see the dates of the exams). Tangential diopter difference is 0 (green), meaning that no changes have occurred in that period of time. The first impression is that the guy never had good refraction, but new topographic exams will be performed 6 months and one year later, before refractive surgery is decided, so as to make sure that no keratoconic formation is on the way

BIBLIOGRAPHY

1. Applegate RA, Nunez R, Buettner J, Howland HC. How accurately can videokeratographic systems measure surface elevation? Optom Vis Sci 1995; 72:785-92.
2. Arffa RC, Warnicki JW, Rehkopf PG. Corneal topography using rasterstereography. Refract Corneal Surg 1989; 5: 414-17.
3. Belin MW, Litoff FK, Strods SJ, Winn SS, Smith RS. The PAR technology corneal topography system. Refract Corneal Surg 1992;8: 88–96.
4. Belin MW, Zloty P. Accuracy of the PAR corneal topography system with spatial misalignment. CLAO J 1993; 19: 64-8.
5. Belin MW, Ratliff CD. Evaluating data acquisition and smoothing functions of currently available videokeratoscopes. J Cataract Refract Surg 1996; 22: 421-6.
6. Borderie VM, Laroche L. Measurement of irregular astigmatism using semimeridian data from video-keratographs. J Refract Surg 1996;12: 595–600.
7. Brancato R, Carones F. Topografia corneale computerizzata. Milano, Italy: Fogliazza, ed. 1994.
8. Cantera E, Carones F, Brancato R, Cantera I, Neuschuler R. Evaluation of a new autofocus device for computer-assisted corneal topography. Invest Ophthalmol Vis Sci 1994; 35 (Suppl): 2063.
9. Cohen KL, Tripoli NK, Holmgren DE, Coggins JM: Assessment of the height of radial aspheres reported by a computer-assisted keratoscope. Invest Ophthalmol Vis Sci 1993;34 (Suppl): 1217.
10. Cohen KL, Tripoli NK, Holmgren DE, Coggins JM. Assessment of the power and height of radial aspheres reported by a computer-assisted keratoscope. Am J Ophthalmol 1995; l l9: 723-32.

11. Corbett MC, O'Brart DPS, Stultiens Bath, Jongsma FHM, Marshall J. Corneal topography using a new Moiré image-based system. Eur J Implant Ref Surg 1995;7: 353-70.

12. Corbett MC, Rosen ES, O'Brart DPS. Corneal topography: principles and applications. BMJ books, Great Britain, 1999.

13. Chan WK, Carones F, Maloney RK. Corneal topographic maps: a clinical comparison. International Society of Refractive Keratoplasty 1994-Abstract book.

14. Dekking HM. Zur Photographie der Hornhautoberfl-Eche. Graefe's Arch Ophtalmol 1930; 124:708-30.

15. Dingeldein SA, Klyce SD, Wilson SE. Quantitative descriptors of corneal shape derived from the computer-assisted analysis of photokeratographs. Refract Corneal Surg 1989;5:372–8.

16. Doss JD, Hutson RL, Rowsey JJ, Brown DR. Method for calculation of corneal profile and power distribution. Arch Ophthalmol 1981; 99: 1261-5.

17. Duke Elder S. System of Ophthalmology. St Louis: CV Mosby Co, 1970;V, 96-101.

18. Ediger MN, Pettit GH, Weiblinger RP. Noninvasive monitoring of excimer laser ablation by time-resolved reflectometry. Refract Corneal Surg 1993;9: 268–75.

19. el-Hage SG. The computerized corneal topographer EH-270. In Shanzlin DJ, Robin JB (Eds): Corneal topography: measuring and modifying the cornea. New York: Springer-Verlag 1991:l 1-24.

20. el-Hage SG. Suggested new methods for photokeratoscopy: a comparison of their validities. I. Am J Optom Arch Am Acad Optom 1971; 48 :897-912.

21. Eghbali F, Yeung KK, Maloney RK. Topographic determination of corneal asphericity and its lack of effect on the outcome of radial keratotomy. Am J Ophtha1mol 1995;119: 275–80.

22. Fleming JF. Should refractive surgeons worry about corneal asphericity? Refract Corneal Surg 1990; 6: 455–7.

23. Friedman NE, Zadnik K, Mutti DO, Fusaro RE. Quantifying corneal toricity from videokeratography with Fourier analysis. J Refract Surg 1996;12: 108–13.

24. Gardner BP, Klyce SD, Thompson HW, et al. Centration of photorefractive keratectomy: topographic assessment. Invest Ophthalmol Vis Sci 1993;35: 803.

25. Greivenkamp JE, Mellinger MD, Snyder RW, Schwiegerling JT, Lowman AE, Miller JM. Comparison of three videokeratoscopes in measurement of toric test surfaces. J Refract Surg 1996; 12: 229-39.

26. Grimm BB. Communicating with keratography. J Refract Surg 1996;12: 156–9.

27. Hannush SB, Crawford SL, Waring GO III, Gemmill MC, Lynn MJ, Nizam A. Accuracy and precision of keratometry, photokeratoscopy and corneal modeling on calibrated steel balls. Arch Ophtalmol 1989; 107:1235-9.

28. Holladay J, Warring GO. Optics and topography in radial keratotomy. In Warring GO (Ed): Refractive Keratectomy for Myopia and Astigmatism. Mosby- Year book, Inc. 1992; 37- 144.

29. Holladay JT, Cravy TV, Koch DD. Calculation of surgically induced refractive change following ocular surgery. J Cat Refract Surg 1992;18: 429–43.

30. Holladay JT. Corneal topography using the Holladay diagnostic summary. J Cat Refract Surg 1997; 23: 209-21.

31. Holladay JT. The Holladay diagnostic summary. In James P Gills (Ed): Corneal Topography: The State of Art. Slack Inc., 1995; 309-323.

32. Huber C, Huber A, Gruber H. Three-dimensional representations of corneal deformations from kerato-topographic data. J Cat Refract Surg 1997; 23: 202–8.

33. Johnson DA, Haight DH, Kelly SE, et al. Reproducibility of videokeratographic digital subtraction maps after excimer laser photorefractive keratectomy. Ophthalmology 1996;103: 1392–8.

34. Jongsma FHM, Laan FC, Stultiens BATH. A Moiré-based corneal topographer suitable for discrete Fourier analysis. Proc Ophthal Tech 1994;2126: 185-92.

35. Kawara T. Corneal topography using Moiré contour fringes. Appl Optics 1979; 18: 3675-8.

36. Kelman SE. Introduction of neural networks with applications to ophthalmology. In Masters BR (Ed): Non-invasive Diagnostic Techniques in Ophthalmology. New York: Springer-Verlag, 1990.

37. Klein SA, Mandell RB. Axial and instantaneous power conversion in corneal topography. Invest Ophthalmol Vis Sci 1995; 36: 2155-9.

38. Klein SA. A corneal topography algorithm that produces continuous curvature. Optom Vis Sci 1992; 69: 829-34.

39. Klyce SD. Computer-assisted corneal topography: high resolution graphic presentation and analysis of keratoscopy. Invest Ophthalmol Vis Sci 1984;25: 1426-35.

40. Klyce SD, Wang JY. Considerations in corneal surface reconstruction from keratoscope images. In Masters BR (Ed): Noninvasive Diagnostic Techniques in Ophthalmology. New York: Springer-Verlag, 1990: 76.

41. Klyce SD, Dingeldein SA. Corneal topography. In Masters BR (Ed): Noninvasive Diagnostic Techniques in Ophthalmology. New York: Springer-Verlag 1990: pp 78-91.

42. Le Geais JM, Ren Q, Simon G, Parel JM. Computer Assisted corneal topography: accuracy and reproducibility of the topographic modeling system. Refract Corneal Surgery 1993;9:347-357.

43. Leroux Les Jardins, Pasquier N, Bertrand I. Topographie cornéenne computérisée: résultats apres kératotomie Radiaire et "T-Cuts". Bull Soc Opht France, 1991:8-9:XCL, 729-734.
44. Leroux Les Jardins, Pasquier N, Bertrand I. Modification de la chirurgie de l'astigmatisme en fonction des résultats de la topographie cornéenne computérisée. Bull Soc Opht France, 1991;12:XCLS, 1097-1104.
45. Koch DD, Foulks GN, Moran CT, Wakil JS. The corneal EyeSys System: accuracy analysis and reproducibility of first-generation prototype. J Refract Corneal Surg 1989; 5: 424-9.
46. Lundergan MK. The Orbscan corneal topography system: verification of accuracy. International Society of Refractive Keratoplasty 1994-Abstract book.
47. Maeda N, Klyce SD, Smolek MK, Thompson HW. Automated keratoconus screening with corneal topography analysis. Invest Ophthalmol Vis Sci 1994, 35: 2749 57.
48. Maeda M, Klyce SD, Smolek MK. Neural network classification of corneal topography. Invest Ophthalmol Vis Sci 1995;36: 1327-35.
49. Maguire LJ, Singer DE, Klyce SD. Graphic presentation of computer analysed keratoscope photographs. Arch Ophthalmol 1987;105: 223-30.
50. Maguire LJ, Wilson SE, Camp JJ, Verity S. Evaluating the reproducibility of topography systems on spherical surfaces. Arch Ophthalmol 1993; 111: 259-62.
51. Maloney RK, Bogan SJ, Waring GO III. Determination of corneal image-forming properties from corneal topography. Am J Ophthalmol 1993; 115: 31-41.
52. Mandell RB, Horner D. Alignment of videokeratoscopes. In Sanders DR, Koch DD (Eds): An Atlas of Corneal Topography. Thorofare NJ: Slack, 1993; pp 197-206.
53. Mandell RB. Contact lens practice, 4th edn. Springfield, IL: Charles C.Thomas, 1988;pp 107-35.
54. Mandell RB. Keratometry and contact lens practice. Optometric Wkly, 1965; May 6: 69-75.
55. Munger R, Priest D, Jackson WB, Casson EJ. Reliability of corneal surface maps using the PAR CTS. Invest Ophthalmol Vis Sci 1996; 37: s562.
56. Mattioli R, Carones F. How accurately can corneal profiles heights be measured by Placido-based videokeratography? Invest Ophthalmol Vis Sci 1996; 37: s932.
57. Mattioli R, Carones F, Cantera E. New algorithms to improve the reconstruction of corneal geometry on the Keratron™ videokeratographer. Invest Ophthalmol Vis Sci 1995; 36:s302.
58. Mattioli R, Tripoli NA. Corneal geometry reconstruction with the Keratron videokeratographer. Optom Vis Sci 1997; 74:881-894.
59. Merlin U. I cheratoscopi: caratteristiche e attendibilita. In Buratto L, Cantera E, Dal Fiume E, Genisi C, Merlin U (Eds): Topografia Corneale. Milano Italy: CAMO, 1995; 43-56.
60. Mishima S. Some physiological aspects of the precorneal tearfilm. Arch Ophthalmol 1965;73: 233.
61. Naufal SC, Hess JS, Friedlander MH, Granet NS. Rasterstereography-based classification of normal corneas. J Cat Refract Surg 1997;23: 222–30.
62. O'Bart DPS, Corbett MC, Rosen ES. The topography of corneal disease. Eur J Implant Ref Surg 1995; 7:173-183
63. Olsen T, Dam-Johansen M, Beke T, Hjortdal JO. Evaluating surgically induced astigmatism by Fourier analysis of corneal topography data. J Cat Refract Surg 1996;22: 318–23.
64. Parker PJ, Klyces SD, Ryan BL, et al. Central topographic islands following photorefractive keratectomy. Invest Ophthalmol Vis Sci 1993;34:803.
65. Prydal JI, Campbell FW. Study of precorneal tear film thickness and structure by interferometry and confocal microscopy. Invest Ophthalmol Vis Sci 1992;33:1996–2005.
66. Rabinowitz YS, McDonnell PJ. Computer-assisted corneal topography in keratoconus. Refract Corneal Surg 1989;5:400-8.
67. Rabinowitz YS, Garbus JJ, Garbus C, McDonnell PJ. Contact lens selection for keratoconus using a computer assisted videokeratoscope. CLAO J 1991; 17:88-93.
68. Roberts C. The accuracy of power maps to display curvature data in corneal topography systems. Invest Ophthalmol Vis Sci 1994; 35: 3524- 3532.
69. Roberts C. Characterization of the inherent error in a spherically-biased corneal topography system in mapping a radially aspheric surface. J Refract Corneal Surg 1994; 10: 103-116.
70. Rowsey JJ, Reynolds AE, Brown DR. Corneal Topography: Corneascope. Arch Ophthalmol 1981;99: 1093-100.
71. Ruiz-Montenegro J, Mafra CH, Wilson SE, et al. Corneal topography alterations in normal contact lens wearers. Ophthalmology 1993;100:128-134.
72. Salabert D, Cochener B, Mage F, Collin J. Kératocone et anomalies topographiques cornéennes familiales. J Fr Ophtalmol 1994;17(II): 646-56.

29

73. Sanders RD, Gills JP, Martin RG. When keratometric measurements do not accurately reflect corneal topography. J Cat Refract Surg 1993;19 (Suppl): 131–5.
74. Seiler T, Reckmann W, Maloney RK. Effective spherical aberration of the cornea as a quantitative descriptor in corneal topography. J Cat Refract Surg 1993;19 (Suppl): 155-65.
75. Takeda M, Ina H, Kobayashi S. Fourier-transform method of fringe-pattern analysis for computer-based topography and interferometry. J Optical Soc Am 1982;72: 156–60.
76. Taylor CT, Sutphin JE. Accuracy and precision of the Orbscan topography unit in measuring standardized radially aspheric surfaces. Invest Ophthalmol Vis Sci 1996; 37: s561.
77. Thall EH, Lange SR. Preliminary results of a new intraoperative corneal topography technique. J Cat Refract Surg 1993;19 (Suppl): 193-7.
78. Tripoli NK, Cohen KL, Holmgren DE, Coggins JM. Assessment of radial aspheres by the arc-step algorithm as implemented by the Keratron keratoscope. Am J Ophthalmol 1995; 120: 658-64.
79. Tripoli NK, Cohen KL, Obla P, Coggins JM, Holmgren DE. Height measurement of astigmatic test surfaces by a keratoscope that uses plane geometry reconstruction. Am J Ophthalmol 1996; 121; 668-76.
80. Vass C, Menapace R. Computerised statistical analysis of corneal topography for the evaluation of changes in corneal shape after surgery. Am J Ophthalmol 1994;118:177–84.
81. Vass C, Menapace R, Rainer G, Schulz H. Improved algorithm for statistical batch-by-batch analysis of corneal topographic data. J Cat Refract Surg 1997;23:903–12.
82. Vass C, Menapace R, Amon M, Hirsch U, Yousef A. Batch-by-batch analysis of topographic changes induced by sutured and sutureless clear corneal incisions. J Cat Refract Surg 1996; 22: 324–30.
83. Wang J, Rice DA, Klyce SD. A new reconstruction algorithm for improvement of corneal topographical analysis. J Refract Corneal Surg 1989; 5:379-87
84. Warnicki JW, Rehkopf PG, Arrra RC, Stuart JC. Corneal topography using a projected grid. In Schanzlin DJ, Robin JB (Eds): Corneal Topography. Measuring and Modifying the Cornea. New York: Springer-Verlag, 1992.
85. Warnicki JW, Rehkopf PG, Curtin DY, Burns SA, Arffa RC, Stuart JC. Corneal topography using computer analyzed rasterstereographic images. Appl Optics 1988;27: 1135–40.
86. Warning GO, Hannush SB, Bogan SJ, Maloney RK. Classification of corneal topography with videotopography. In Shanzlin DJ, Robin JB (Eds): Corneal Topography: Measuring and Modifying the Cornea. New York: Springer-Verlag, 1992;47-73.
87. Wilson SE, Klyce SD, Husseini ZM. Standardized color-coded maps for corneal topography. Ophthalmology 1993;100: 1723-7.
88. Wilson SE, Wang JY, Klyce SD. Quantification and mathematical analysis of photokeratoscopic images. In Shanzlin DJ, Robin JB (Eds): Corneal Topography: Measuring and Modifying the Cornea. New York: Springer-Verlag, 1991; 1-81.
89. Wilson SE, Klyce SD. Quantitative descriptors of corneal topography: a clinical study. Arch Ophthalmol 1991;109:349-53.
90. Wilson SE, Verity SM, Conger DL. Accuracy and precision of the corneal analysis system and the topographic modeling system. Cornea 1992; 11: 28-35.
91. Young JA, Siegel IM. Isomorphic corneal topography: a clinical approach to 3-D representation of the corneal surface. Refract Corneal Surg 1993;9: 74–8.
92. Young JA, Siegel IM. Three-dimensional digital subtraction modeling of corneal topography. J Refract Surg 1995; 11: 188–93.

Chapter 2

Special Topographic Conditions

Guillermo L Simón Castellvi
Sarabel Simón
José Mª Simón
Cristina Simón

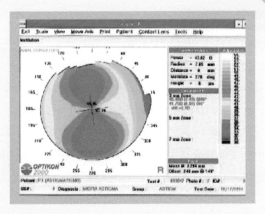

MAP OF A NORMAL ROUND CORNEA

There is a **wide spectrum of normality**. No human cornea demonstrates the kind of regularity found in the calibration spheres of a topographer: the eye is not polished glass-made. Normal corneal topography can take on many topographic patterns: Figure 2.1 shows the axial map of a right *eye* normal **round cornea**, with concentric green rings in an absolute scale. Notice that the nasal side of this healthy corneal map becomes blue more quickly than temporal side, indicating that the nasal cornea is flatter than the temporal. In the central 3 mm zone, there is a small amount of astigmatism (1 D displayed), which is within normal limits, and does not mean that the patient needs to be corrected with this astigmatism.

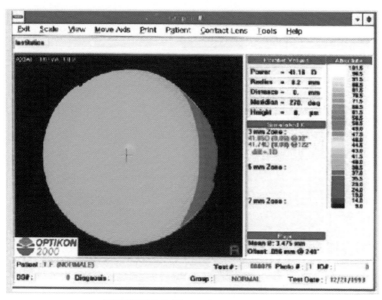

FIGURE 2.1: Normal round cornea

NORMAL CORNEA WITH ASTIGMATISM ACCORDING TO THE RULE

Regular astigmatism (**with-the-rule**) gives an oval axial corneal map, being the most common deviation from optically perfect spherical (round) cornea. In Figures 2.2 and 2.3, observe that the bow tie is vertical (the long axis is near the vertical meridian) in an axial map, representing a cornea having with-the-rule-astigmatism. Figure 2.2 displays an axial curvature map of a –3.7 D regular astigmatism in an adjustable scale. Always check the scale in which the map is offered: color differences do not always mean a difference in dioptric or radial values, but can mean a difference in the scale used by the explorer. Notice that a simulated keratometric overlay is displayed at the center of the bow tie.

Modern topographers run under Windows™ operating system, and are easy to use. Most software enables to enlarge desired areas for better explanation to the patient and to better view the details. Figure 2.3 shows an enlarged area of a with-the-rule astigmatism with an absolute scale.

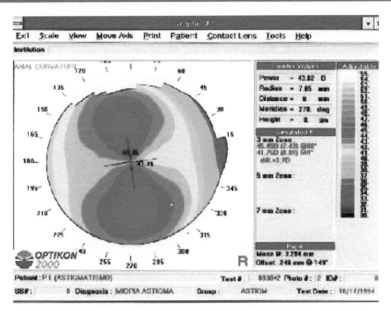

FIGURE 2.2: Normal cornea with astigmatism

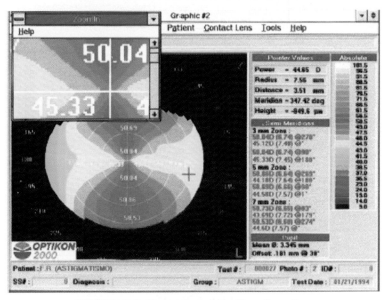

FIGURE 2.3: Normal cornea with astigmatism

TOPOGRAPHIC MAP OF ASTIGMATISM EXPRESSED IN HEIGHTS

Representation of the topographic map of an astigmatism (–3.75 D at 176°) expressed in height (in microns) (Figure 2.4). The yellow area corresponds to a sphere with a defined radius, while orange-red and green-blue areas correspond to either elevation or flattening of the cornea. Notice that color scale may confuse the explorer.

KERATOCONUS

An important indication of corneal topography is the screening of candidates for refractive surgery. It is very important to identify patients with corneal ectasia, since surgical outcomes are uncertain in most

33

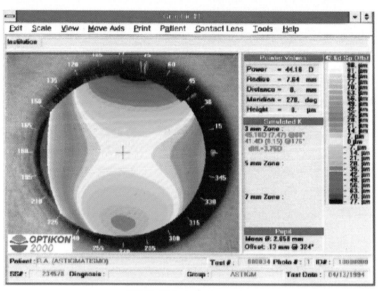

FIGURE 2.4: Astigmatism

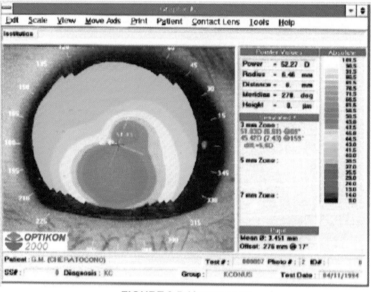

FIGURE 2.5: Keratoconus

cases. Early detection of a subclinical keratoconus can save the patient of a refractive procedure (incisional or photoablative) that likely will not result in the desired visual outcome, and may result in dangerous corneal thinning. The most frequent ectatic corneal disorder is keratoconus. This condition is characterized by a corneal stromal thinning. It typically presents in early adulthood, is almost always bilateral (although can be very asymmetric), and progresses slowly over the years. Mild keratoconus cannot be detected easily at the slit-lamp, and only corneal topography can help detecting them. Some other conditions, like corneal warpage of RGP contact lenses may mimic mild keratoconus corneal maps. In most cases, the corneal thinning occurs just inferior to the corneal center. Protrusion of this region gives the cornea an exaggerated prolapsing shape. The point of maximum protrusion is called

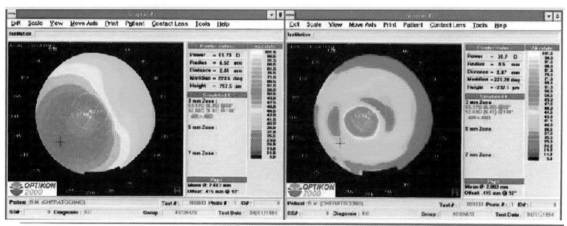

FIGURE 2.6: Keratoconus

the apex of the cone. Figures 2.5 and 2.6 display a typical map of a moderate keratoconus (–5.6 D), showing a corneal steepening inferior to corneal vertex (orange-red, in absolute scale, in the shape of a pear fruit). Notice the high corneal central power (around 50 D), the inferior cornea (orange) steeper than superior cornea (green), and the large difference between the power of the corneal apex and that of the periphery.

A topographic classification of keratoconus can been established (Table 2.1).

Severity	Site of the cone	Shape of the cone	Slit-lamp detectable
Subclinical	Inferior	like a pear fruit	No
Clinical: Mild	Inferior	Typical, oval like a pear fruit	Sometimes needs a trained explorer
Moderate	Central	Globus +/– Inferior	Yes
Severe	Superior	Nipple	Yes, visible without slit-lamp

TABLE 2.1: Topographic classification of keratoconus

The comparison of representation of dioptric powers, axial (left) and local (right), of the same eye with an inferotemporal keratoconus is surprising: notice the minimal extension of the corneal surface involved in the pathology, and the flattening of the adjacent area.

CORNEAL ULCER

By quantifying the irregularity of the cornea, topography helps to determine the proportion of the visual loss of a patient suffering from a corneal ulceration or epithelial disruption close to the visual axis. It also helps to follow-up a corneal abscess or ulceration. Figure 2.7 shows the true curvature map of a corneal inferior ulceration. Notice the local flattening of the corneal surface (in blue), resulting from the localized depression of the ulcer, surrounded by a ring of edematous elevated tissue (in red).

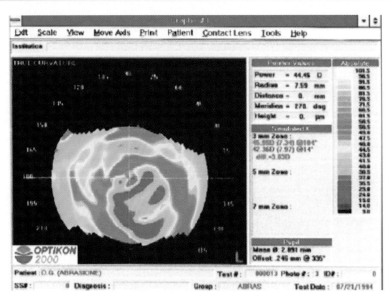

FIGURE 2.7: Corneal ulcer

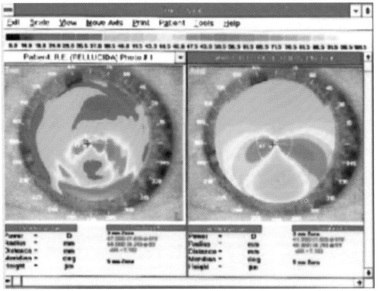

FIGURE 2.8: Marginal pellucid degeneration

MARGINAL PELLUCID DEGENERATION

Stromal corneal disease includes a variety of inflammatory and non-inflammatory disorders, like Terrien's marginal degeneration, Mooren's ulceration, pellucid marginal degeneration and others. Figure 2.8 displays true elevation map (left) and axial map (right) of a pellucid marginal degeneration, a narrow band of corneal thinning located 1 to 2 mm from the inferior limbus. Observe the flattening of the central cornea (true elevation and axial maps) along the vertical axis. Extensive peripheral guttering leads to irregular against-the-rule astigmatism, such as this arching inferior bow tie visible in the axial map. These topographic findings are characteristic: they help establishing diagnosis even in patients without slit-lamp typical findings.

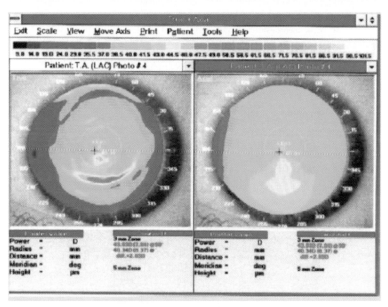

FIGURE 2.9: Contact lens warpage

CONTACT LENS OVERUSE (WARPAGE)

Different types of contact lenses have different impact on corneal surface and different indications. We can classify them into three main groups: soft, rigid gas-permeable (RGP) and hard (PMMA). The last are no longer considered suitable for making contacts, and are only prescribed in special cases. Rigid gas-permeable contact lenses are relatively popular: they offer good visual performance, they can be polished, they tolerate most known cleaning solutions, and custom designs are possible. The bad side also exists, since they require individualized fitting (by means of K-readings, topographic maps, …), they are not easily tolerated at first, and induce with relative ease changes of the shape of the cornea: the process of changes is termed warpage. It is thought due to mechanical pressure on the cornea, although other factors like oxygen deficiency have not been excluded. Many topographic patterns may result, like the one in Figure 2.9, depending upon the fit (size, curvature, …) and position of the lens. In this case, observe the inferior steepening in the axial map causing meridian asymmetry as a result of superior riding contact lens. The true elevation map shows corneal surface irregularity (orange).

Cessation of the lens wear and good ocular lubrication result in return to corneal former shape.

CURVED ARCUATE KERATOTOMIES (ASTIGMATIC KERATOTOMIES)

Most refractive efforts have concentrated on altering the shape of the cornea, which is the main diopter of the eye. Topography is valuable in the preoperative assessment and planning of the surgery. Figure 2.10 displays both true elevation (left) and axial maps (right) of an astigmatic patient who underwent astigmatic keratotomies. Two paired circumferential relaxing incisions centered on the steep axis result in focal steepening (orange-red in true elevation map) and central flattening in that meridian (blue). The final result is 0.13 D of astigmatism in the 3 mm central cornea.

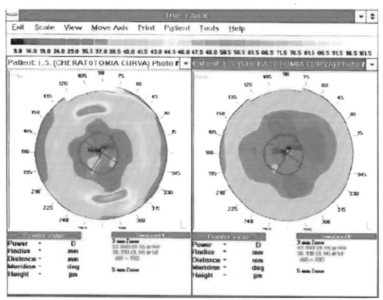

FIGURE 2.10: Astigmatic keratotomy

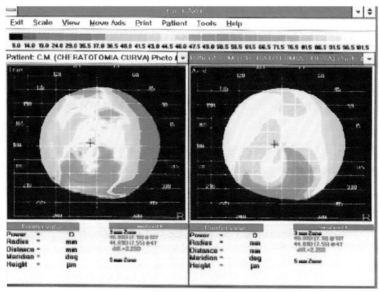

FIGURE 2.11: Keratotomy with resulting ectasia

KERATOTOMY WITH RESULTING ECTASIA

Every surgical procedure has some risks the patient must be aware of. Any kind of keratotomy (radial, astigmatic or other) may perforate the globe or result in an ectasia like the one shown in Figure 2.11. The inferior ectasia simulates an irregular keratoconus, in both true elevation (left map) and axial (on the right) maps.

PHOTOREFRACTIVE KERATECTOMY PRK

To correct myopia, the excimer laser removes more tissue from the center than the periphery of the treatment zone (ablation zone). The ablation profile is different for every model of laser. In Figure 2.12,

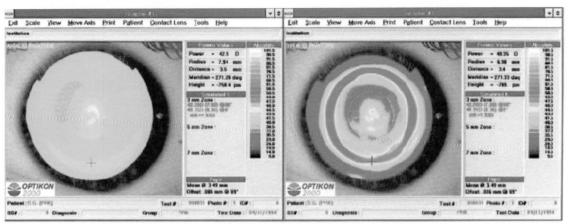

FIGURE 2.12: PRK

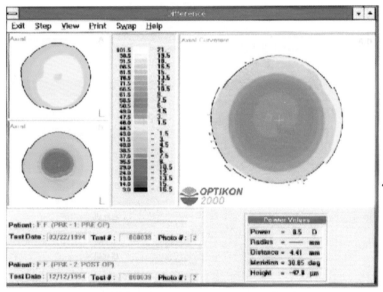

FIGURE 2.13: Subtraction map in PRK

map on the left represents the spherical approach (axial curvature) of a patient who suffered myopic photorefractive keratectomy. Only the "true elevation" map (on the right) shows the transition area, where dioptric powers are very high (ring in red).

SUBTRACTION MAP IN A PRK

The most effective way of displaying the changes in a cornea that undergoes a refractive procedure are difference maps (Figure 2.13). The change induced by surgery is obtained by subtracting the preoperative map (upper small axial map) from the postoperative map (lower small axial map). The image on the right shows the result (in terms of dioptric variation, axial curvature) of a myopic PRK. In red, the ablation zone. In orange, the transition zone, which is easily delineated in the postoperative axial map which shows that the central cornea has been flattened (lower small axial map on the left).

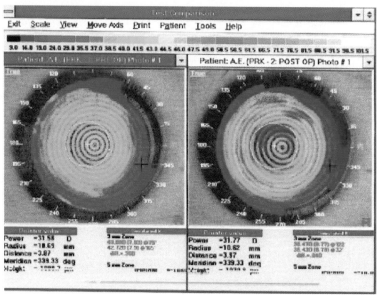

FIGURE 2.14: True curvature analysis in PRK

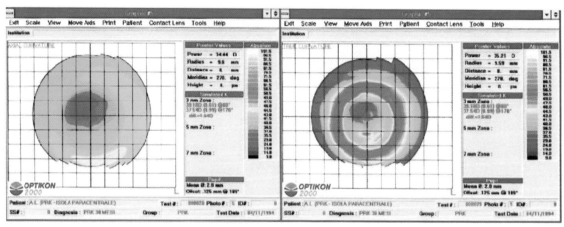

FIGURE 2.15: Paracentral island

TRUE CURVATURE ANALYSIS IN PRE/POST PRK

The comparison between preoperative and postoperative true curvature analysis of the same PRK patient shows no variations of the peripheral cornea after surgery (Figure 2.14).

PARACENTRAL ISLAND

Many are the potential complications of laser refractive surgery. Some may be attributable to the ablative pattern of each model of excimer laser, like central or paracentral islands, although the origin is uncertain. They are defined as any area within the ablation zone surrounded by areas of lesser curvature on more than 50 percent of its boundaries. They are a topographic pattern in PRK and LASIK patients, not always obvious. Figure 2.15 displays a paracentral island after myopic PRK: it can be identified down inside the ablation red ring as a yellow-orange spot. Notice that only with the calculation method of local

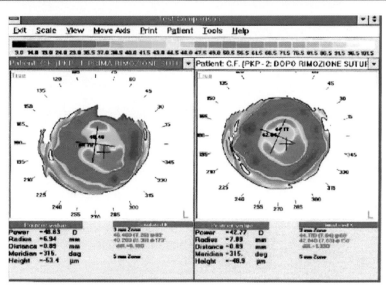

FIGURE 2.16: Effect of suture removal after keratoplasty

powers (true curvature map on the right), this small abnormality is made visible, remaining invisible in the axial map (on the left).

EFFECT OF SUTURE REMOVAL AFTER KERATOPLASTY

Serial topographic exams after a penetrating keratoplasty reveal large configurational changes in the first two months, which remain stable until suture removal. Topography is then used to determine the suture to be removed in order to lower suture-induced astigmatism and enhance visual recovery. Figure 2.16 shows a test comparison: left map displays high astigmatism after a penetrating keratoplasty (–6.18 at 173°), right map displays the reduction to 1.33 D after suture removal. Notice the asymmetry of power between the two hemi-meridians, that improves after suture removal. Observe the red areas of high power (and elevation) near the wound.

Topographer is preferred over keratometer as most changes do occur outside the 3 mm area measured by the keratometer.

SOFTWARE ADJUSTMENT OF A DE-CENTERED AXIS

The Keratron™ Corneal Topographer (Optikon 2000® S.p.A, Italy-Europe) offers some interesting features like the possibility of replacing the optical axis when the patient's fixation is not as desired or corneal centration is not perfect. The system is able to recalculate the optical power values for the whole cornea (Figure 2.17). Notice that values at the optical axis differ from the original map with geometric axis calculations (on the left) and the recalculated map with the new visual axis position (map on the right).

MYOPIC AND HYPEROPIC KERATOMILEUSIS (LASIK)

In Figure 2.18, two "true curvature" maps of both myopic (left) and hyperopic (right) keratomileusis are shown. To correct myopia, excimer laser removes a central disk of corneal stroma, resulting in

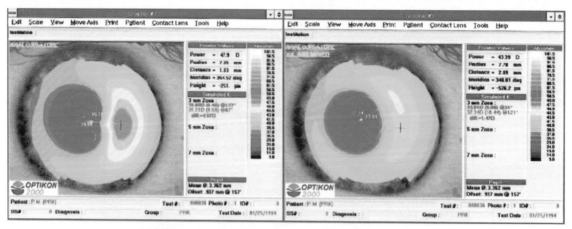

FIGURE 2.17: Software adjustment of a de-centered axis

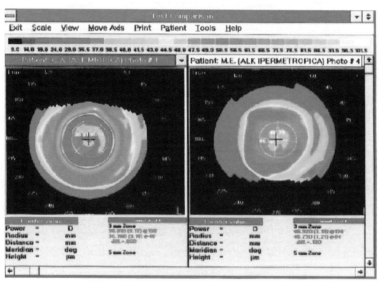

FIGURE 2.18: LASIK

central flattening (blue) and the presence of a relative peripheral steepening ring (red). Corneal topographic changes similar to those seen after photorefractive keratectomy (PRK) occur after LASIK for myopia.

To correct hyperopia, the excimer laser does just the opposite: it removes an annulus or ring of tissue from the midperiphery (blue) to steepen the central cornea (red).

INTRASTROMAL SEGMENTED GRAFT FOR THE CORRECTION OF HIGH MYOPIAS

Figure 2.19 shows a "true curvature" map of a left eye cornea that received an intrastromal segmented graft for the correction of high myopia. The map is similar to that of a myopic LASIK, but less regular.

FLUORESCEIN SIMULATION IN RGP CONTACT LENS

Contact lens fitting applications are used to help choosing the best lens for every case, by simulating the fluorescein film pattern and contact lens position of rigid contact lenses (RGP and PMMA). The simulated

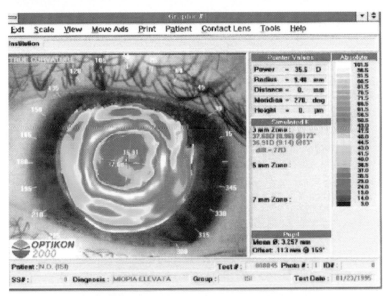

FIGURE 2.19: Intrastromal segmented graft

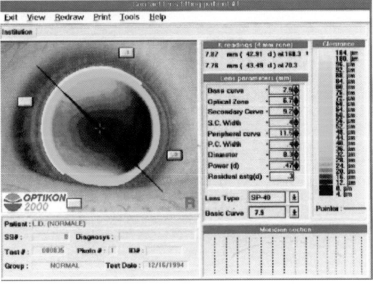

FIGURE 2.20: Fluorescein stimulation in RGP contact lens

fluorescein feature is intended to reduce fitting time by viewing the effect of changing lens parameters on a personalized basis, depending on the patient's corneal exam (Figure 2.20). Let us notice that the true *in vivo* result of any computerized fluorescein test may vary due to differences caused by lid action on the lens (aperture and weight).

ACKNOWLEDGMENTS

All maps have been taken with a KERATRON™ Corneal Topographer (Optikon 2000® S.p.A, Italy-Europe). The corneal maps are courtesy of:
• Instituto Scientifico Ospedale San Raffaele-Milano (Prof Brancato-Dr Carones)

- Ospedale Fatebenefratelli-Roma (Prof Neuschüller-D.ssa Cantera)
- Centro Oculistico-Rovigo (Prof Merlin-Dr Camellin)
- Clinica Oculistica Universitaria-Padova (Prof Bisantis)
- University of North Carolina-Chapel Hill (Prof Cohen-D.ssa Tripoli)
- University of California-Jules Stein Institute-Los Angeles (Dr Maloney)

We want to specially thank them as well as the manufacturer of the Keratron™ videokeratoscope, Opticon 2000® S.p.A., for the permission to reproduce them.

Topographic Machines

Guillermo L Simón Castellvi
Sarabel Simón
José Mª Simón
Cristina Simón

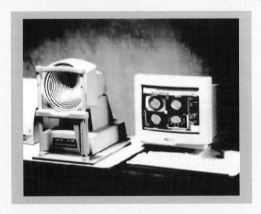

ZEISS HUMPHREY SYSTEMS® ATLAS™ CORNEAL TOPOGRAPHY SYSTEM MODELS 993 AND ECLIPSE 995 (FIGURE 3.1)

Zeiss Humphrey Systems® ATLAS™ Corneal Topography System Models 993 and Eclipse 995 are best sellers in the USA (Table 3.1). They measure true elevation data (Figure 3.2), through an advanced **arc-step algorithm** (similar to Optikon 2000® Keratron™), by means of 20 to 22 ring conical Placido disk. The Atlas Eclipse 995 offers ultra-low illumination and increased peripheral coverage (limbus to limbus). They also offer automatic pupil measurement. Software displays are viewed in a 10.4" TFT 640 × 480 pixel resolution in 18 bit color; they include: photokeratoscope view, axial map, tangential map, numeric view, and profile view. Very interesting optional software packages are available at a price: MasterFit™ contact lens module, corneal elevation map, corneal irregularity map, refractive power map, keratoconus detection map, VisioPro™ ablation planing software and Healing Trend/STARS™ display.

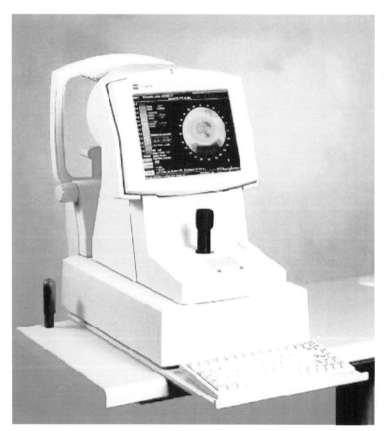

FIGURE 3.1: Zeiss Humphrey ATLAS™ corneal topography system

TECHNOMED® COLOR ELLIPSOID TOPOMETER

The reproducibility of videokeratography measurements is mainly dependent on the accuracy of manual adjustment in the focal plane. Videokeratoscopes having small Placido cones show a

TABLE 3.1: Zeiss Humphrey systems® ATLAS™ corneal topography system models 993 and Eclipse 995

	Technical specifications	
	ATLAS 993	*ATLAS ECLIPSE 995*
Working distance	70 mm	70 mm
Field of view	11.4 mm	12.5 mm
Number of rings	20	22 (18 superiorly)
Dioptric range	9 to 108 D	9 to 108 D
Optics	High-res CCD camera	High-res CCD camera
Repeatability (test object)	± 0.1 D	± 0.1 D
Repeatability (normal corneas)	± 0.25 D	± 0.25 D
Luminosity	Visible light	**Infrared** (very low-light)
Voltage	100/120/220/240 V AC	100/120/220/240 V AC
Size (Width x Depth x Height) mm	313 x 466 x 457 mm	313 x 466 x 457 mm
Weight	17 kg	20 kg

* Hardware is included: configuration may vary (450 MHz microprocessor, 64 MB RAM memory, 20 GB hard disk drive, 3.5 "floppy disk drive, USB and Ethernet sockets, 10.4" TFT flat panel monitor display, one button joystick control, compact keyboard, Glidepoint™ touchpad. Model 955 incorporates infrared chin rest sensors in the patented chin rest design

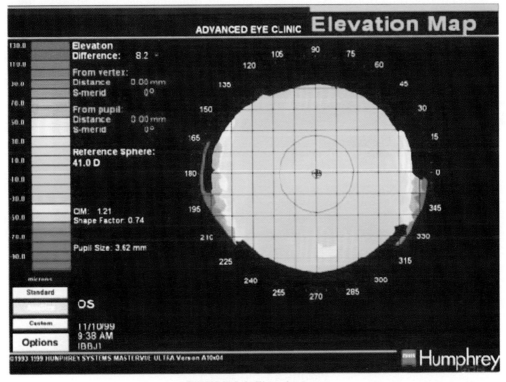

FIGURE 3.2: Elevation map

considerable amount of error when the required working distance between cornea and keratoscope is not maintained. The advantages of small cones (optimal illumination and the reduction of anatomically caused shadows) are in no proportion to the disadvantage, poor depth of focus, resulting in poor reproducibility.

The Color Ellipsoid Topometer compensates defocusing errors with software and hardware, by means of a triangulation measurement, enhancing precision and theoretically avoiding measuring artifacts. It is the only Placido (30 ring) system with color-coded rings (three colored rings). By means of a laser, it measures 10800 points, providing real height values and has ray tracing software. A new module enables topography-driven laser ablation. This unit is specially useful in diagnosing postoperative problems in a refractive practice, specially in those cases with a loss of vision that cannot be explained. The Color Ellipsoid Topometer can predict the quality of vision based on the shape of the cornea and pupil.

DICON ® CT200 (FIGURE 3.3)

The reproducibility of videokeratography measurements is mainly dependent on the accuracy of manual adjustment in the focal plane. The DICON® CT200 is a cheap easy-to-use instrument with **autofocus** and **autoalignment** that eliminate joystick and explorer subjectivity, thus improving repeatability (Table 3.2). The big Placido disk cone in managed from the computer by means of the mouse. Final alignment (up and down) and focusing (forwards and backwards) are automatically performed by the motorized instrument head.

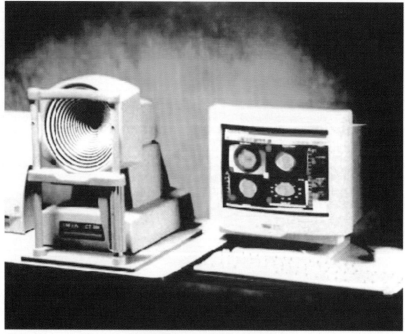

FIGURE 3.3: DICON® CT200

It **can explore the whole cornea** (apex and limbus to limbus) thanks to an offset fixation (Figure 3.4). The patient can fixate different green lights, to allow complete cornea coverage. Offset-fixation mapping allows for more precise mapping of the central 3 mm of the cornea. More true data points from the apex and true limbus-to-limbus measurements over a large corneal area provide for better coverage without extrapolation.

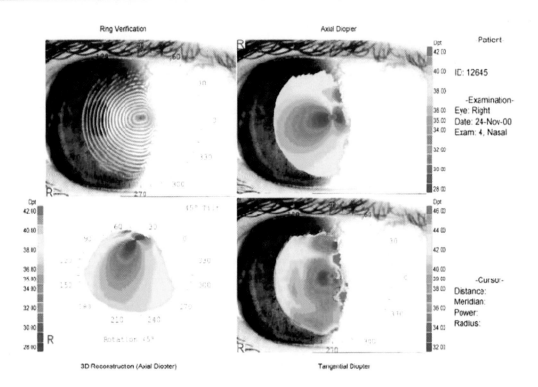

FIGURE 3.4: Dicon's CT-200™ can explore the whole cornea (apex, and limbus to limbus) thanks to an offset fixation. The patient fixates different green lights: shown is a quadruple view of right eye corneal maps display a nasal fixation, including 3-D reconstruction with a 45° tilt (left and down). Optional software (Multiview™) provides total cornea coverage using the mentioned multiple fixation targets. Limbal measurements are not always reliable, being subject to many artifacts.

Nevertheless, we miss a different chin rest to allow faster exams by eliminating the need for patient's head re-centration from one eye to the other.

The system generates maps in seconds and detailed customized reports can be printed in less than a minute with any color printer running under MS Windows '95™ operating system.

A very interesting feature of this instrument is the **Bull's Eye Targetting**™: the system automatically targets the apex position of a cone (keratoconus or other), providing a numerical index for that cone. An auto-alarm is activated so that any suspicious case of keratoconus (or excessive corneal elevation with an index higher than 10) is automatically detected and acoustically signaled as a peak detection warning window appears in the display after the image capture is complete. New users will appreciate this feature: a low index is not uncommon, and does not always mean that we face a pathologic cornea. High indices in a tangential map almost always mean that we face a keratoconus or another kind of corneal ectasia (Figure 3.5).

Peak detection can be triggered by any suspect peak, including mucus in the tear film, or localized areas of film break-up. In one such case, always have the patient close the eyes for a while and blink a few extra times before retaking the picture. In case of doubt, it is advisable to retake the picture again. The determination of the condition producing the corneal elevation needs to be confirmed by other clinical tests, like slit-lamp examination or others.

49

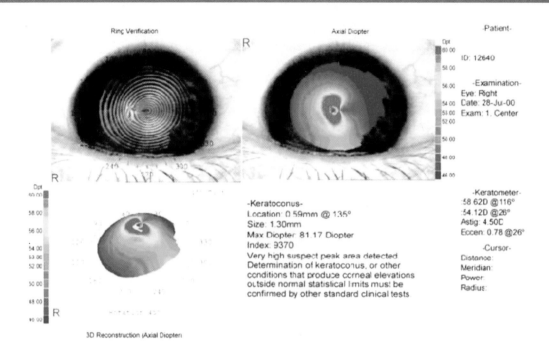

FIGURE 3.5: Shows a quadruple display map of the right eye of a 55-year-old man suffering from progressive bilateral corneal central ectasia. Notice the distortion of the mires in the ring verification map (up and left), the enormous "red" central and paracentral elevation in the axial diopter map (up and right). Statistical information is displayed following the peak detection, identifying the location, size, maximum power, peak index and probability statement ("very high suspect peak area detected"). One such high index (index = 9370) always means that we face a keratoconus or another kind of corneal ectasia. The ectasia was clearly visible at the slit-lamp

The DICON® CT-200™ software includes an optional refractive module that allows single analysis (Figure 3.6), trend analysis of multiple displays and a special package called VISX ® STAR S2™ Ablation Planner.

The VISX® STAR S2™ Ablation Planner is offered as an option and is intended to learn the control system for the Visx® laser. It offers a custom display of the CT 200 Elliptical Elevation Map, and access to the VISX® STAR S2™ control panel. It allows a simulated (not real) image of the before/after laser ablation for better comprehension of the procedure.

Developed by Dr Robert B Mandell is a simplified contact lens fitting software, with fluorescein simulation. You can design unique lenses for each cornea (personalized designs) and send the data directly to the manufacturer (via modem) or print the order sheet for faxing or mailing.

EYE SYS® 2000

Topographers from Premier Laser Systems, **EyeSys Corneal Analysis System 2000** *and* **EyeSys Vista Hand-held corneal topographer,** *have been the leading topographers in the USA for years but might have been discontinued at the moment you may read this chapter due to Premier Laser Systems' bankruptcy. We have included them to honor the topographers we learned with, as most*

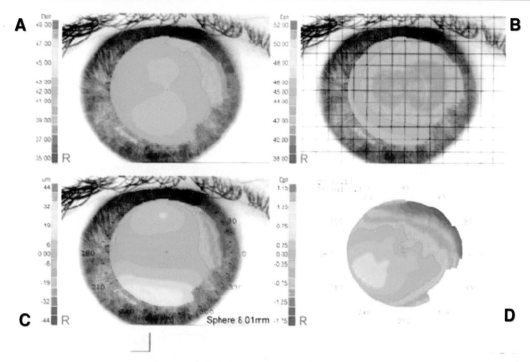

FIGURE 3.6: The "Single Analysis" menu option of the DICON ® CT-200™ displays a single exam with four customizable map views: **A** axial diopter, **B** refractive diopter (shown with a square grid overlay), **C** spherical height and d) irregularity (shown without the eye overlay). The irregularity map, **D** reports an index (Q = –0.10) that measures eccentricity (a measure of asphericity) and the amount of astigmatism that has been subtracted from the original ideal spherical corneal data (in this case, 1.12 D)

topographic texts still refer to them. We hope that new partners in early future or potential buyers help to guarantee the survival of EyeSys topographers in this hard marketplace.

KERATRON™ CORNEAL TOPOGRAPHER (OPTIKON 2000® S.P.A, ITALY -EUROPE) (FIGURE 3.7)

The Keratron™ topographer is one of our preferred systems: it is a must if you are in refractive surgery (Table 3.3). The Keratron Topographers offer automatic image capture. A patented corneal vertex detector system is housed inside a slight protrusion on either side of the cone. If you position the Keratron™ too close or too far, image capture just will not happen. Only when the system detects the vertex in the exact right position, image is automatically captured, thus obtaining more reproducible maps.

Introduced in 1994, the Keratron™ was the first hardware platform designed to get the most of an ARC STEP surface reconstruction, achieving accuracy and sensitivity, without smoothing of data or extrapolating to fill in topographic shadows. The Keratron's **own method of arc-step mapping** accurately maps aspheric surfaces. It uses a small Placido cone of rings.

Its patented infra-red vertex detector sensor determines the exact position of the corneal vertex and begins constructing a web of "Arcs" between the intersections of 26 rings and 256 meridians, from the

TABLE 3.2: DICON® CT-200™	
Technical specifications	
Videokeratoscope	
Tested area	
Keratoscope cone	Big cone, 16 bright Placido rings and 16 dark rings
Measured points	11,500
Corneal coverage	Total, by means of different fixation targets with standard software (optional Multiview™ software provides total corneal coverage)
Range of dioptric powers	
Resolution	
Focusing	Autofocus, autoalignment for X, Y and Z
Camera	High-resolution video system
Voltage	110 or 230 V, 50/60 Hz
Computer	Included with the system (may vary), separate
Processor	Intel® PENTIUM™
Main memory	32 MB RAM (minimum)
Hard disk	4.3 GB (minimum)
Floppy disk drive	3 ½"-1.44 MB
Monitor	Color 14" Super VGA
Video Mode	Up to 1024x768 and 256 colors
Mouse	Included, 100% Microsoft compatible
Printer	Any color printer running under Windows
Modem	Internal (in some countries)
Software	32-bit programs (Eye 3.40 and Backup software on CD), running under Windows ™ 95
Color maps	
Color scales	Absolute, normalized, adjustable, mm or D
Keratometric data	simulated K-reading, mm or D
Pupil	Edge mapping, diameter and offset
Available maps	Axial, spherical height , tangential, refractive, numerical display, meridional, 3-D reconstruction map, Elliptical elevation
Printouts	Full color, customizable reports
Special functions	Profile, map difference, map comparison, PRK-LASIK simulation Simultaneous screen displays for rapid analysis and ease of use Keratoconus detection Irregularity index to measure corneal distortion which affects quality of vision Delta map to determine changes between exams
Surgical modules	Advanced surgical module for healing trend analysis with difference maps (optional) VISX® STAR S2™ Ablation Planner
On-line help	Available
Contact lens fitting	Fluorescein simulation of any RGP CL geometry or major CL producers (customizable lens design) Mandell contact lens module "Easy-Fit™" (standard) Mandell contact lens module "Advanced-Fit™" (optional)
Internet connection	Possible
Direct faxing	Possible as standard for contact lens ordering or sending reports, through operating system
LAN operations	Possible, through operating system

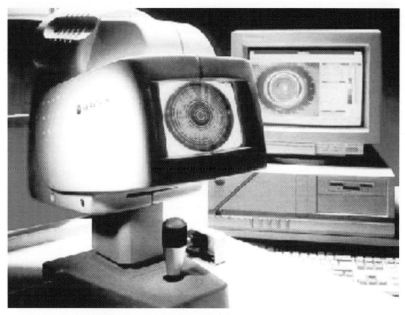

FIGURE 3.7: Keratron™ corneal topographer

vertex to the periphery. Defining corneal vertex position and starting measurements from it provide this topographer with high accuracy. Curvature and height are simultaneously derived from the length and shape of each arc. Mapping beginning at the corneal vertex, this instrument easily detects up central islands or minor defects. Each data point of the "web" is related to another one, thus eliminating inaccuracies of traditional Placido "concentric rings method" which take measurement of each point independently from one another, resulting in possible errors.

While most topographers first create an axial map and then convert the axial data into different maps, every Keratron's map is calculated separately without conversions, thus decreasing probability of errors. Since the Keratron does not convert data, map error is minimal in all maps.

True corneal elevation (height) in microns as well as the traditional curvature maps are created. This system enables to map the image of a patient with bad fixation—through mathematics reconstruction. The system is fast and easy to use, working under MS Windows™ environment. The powerful software is the gem of the system: novice will find some difficulty; but once you master it, you will not want to get rid of this topographer.

You can design unique lenses for each cornea (personalized designs) and send the data directly to the manufacturer (via modem). A recently developed software by Jim Edwards, OD *(patents pending)* called WAVE uses a unique but logical approach to contact lens design by effectively creating a mirror image of the peripheral cornea in the lens design process. Contact lenses designed with wave drape the cornea in a manner similar to a soft lens. As the lens periphery matches the peripheral cornea, lens centration should be unsurpassed, even with reverse geometry lenses.

Optikon 2000® has made a small portable topographer called **scout portable topographer** with the same features as the full size device: at the moment these lines are written, it suffers from some youth

TABLE 3.3: KERATRON™ Corneal Topographer

Technical specifications

Videokeratoscope

Tested area	10 mm x 14 mm (visible on the monitor)
Keratoscope cone	28 equally spaced borders of black and bright Placido rings
Tested points	More than 80,000
Measured points	7,168
Corneal coverage	From 0.33 mm (first ring) to about 90% of a normal cornea
Range of dioptric powers	From I to 127 D
Resolution	+/– 0.01D; 1 micron
Focusing	Infrared automatic, Eye Position Control System (patented)
Camera	High-resolution (C.C.I.R. system)
Monitor	6" black and white

Computer (minimal requirements)

Processor	Intel™ PENTIUM®
Main memory	32 MB RAM (minimum)
Hard disk	2 GB (minimum)
Floppy disk drive	3½"-1.44 MB
Monitor	Color 14" Super VGA
Video mode	Up to 1280 × 1024 and up to 16 million colors
Mouse	Any 100% Microsoft compatible
Printer	Any color printer running under Windows™
Software	Microsoft® Windows™ 3.11, '95 or '98

Color maps

Color scales	Absolute, normalized, adjustable, spherical offset, mm or D
Keratometry	K-reading, meridians, Emi-meridians, Maloney indices
Pupil	edge mapping, diameter and offset
Zones	3, 5 and 7 mm
Maps representations	Local true curvature, axial and refractive powers (All with arc-step algorithm)
Eye/map orientation	Video-keratoscope axis, or moved to the entrance pupil or to any chosen axis
Printouts	Large and small size with the patient's form, list of the filed examinations
Special functions	Profile, map difference, map comparison, PRK simulation
On-line help	Available from any screen
Contact lens fitting	Simulation of any RGP CL geometry or major CL producers
	Tilting and displacement of the lens
	Eccentricity and apical radius measurements at 6/8 mm of the main axes, or locally on any axis
	Autofit programs (curvature classical and height fitting) with personalized protocols
	Adjustable clearance scale
	Optional Wave Contact Lens Design software (available in the USA)
Internet connection	Possible with personalized template letter
LAN operations	Possible
Image capture	Possible from an external slit-lamp TV camera, with KeraCap software (included) and a generic frame capture board

design defects that will be soon addressed by Opticon 2000®. It is available as slit-lamp model, hand-held model, table top model or surgical microscope model.

ET-800 CORNEAL TOPOGRAPHY SYSTEM

Euclid Systems Corporation® ET-800 CTS is another interesting product in this round-up, since it uses a completely different method of topography called **Fourier profilometry**.

The technique uses the projection of 2 identical sine wave patterns onto the surface of the eye. The projection is done using filtered blue light that induces fluorescence of a liquid (fluorescein) that has been applied to the tear film before the examination. The resulting image is captured by a CCD camera. Two-dimensional Fourier transform mathematics are used to calculate the phase shift of the projected wave pattern. The phase shift is directly related to the height information. This method analyses over 300,000 data points to achieve true elevation co-ordinates, with each point accurate to approximately the thickness of the tear film (about one micron). The problem is that thickness of the tear film varies with the daytime, and is not the same for each patient.

The system uses no rings or Placido disk. It is quite fast (processing time: 4 seconds). The focusing mechanism is a live TV camera. It provides full scleral and corneal coverage up to 22×17 mm (useful to assess pterygium evolution). It is sold as the "only" topographer to measure true corneal elevation. Let us observe again that most topographers measure corneal elevation by extrapolating from corneal reflex (thus interfered by tear film layer quality). It might well be the most precise method, each of the 300,000 data points being accurate to about 1 micron; but unfortunately, it is not widespread enough to become a reference system. It still needs clinical validation.

This ***projection technique*** visualizes the surface directly while a reflection technique amplifies the corneal topographic distortions. It measures with low light level for patient, offering full K analysis, "e" value analysis, cross sections, ellipsoidal difference map, full patient and radiological histories, and an easy to-use four-click exam wizard.

EYE MAP EH-290 ALCON® CORNEAL TOPOGRAPHY SYSTEM

Alcon® EH-290 Eye Map Corneal Topography System is a large 23 narrow modified Placido disk system. The modified patented Placido cone design is supposed to be very accurate and sensitive (Table 3.4). Easy and intuitive to use (software runs under Windows™), it offers advanced contact lens software, keratoconus detection, corneal statistics information and advanced communication software.

TOMEY® AUTOTOPOGRAPHER

Tomey® autotopographer is a cheap, small and portable fully automatic self-topographer that requires no operator alignment (Table 3.5). The patient places his or her face on an ergonomically designed face rest and the automated topographer is activated by proximity sensors, automatically taking the

TABLE 3.4: Alcon® EH-290 Eye Map Corneal Topography System
Technical specifications

Measuring System:
- Aspheric measuring system
- Placido disk images
- Over 8,000+ data reference points
- 23 non-linear rings
- Fully automated (centring/focusing/image capture), with 20 step image focusing process
- Microsoft™ Windows™ operating system—produces a graph in less than 30 seconds
- Linear analysis verification graph
- True tangential measuring algorithms
- 3D data calculations
- Large image view

System Hardware

Separate optical head and computer system (computer system may vary in different countries). Storage capacity of over 31,000 + patient files (w/o images)

EyeMap EH-290 Specifications
- Power requirements: 110/120 volts AC, 60 Hz, 220/250 volts AC, 50 Hz
- Processing time: 7 seconds
- Fixation point distance: Optical infinity/on axis
- Area of coverage: <4.6 mm diameter to 10>mm diameter depending on the surface curvature
- Photokeratoscope: patented Visioptic design (US Patent No. 4,978,213)
- Optical Head: 23 non-linear spaced rings
- Positioning system: EyeMap EH-290 software driven auto-position system
- Camera: High resolution CCD Video Camera
- Monitor: Color monitor
- Keyboard: 101 key enhanced keyboard
- Hard disk: 540 megabytes
- Removable hard disk: 1,5 gigabytes
- Floppy disk: 1,44 megabytes

TABLE 3.5: TOMEY ™ autotopographer
Technical specifications

Area measured	0,19 to 11,5 mm
Dioptric range:	9 to 101,5 diopters
Number of rings:	31, low level light
Evaluated points:	7.936
Dimensions:	384 (height) × 230 (width) × 358 (depth) mm
Power:	100/120/220/240 VAC, 50/60 Hz
Weight:	5,5 kg/12 lbs
PC minimum requirements:	Intel® Pentium™ 133
	Microsoft® Windows™ 95 or better,
	32 MB RAM, 100 MB hard disk drive free space
	800 × 640 SVGA color monitor
	bi-directional parallel port
	3.5" floppy disk drive

measurements. The software, that can be installed in a pre-owned PC, runs under Windows™ operating system. The software is very complete and comprehensive, and includes a contact lens wizard with interactive fluorescein displays. Optional software packages include: height and height change maps,

Klyce corneal statistics, keratoconus screening and the contact kens wizard. The low level lights cone is intended to produce minimal glare and disturbance for the patient.

OCULUS® KERATOGRAPH™ AND HAAG-STREIT® KERATOGRAPH CTK 922

OCULUS® Keratograph (Figure 3.8) and Haag-Streit® Keratograph CTK 922 (Figure 3.9) are very similar instruments sold under different brand names and different packaging (Table 3.6). They are compact systems that can fit any refractive unit and include built-in keratometer in connection with the topography system. The software runs under Windows™ operating system and is easy to use, with automatic measurement. The Oculus® can be an integrated computerized system (Keratograph C, in the Figure) or an independent system linked to a pre-owned computer. A non-contact measurement large Placido system with 22 rings in a hemisphere and 22.000 measuring points try to guarantee a high resolution.

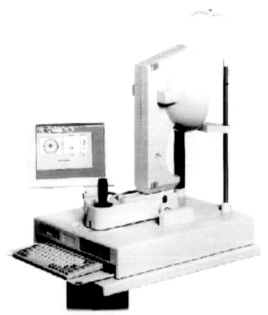

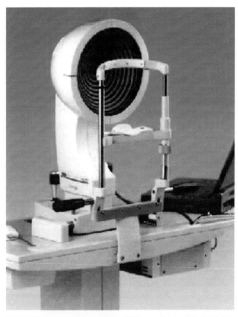

FIGURE 3.8: OCULUS® keratograph   **FIGURE 3.9:** Haag-Streit® keratograph CTK 922

The working distance of 80 mm is enough to make the patient feel comfortable. The light system (warm colored) is intended to produce minimal glare and disturbance for the patient.

They have an interesting software that allows contact lens-fitting in three simple steps: automated contact lens recommendation with a database that includes 20.000 lens geometries from all major contact lens manufacturers, and can be easily enlarged, and realistic fluo-image simulation of contact lens adaptation (Figure 3.10). There is a possibility of measuring the back surface of rigid gas-permeable contact lens through optional Lens Check software.

There is also an optional statistics software package called Datagraph, intended for refractive surgeons. This system allows wonderful comprehensive kinetic three-dimensional analysis of corneal topography

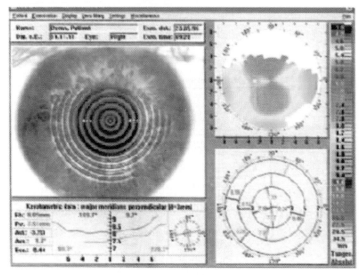

FIGURE 3.10A

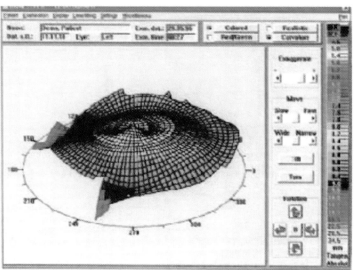

FIGURE 3.10B

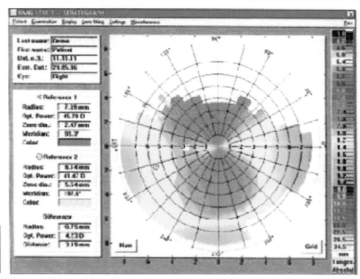

FIGURE 3.10C

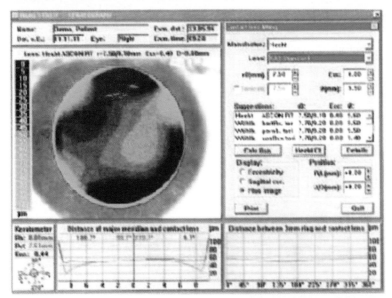

FIGURE 3.10D

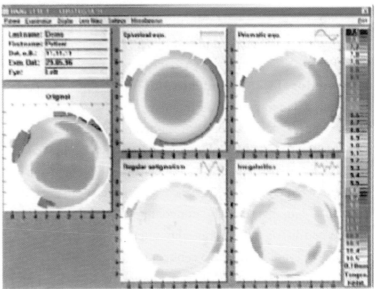

FIGURE 3.10E

FIGURES 3.10A to E: Haag-Streit® KERATOGRAPH CTK 922™ output modalities include: **A.** Overview image with simulated keratometer (right and down), **B.** comprehensive kinetic three-dimensional (3-D) analysis of corneal topography for simple explanation to the patient, **C.** zoom-up image of a map, **D.** fluorescein image simulation for contact lens fitting, and **E.** Fourier expressive analysis (Published with permission from HAAG-STREIT® AG International)

for simple explanation to the patient (Figure 3.11). Fourier surface analysis (Figure 3.12) is available and new software is under development for refractive surgery and contact lens fitters.

Also optional is the Topolink software, that integrates the corneal topography data and some but not all excimer laser software.

TABLE 3.6: OCULUS® keratograph™ and HAAG-STREIT® keratograph™ CTK 922

Technical specifications	
Measuring:	3 to 38 mm
	9 to 99 Diopters
Accuracy:	± 0,1 D
Reproducibility:	± 0,1 D
Number of rings:	22
Evaluated points:	**22.000**
Dimensions:	510 (height) × 300 (width) × 280 (depth) mm
Weight:	2,3 kg
PC requirements:	Intel® Pentium™ 100
	Windows 3.1 or higher
	16 MB of RAM memory
	1 MB graphics VGA card with at least 256 colors

ORBSCAN IIZ™ - BAUSCH & LOMB® SURGICAL, INC. (USA) (FIGURE 3.13)

This is a truly revolutionary instrument for the study of the cornea. It combines a slit-scanning system and a Placido disk (with 40 rings) to measure the **anterior elevation and curvature** of the cornea and the **posterior elevation and curvature** of the cornea (Table 3.7). It offers a **full corneal pachymetry map** with white-to-white measurements.

Orbscan IIz™ takes a series of slit-beam images of two scanning slit-lamps projected beams at 45 degrees, to the right or left of the instrument axis. During the exam, the patient fixates on a blinking red light coaxial with the imaging system. Forty images are taken by the system, 20 with slit-beams projected from the right and 20 from the left. The 20 images are acquired in 0.7 seconds each. Simultaneously, a tracking system measures the nonvoluntary movements of the eye during the exam.

Orbscan IIz™ is able to measure anterior chamber depth, angle kappa, pupil diameter, simulated keratometry readings (3 and 5 central mm of the cornea), and the thinnest corneal pachymetry reading. (Figures 3.14 and 3.15). It offers every traditional map apart from those of posterior corneal surface. Elevation topography of the anterior cornea enables clinicians to more accurately visualize the shape of abnormal corneas, which should lead to more accurate diagnoses and better surgical results. It has proven to be an extraordinary tool for research and for the refractive surgeon.

The system is able to acquire over 9,000 data points in 1.5 seconds, which is fast, but not enough for the patient to feel comfortable. Not every patient can avoid blinking; and in some cases, measurements have to be repeated. A faster processing speed would be desirable, although we feel very comfortable with the system.

Easy to use and running under Microsoft® Windows™ NT 4.0 operating system, the major disadvantage is the high price, that makes it not affordable for most ophthalmologists. Any color printer running under NT 4.0 can be used. Three-dimensional views of the different maps are available (see Figure 3.16).

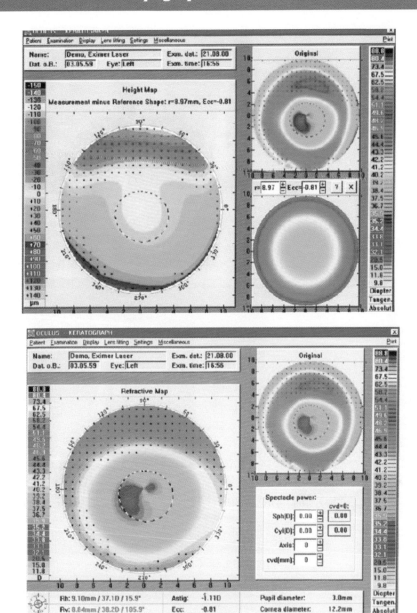

FIGURES 3.11 and 3.12: Oculus® Keratograph™ screen shots with elevation (height) map and refractive map (Published with permission from OCULUS Optikgeraete GmbH)

Figure 3.14 displays different preoperative and postoperative maps of the right eye of a patient who underwent a refractive myopic Zyoptics™ LASIK procedure. Images were taken with Orbscan IIz™-Bausch & Lomb® Surgical, Inc. (USA) topographer.

The anterior best fit sphere (BFS) is calculated to best match the anterior corneal surface. The Elevation BFS map subtracts the calculated best fit sphere size against the eye surface in millimeters (mm). The difference between the sphere and the eye surface is expressed in distance, in a radial way, from the center of the sphere as shown in Figure 3.14 (map Anterior Float BFS). The shape of a sphere

61

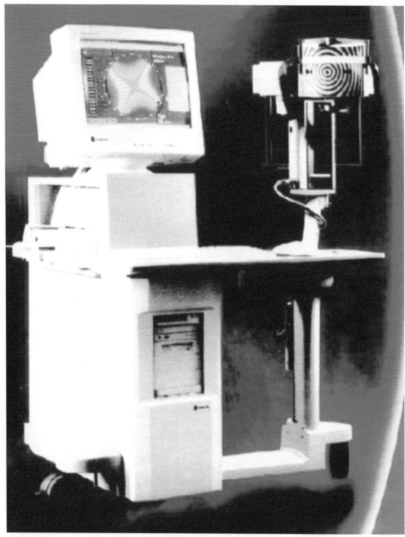

FIGURE 3.13: Orbscan IIz

TABLE 3.7: Measurable parameters with Bausch and Lomb Surgical® Orbscan IIz™

- *Measurable ocular surfaces:*
  - — Anterior corneal surface
  - — Posterior corneal surface
  - — Anterior surface of the iris (anterior chamber depth)
  - — Crystalline lens
- *Geometry and shape maps:*
  - — Relative elevation
  - — Inclination
  - — Surface curvature
- *Distance maps between surfaces:*
  - — Full-corneal pachymetry
  - — Anterior lens depth
- *Optical function maps:*
  - — Optical power
  - — Point spread function
  - — Optical effectiveness

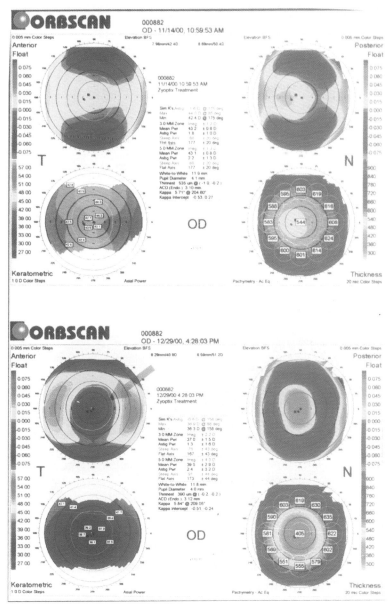

FIGURE 3.14: Myopic LASIK pre/postoperative with
ZYOPTICS™ excimer laser

being easily imagined by the explorer, deviation from that spherical surface in a special case helps to appreciate the true shape of the eye and its deviation from symmetry (asymmetry). The map has 35 default color steps, the size of each step being measured at the bottom of each color (five microns is the default for the BFS map). The best fit between eye surface and sphere is represented in green. Areas under this spherical ideal surface are represented in blue, while warmer colors (orange-red) identify areas above this ideal sphere.

The box in the middle of the displays shows patient information of interest like patient's name, examination date, diameter (mm) and power (D) of the ideal sphere, diagnosis, simulated keratometry

63

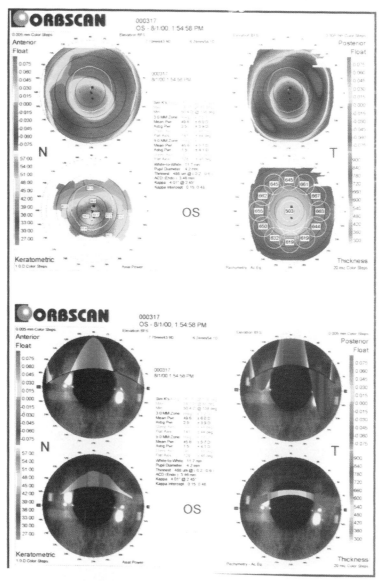

FIGURE 3.15: Displays different maps of the left (OS) eye of a patient with a keratoconus. Images were taken with ORBSCAN IIz™-Bausch and Lomb® Surgical, Inc. (USA) topographer. Notice the central elevation in both anterior and posterior surfaces of the cornea, with reduced corneal thickness (comparing to a normal eye) and high astigmatism. The four inferior maps display different cross section along the 0° to 180° meridian that demonstrate how the cornea is higher than the best fit sphere centrally (reddish central mountain overlaid on the corneal display) and lower in the midperiphery (bluish depression at both sides of the mountain) (Courtesy of Dr Andreu Coret, Institut Oftalmològic de Barcelona, Barcelona-Spain)

readings, white-to-white distance, pupil diameter, thinnest measurement for that cornea, anterior chamber depth (either from epithelium or endothelium), angle kappa, and kappa intercept.

The *posterior best fit sphere* (BFS) is calculated to best match the posterior corneal surface.

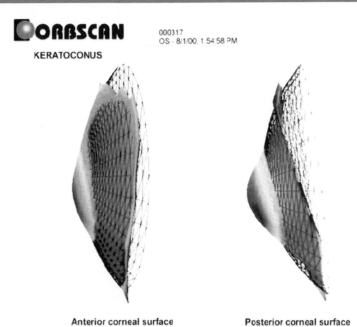

ORBSCAN

KERATOCONUS

000317
OS - 8/1/00, 1 54 58 PM

Anterior corneal surface   Posterior corneal surface

FIGURE 3.16: 3-D imaging of both surfaces of the cornea with Orbscan IIz™ software is really meaningful for the patient. Notice that central protrusion is higher in posterior than in anterior surface of the cornea: in between, corneal thickness is reduced. (Courtesy of Dr Andreu Coret, Institut Oftalmològic de Barcelona, Barcelona-Spain)

The keratometric simulates keratometric values at special areas.

The thickness map (pachymetry map) shows the differences in elevation between the anterior and posterior surfaces of the cornea. By moving the mouse over the map, the explorer can obtain measurements of the thickness at each point. This map can be overlaid by the average measurements that would be taken with a traditional ultrasound pachymeter (encircled values). This map is invaluable for preoperative assessment of the refractive patient, and to determine the true ablated tissue depth in the postoperative period of PRK and refractive patients. Thickness maps clearly demonstrate that ablation zone (arrow) has decreased in thickness from 544 to 405 microns. Notice that corneal thickness increases as we get closer to the limbus.

Chapter

4

Orbscan

J Agarwal
Amar Agarwal
Athiya Agarwal
Sunita Agarwal

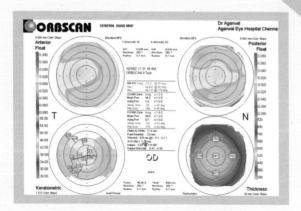

INTRODUCTION

Keratometry and corneal topography with placido discs systems were originally invented to measure anterior corneal curvature. Computer analysis of the more complete data acquired by the latter has in recent years has been increasingly more valuable in the practice of refractive surgery. The problem in the placido disc systems is that one cannot perform a slit scan topography of the cornea. This has been solved by an instrument called the Orbscan that combines both slit scan and placido images to give a very good composite picture for topographic analysis. Bausch and Lomb manufacture this.

PARAXIAL OPTICS

Spectacle correction of sight is designed only to eliminate defocus errors and astigmatism. These are the only optical aberrations that can be handled by the simplest theory of imaging, known as paraxial optics, which excludes all light rays finitely distant from a central ray or power axis. Ignoring the majority of rays entering the pupil, paraxial optics examines only a narrow thread-like region surrounding the power axis. The shape of any smoothly rounded surface within this narrow region is always circular in cross-section. Thus from the paraxial viewpoint, surface shape is toric at most: only its radius may vary with meridional angle. As a toric optical surface has sufficient flexibility to null defocus and astigmatism, only paraxial optics is needed to specify corrective lenses for normal eyes. Paraxial optics is used in keratometers and two-dimensional topographic machines.

RAYTRACE OR GEOMETRIC OPTICS

The initial objective of refractive surgery was to build the necessary paraxial correction in to the cornea. When outcomes are less than perfect, it is not just because defocus correction is inadequate. Typically, other aberrations (astigmatism, spherical aberration, coma, etc) are introduced by the surgery. These may be caused by decentered ablation, asymmetric healing, biomechanical response, poor surgical planning, and inadequate or misinformation. To assess the aberrations in the retinal image all the light rays entering the pupil must properly be taken in account using raytrace (or geometric) optics. Paraxial optics and its hypothetical toric surfaces must be abandoned as inadequate, which eliminates the need to measure surface curvature. Raytrace optics does not require surface curvature, but depends on elevation and especially surface slope. The Orbscan uses raytrace or geometric Optics.

ELEVATION

Orbscan measure elevation, which is not possible in other topographic machines. Elevation is especially important because it is the only complete scalar measure of surface shape. Both slope and curvature can be mathematically derived from a single elevation map, but the converse is not necessarily true. As both slope and curvature have different values in different directions, neither can be completely represented by a single map of the surface. Thus, when characterizing the surface of non-spherical test objects used to verify instrument accuracy, elevation is always the gold standard.

67

Curvature maps in corneal topography (usually misnamed as power or dioptric maps) only display curvature measured in radial directions from the map center. Such a presentation is not shift-invariant, which means its values and topography change as the center of the map is shifted. In contrast, elevation is shift-invariant. An object shifted with respect to the map center is just shifted in its elevation map. In a meridional curvature view it is also described. This makes elevation maps more intuitively understood, making diagnosis easier.

To Summarize

1. Curvature is not relevant in raytrace optics.
2. Elevation is complete and can be used to derive surface curvature and slope.
3. Elevation is the standard measure of surface shape.
4. Elevation is easy to understand.

The problem we face is that there is a cost in converting elevation to curvature (or slope) and vice versa. To go from elevation to curvature requires mathematical differentiation, which accentuates the high spatial frequency components of the elevation function. As a result, random measurement error or noise in an elevation measurement is significantly multiplied in the curvature result. The inverse operation, mathematical integration used to convert curvature to elevation, accentuates low-frequency error. The Orbscan helps in good mathematical integration. This makes it easy for the ophthalmologist to understand as the machine does all the conversion.

ORBSCAN I AND II

Previously, Orbscan I was used. This had only slit scan topographic system. Then the placido disc was added in Orbscan I. Hence Orbscan II came into the picture.

SPECULAR VS BACK-SCATTERED REFLECTION

The keratometer eliminates the anterior curvature of the pre-corneal tear film. It is an estimate because the keratometer only acquires data within a narrow 3 mm diameter annulus. It measures the anterior tear-film because it is based on specular reflection (Figure 4.1), which occurs primarily at the air-tear interface. As the keratometer has very limited data coverage, abnormal corneas can produce misleading or incorrect results.

Orbscan can calculate a variety of different surface curvatures, and on a typical eye, these are all different. Only on a properly aligned and perfectly spherical surface are the various curvatures equal. The tabulated SimK values (magnitudes and associated meridians) are the only ones designed to give keratometer- like measurements. Therefore it only makes sense to compare keratometry reading with SimK values.

Orbscan uses slit-beams and back-scattered light (Figure 4.2) to triangulate surface shape. The derived mathematical surface is then raytraced using a basic keratometer model to produce simulated keratometer (SimK) values. So, it is the difficulty of calculating curvature from triangulated data, the repeatability of

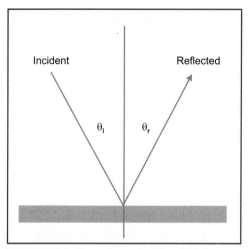

FIGURE 4.1: Specular reflection. This is used in keratometers. This is angle-dependent

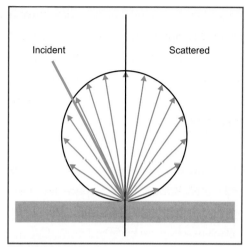

FIGURE 4.2: Back-scattered reflection. This is used in orbscan. This is omni-directional

Orbscan I SimK values is usually not as good as a clinical keratometer. But when several readings of the same eye are averaged, no discernable systematic error is found.

So, if one reading is taken and a comparison is made, the difference may be significant enough to make you believe the instrument is not working properly. So, when the placido illuminator was added to Orbscan II to increase its anterior curvature accuracy, it also provided reflected data similar to that obtained with a keratometer. This reflective data is now used in SimK analyses, resulting in repeatabilities similar to keratometers and other placido based corneal topography instruments.

Keratometry measures the tear-film, while slit-scan triangulation (Figure 4.3) as embodied in Orbscan sees through the tear- film and measures the corneal surface directly. Thus an abnormal tear-film can produce significant differences in keratometry but not in Orbscan II.

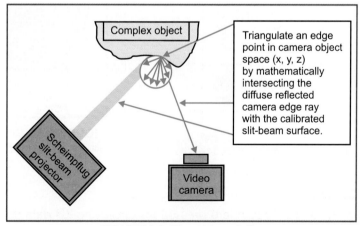

FIGURE 4.3: Direct triangulation

Curvature measures the geometric bending of a surface, and its natural unit is reciprocal length, like inverse millimeters (1/mm). When keratometry was invented this unfamiliar unit was replaced by a dioptric interpretation, making keratometry values equivalent on average (i.e., over the original population) to the paraxial back-vertex power of the cornea. As it has become increasingly more important to distinguish optical from geometric properties, it is now more proper to evaluate keratometry in "keratometric diopters". The keratometric diopter is strictly defined as a geometric unit of curvature with no optical significance. One inverse millimeter equals to 337.5 keratometric diopters.

IMAGING IN THE ORBSCAN

In the Orbscan, the calibrated slit, which falls on the cornea, gives a topographical information, which is captured and analyzed by the video camera (Figure 4.4). Both slit beam surfaces are determined in camera object space. Object space luminance is determined for each pixel value and framegrabber setting. Forty slit images are acquired in two 0.7-second periods. During acquisition, involuntary saccades typically move the eye by 50 microns. Eye movement is measured from anterior reflections of stationary slit beam and other light sources. Eye tracking data permits saccadic movements to be subtracted form the final topographic surface. Each of the 40 slit images triangulates one slice of ocular surface (Figure 4.5). Before an interpolating surface is constructed, each slice is registered in accordance with measured eye movement. Distance between data slices averages 250 microns in the coarse scan mode (40 slits limbus to limbus). So Orbscan exam consists of a set of mathematical topographic surfaces (x, y), for the anterior and posterior cornea, anterior iris and lens and backscattering coefficient of layers between the topographic surfaces (and over the pupil) (Figure 4.6).

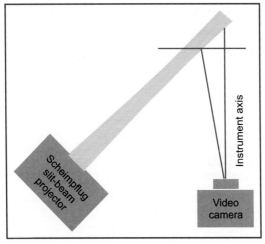

FIGURE 4.4: Beam and camera calibration in the orbscan

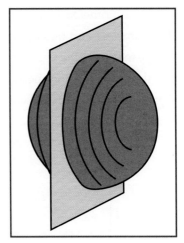

FIGURE 4.5: Ocular surface slicing by the orbscan slit

MAP COLORS CONVENTIONS

Color contour maps have become a standard method for displaying 2D data in corneal and anterior segment topography. Although there are no universally standardized colors, the spectral direction (from blue to red) is always organized in definite and intuitive way.

Blue = low, level, flat, deep, thick, or aberrated.

Red = high, steep, sharp, shallow, thin, or focused.

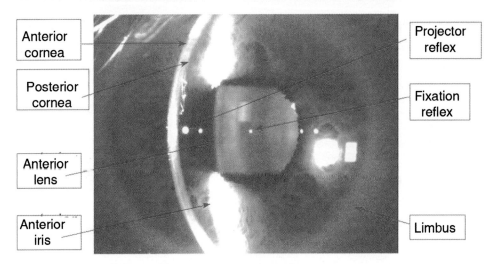

FIGURE 4.6: Detailed orbscan examination

ANALYSIS OF THE NORMAL EYE BY THE ORBSCAN MAP

The general quad map in the Orbscan of a normal eye (Figure 4.7) shows 4 pictures. The upper left is the anterior float, which is the topography of the anterior surface of the cornea. The upper right shows the posterior float, which is the topography of the posterior surface of the cornea. The lower left map shows the keratometric pattern and the lower right map shows the pachymetry (thickness of the cornea). The Orbscan is a three-dimensional slit scan topographic machine. If we were doing topography with a

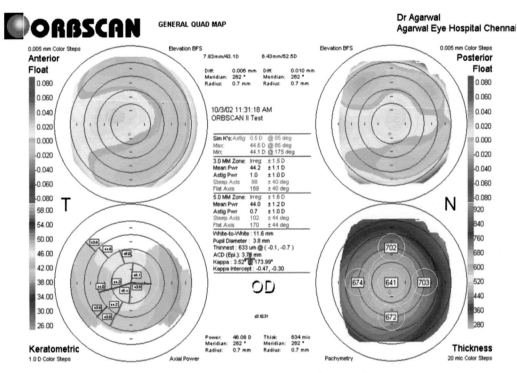

FIGURE 4.7: General quad map of a normal eye

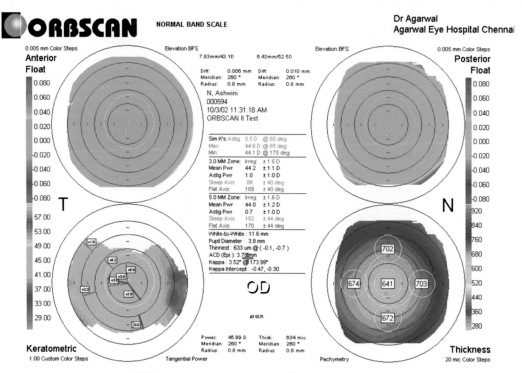

FIGURE 4.8: Normal band scale filter on a normal eye

machine, which does not have slit scan imaging facility, we would not be able to see the topography of the posterior surface of the cornea. Now, if the patient had an abnormality in the posterior surface of the cornea, for example as in primary posterior corneal elevation this would not be diagnosed. Then if we perform Lasik on such a patient we would create an iatrogenic keratectasia. The Orbscan helps us to detect the abnormalities on the posterior surface of the cornea.

Another facility, which we can move onto once we have the general quad map, is to put on the normal band scale filter (Figure 4.8). If we are in suspicion of any abnormality in the general quad map then we put on the normal band scale filter. This highlights the abnormal areas in the cornea in orange to red colors. The normal areas are all shown in green. This is very helpful in generalized screening in pre-operative examination of a Lasik patient.

CLINICAL APPLICATIONS

Let us now understand this better in a case of a primary posterior corneal elevation. If we see the general quad map of a primary posterior corneal elevation (Figure 4.9) we will see the upper left map is normal. The upper right map shows abnormality highlighted in red. This indicates the abnormality in the posterior surface of the cornea. The lower left keratometric map is normal and if we see the lower right map, which is the pachymetry map one will see slightly, thin cornea of 505 microns but still one cannot diagnose the primary posterior corneal elevation only from this reading. Thus we can understand that if not for the upper right map, which denotes the posterior surface of the cornea, one would miss this condition. The Orbscan can only diagnose this.

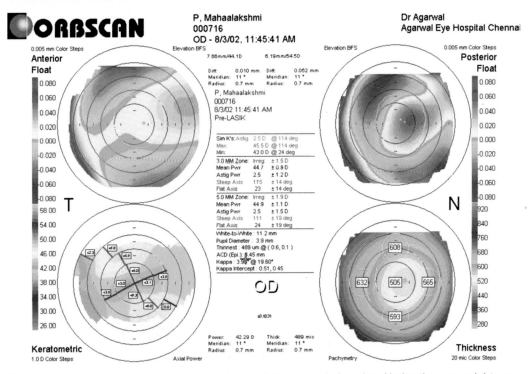

FIGURE 4.9: General quad map of a primary posterior corneal elevation. Notice the upper right map has an abnormality whereas the upper left map is normal. This shows the anterior surface of the cornea is normal and the problem is in the posterior surface of the cornea

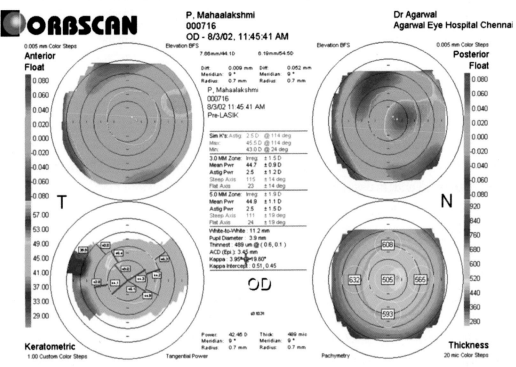

FIGURE 4.10: Quad map of a primary posterior corneal elevation with the normal band scale filter on. This shows the abnormal areas in red and the normal areas are all green. Notice the abnormailty in the upper right map

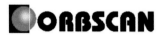

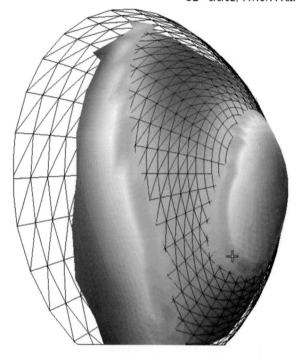

FIGURE 4.11: Three-dimensional map of primary posterior corneal elevation. This shows a marked elevation in respect to a normal reference sphere highlighted as a black grid. Notice the red color protrusion on the black grid. This picture is of the posterior surface of the cornea

Now, we can put on the normal band scale filter on (Figure 4.10) and this will highlight the abnormal areas in red. Notice in Figure 4.10, the upper right map shows a lot of abnormality denoting the primary posterior corneal elevation. One can also take the three-dimensional map of the posterior surface of the cornea (Figure 4.11) and notice the amount of elevation in respect to the normal reference sphere shown as a black grid. In a case of a keratoconus (Figure 4.12) all four maps show an abnormality, which confirms the diagnosis.

If we take a Lasik patients topography we can compare the pre- and the post-Lasik (Figure 4.13). This helps to understand the pattern and amount of ablation done on the cornea. The picture on the upper right is the pre-op topographic picture and the one on the lower right is the post-Lasik picture. The main picture on the left shows the difference between the pre- and post-Lasik topographic patterns. One can detect from this any decentered ablations or any other complication of Lasik surgery.

Corneal topography is *extremely important in cataract surgery. The smaller the size of the incision lesser the astigmatism and earlier stability of the astigmatism will occur.* One can reduce the astigmatism or increase the astigmatism of a patient after cataract surgery. The simple rule to follow is that—*wherever you make an incision that area will flatten and wherever you apply sutures that area will steepen.* One

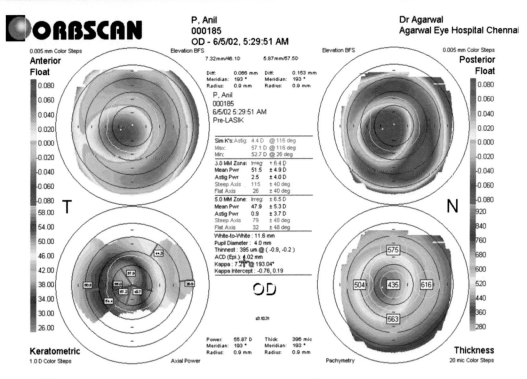

FIGURE 4.12: General quad map of a keratoconus patient showing abnormailty in all four maps

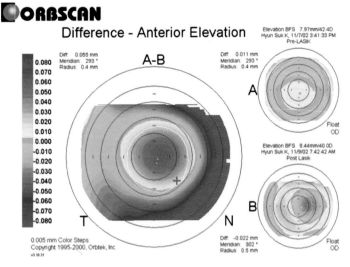

FIGURE 4.13: Difference of pre- and post-Lasik

can use the Orbscan to analyze the topography before and after cataract surgery. For instance in an Extracapsular cataract extraction one can check to see where the astigmatism is most and remove those sutures. In a phaco the astigmatism will be less and in Phakonit where the incision is sub 1.5 mm the astigmatism will be the least.

We can use the Orbscan to determine the anterior chamber depth and also analyze where one should place the incision when one is performing astigmatic keratotomy. The Orbscan can also help in a good fit of the contact lens with a fluorescein pattern.

SUMMARY

The Orbscan has changed the world of topography as it gives us an understanding of a slit scan three-dimensional picture. One can use this in understanding various conditions.

Chapter 5

The Orbscan IIz Diagnostic System and Zywave Analysis

Gregg Feinerman
N Timothy Peters
Kim Nguyen
Marcus Solorzano
Shiela Scott

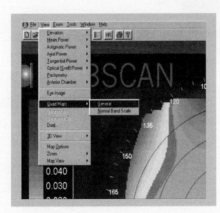

INTRODUCTION

The combination of topographic and wavefront data is the foundation for customized ablation. The Zyoptix™ Diagnostic Workstation seamlessly integrates wavefront and topographical data for customized treatments (Figure 5.1). It is ergonomic and easy to use, and provides surgeons with a platform for comprehensive diagnosis and treatment. The ORBSCAN® IIz uses slit scanning technology to measure corneal curvature. It also provides true three-dimensional elevation based on triangulation and curvature of both anterior and posterior surfaces of the cornea. The ZYWAVE™ II ABERROMETER provides wavefront measurements based on Hartmann-Shack technology. It measures higher order aberrations (HOAs) up to the 5th order.

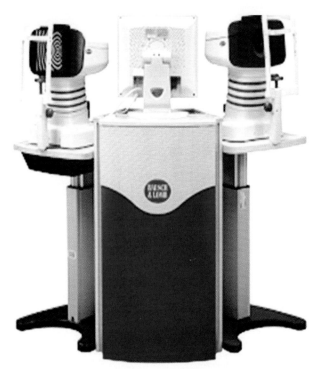

FIGURE 5.1: The Zyoptix™ diagnostic workstation

ORBSCAN

Corneal topography has evolved over time from a manual keratometer to simple placedo disc topographers, to the Orbscan. The Orbscan uses a combination of placedo disc images with 20 slit scans to the left and 20 slits scan to the right. This allows for forty overlapping scans in the central 5 mm zone that then allows for the four basic measurements listed below. The Orbscan measures four essential elements:

1. Corneal power
2. Corneal thickness
3. Anterior corneal elevation
4. Posterior corneal elevation

QUAD MAP

The quad map is the most common and useful way to get an overall view of the cornea. It combines anterior elevation, posterior elevation, corneal power and pachymetry into one view (Figures 5.2 and 5.3).

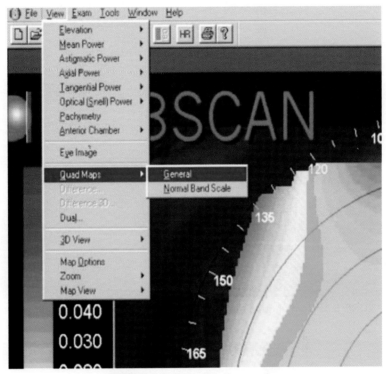

FIGURE 5.2: Selecting the quad map

POWER MAPS

One of the most confusing tasks in refractive diagnostic testing is deciding which corneal power maps to interpret. The Orbscan offers multiple ways to measure corneal power. The type of corneal power map to choose depends on what you are trying to interpret. The default setting is the **mean power map** (Figures 5.4, 5.5 and 5.8). It is most useful for eyes with extreme abnormalities. The mean power map determines the location of a surface abnormality. The **axial power map** is a familiar sagittal map from placido systems (Figures 5.6 and 5.7). It provides a comfortable transition for new Orbscan users; but only uses placido rings. Normal astigmatism appears in a classic bow-tie pattern.

PACHYMETRY MAP

The pachymetry map (Figures 5.9 to 5.11) unquestionably makes the Orbscan diagnostic system unique. The Orbscan measures thickness from the tear film layer to Descemet's membrane, thus its pachymetry readings are thicker than those obtained with ultrasound pachymetry. However, the Orbscan has an adjustment factor called the acoustic factor, which can be set to replicate ultrasound pachymetry. The default setting is 92 percent, but each user may adjust this percentage to mimic what their own ultrasound

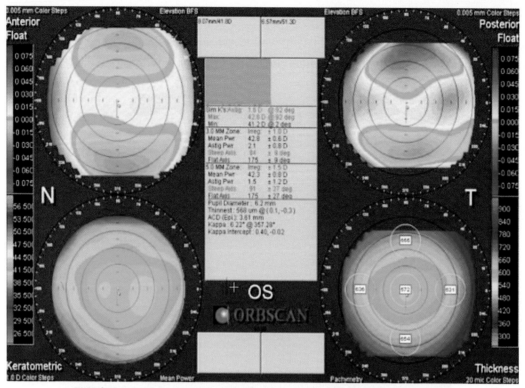

FIGURE 5.3: Normal quad map showing typical with the rule astigmatism

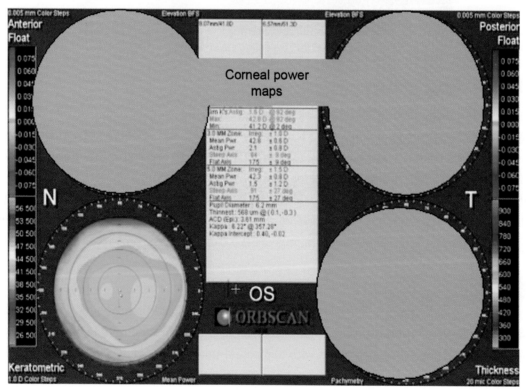

FIGURE 5.4: Mean power map

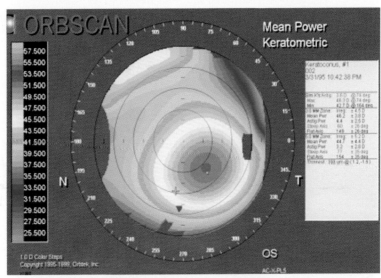

FIGURE 5.5: Mean power map demonstrating keratoconus

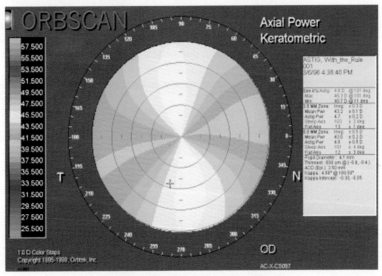

FIGURE 5.6: Axial power map

reading show. The Orbscan not only provides a central pachymetry reading, but it also provides a superior, inferior, nasal, and temporal reading at the 6 mm zone. It also provides a reading showing the thinnest part of the cornea that may not necessarily be the central reading. The extra reading allow for the subtle interpretation of variable corneal thickness in conjunction with other topographic abnormalities, to aid in the detection of forme-fruste keratoconus as well as other corneal disease processes.

READING CORNEAL ELEVATION MAPS

Global Perspective

The map in the upper left of the quad maps (Figure 5.12) is the anterior elevation map. Understanding the usefulness of the map requires some background perspective. Think first from a global perspective.

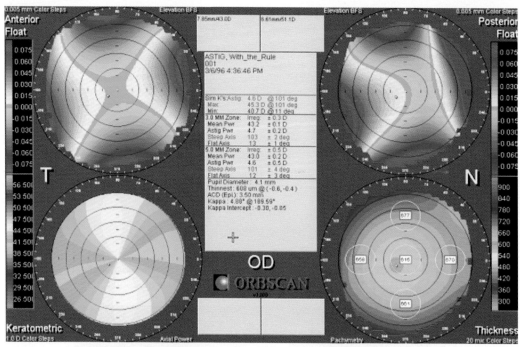

FIGURE 5.7: Axial power map demonstrating regular astigmatism

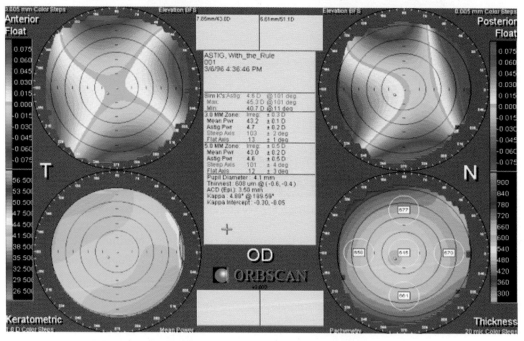

FIGURE 5.8: Mean power map demonstrating regular astigmatism

If we view the surface of the earth from a great distance it losses all of its relevant features and appears totally smooth, but if we change the scale then we can perceive significant height discrepancies. The cornea is the same way. When looking at a proper scale we can see height differences. To understand these differences we have to compare the height of the actual cornea to the heights of a best-fit sphere.

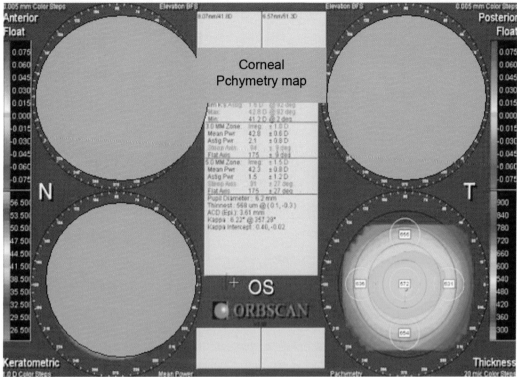

FIGURE 5.9: Pachymetry map

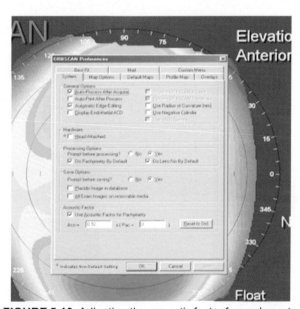

FIGURE 5.10: Adjusting the acoustic factor for pachymetry

A normal prolate cornea is steep in the center, and flat in the periphery (Figures 5.13 and 5.14). When this is overlayed with a best-fit sphere the center of the normal cornea is steeper than the best-fit sphere. Steep colors are red ones, and thus the central cornea is red on a normal elevation map. The mid-periphery of a normal cornea is flatter than our reference best-fit sphere and thus appears blue on an

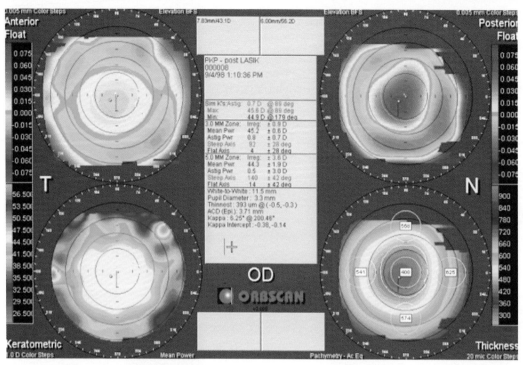

FIGURE 5.11: Pachymetry map of postoperative LASIK

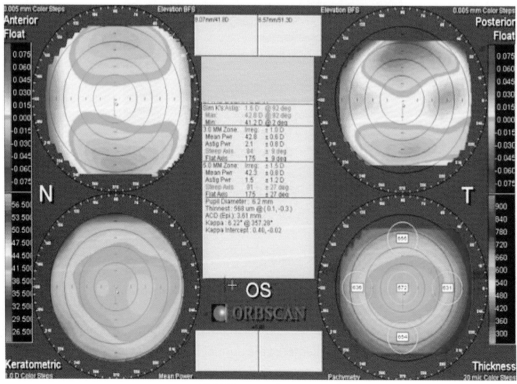

FIGURE 5.12: Quad map

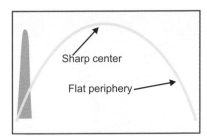

FIGURE 5.13: Elevation topology—
normal cornea

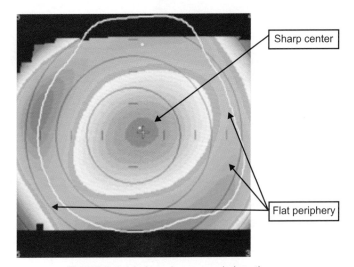

FIGURE 5.14: Anterior corneal elevation map

elevation map. Now consider a post-LASIK elevation profile on a previously myopic patient (Figure 5.15). The reference sphere is best fit to the postablation shape, but the post-LASIK cornea is now oblate with a flatter center. This will appear as a blue central zone. The mid-periphery is now steeper than the reference sphere and appears as a red ring. The untouched peripheral cornea again then becomes flatter than the reference sphere and appears blue on our scale in a normal post-myopic LASIK elevation map. The anterior corneal elevation take home message is that:

- Elevation is measured relative to a "Best Fit Sphere"
- The elevation "is what it is" but may appear different depending how we look at it in relation to the best fit sphere

POSTERIOR CORNEAL ELEVATION MAPS

- The posterior corneal elevation is another unique and defining feature of the Orbscan. As we recall from basic science, the posterior corneal power is negative and much smaller than anterior corneal power (Figure 5.16). Thus the posterior surface reduces corneal power.

  There has been no prior experience with this information, and this surface is simply assumed to be normal by all other topographic systems. When interpreting the posterior float we need to put the

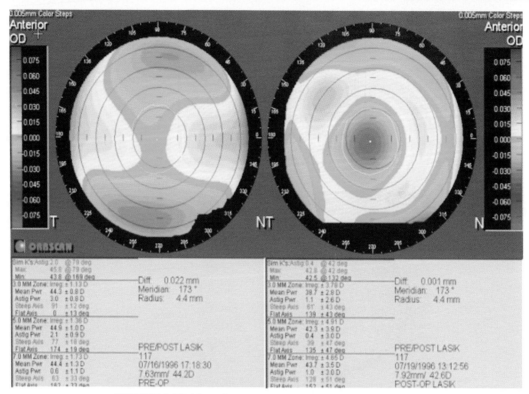

FIGURE 5.15: Elevation map pre- and postoperative LASIK

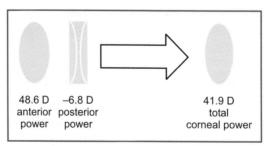

| 48.6 D anterior power | −6.8 D posterior power | 41.9 D total corneal power |

FIGURE 5.16: The posterior corneal surface reduces corneal power

posterior cornea in context. It is important to look for pattern recognition, and to look for related changes on other maps. Similar to the anterior elevation map, the posterior elevation map is related to a best fit sphere. When reading this map two features are of greatest importance. One is the location of the steepest part of the posterior float. This should be relatively central, but is a more concern should it be located away from the center and in an area of corneal thinning. The second is the posterior float difference. This number is given in microns and is the difference between the steepest and flattest part of the posterior elevation. Much debate has centered over the magnitude that constitutes an abnormal reading, but 45 to 50 microns seems to be the maximum difference that is widely accepted. It is also important to keep in mind that while the posterior float difference appears to be clinically relevant, that isolated findings have limited value.

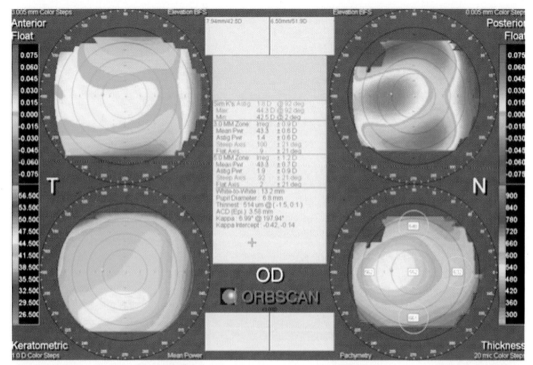

FIGURE 5.17: Caution—One abnormal map

THREE STEP RULE

Dr Karpecki and Moyes have developed what they refer to as the Three Step Rule when interpreting the posterior elevation. If there is one abnormal map (Figure 5.17) then it is ok to perform LASIK with caution. If there are two abnormal maps (Figure 5.18) then it is still okay to proceed, but with concern, and if there are three abnormal maps (Figure 5.19) the LASIK is contraindicated. Below are some quad maps demonstrating the different levels of concern.

PREOPERATIVE LASIK SCREENING

Three Step Rule

- One abnormal map: Caution
- Two abnormal maps: Concern
- Three abnormal maps: Contraindication

This quad map shows three normal maps, but the posterior float is abnormal because the difference reading is greater than 50 microns.

This quad map shows two normal maps, but the posterior difference is again over 50 microns. This quad map, however, also shows an abnormally thin central pachymetry. This thinning has good correlation with the steepest location of the posterior elevation map.

This quad map has three abnormal maps. The posterior difference is greater then 50 microns, there is a well-correlated steep area on the anterior elevation map, and a well correlated area of high power on the mean power map. This is an absolute contraindication for LASIK.

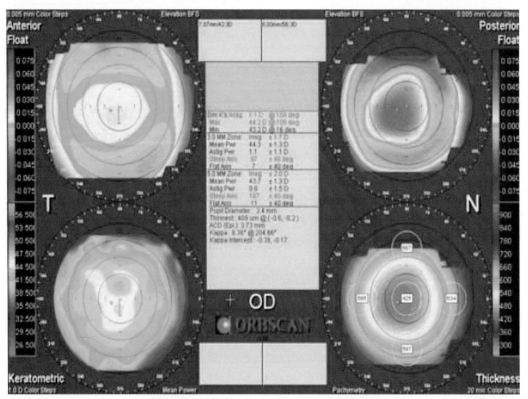

FIGURE 5.18: Concern—Two abnormal maps

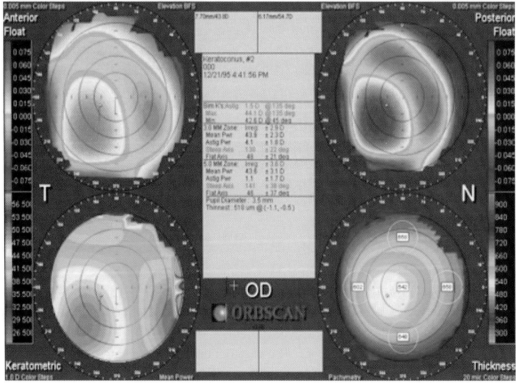

FIGURE 5.19: Contraindication—Three abnormal maps

MIDDLE BOX

When reading the quad maps try not to forget the information in the middle box (Figure 5.20). This box provides standard keratometric readings, white-to-white distance in millimeters, angle kappa readings, and more. The thinnest are of the cornea is displayed here as well as the amount of corneal irregularity within the central 3 and 5 mm zones. These irregularity indicies are considered abnormal if they exceed 1.5 and 2 diopters respectively. This extra information combined with the quad maps provides the most complete screening tool available to detect preoperative corneal abnormalities to reduce the risk of iatrogenic induced keratoectasia. Dr(s) Karpecki and Moyes have compiled a list of Orbscan risk factors for Keratoectasia based on extensive retrospective case reviews. This is a guideline that other users may want to consider when screening LASIK candidates.

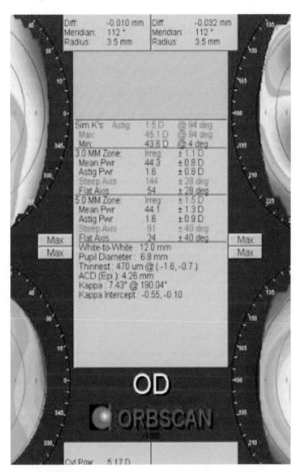

FIGURE 5.20: Orbscan middle box data

ORBSCAN RISK OF ECTASIA INDICES

1. Number of abnormal maps
2. Posterior surface float (difference) >0.050 D
3. 3 mm and 5 mm irregularity

4. Peripheral thickness changes
5. Astigmatism variance between eyes
6. Steep K's—mean power map

The first item is the number of abnormal maps. As stated earlier in the three-step rule, one abnormal map is a caution sign, two is of concern, and three is an absolute contraindication. The second item is the posterior float difference (Figure 5.21). A difference of greater than 50 is generally accepted as abnormal, but other physicians have suggested that 50 is the limit in normal corneas, but in corneas that are thinner than normal to start with a difference over 40 should be considered abnormal.[1] The third item is the amount of irregularity in the central 3 mm and 5 mm zones (Figures 5.22A and B). Greater than 1.5 diopter and 2.0 diopters respectively is considered abnormal and cause for concern. The fourth item is how the central pachymetry reading compares to the peripheral 6 mm reading and to the thinnest reading (Figure 5.23). These numbers are considered abnormal if the peripheral 6 mm readings are not at least 20 microns thicker than the central reading, especially if they are correlated with abnormalities on other quad maps. The thinnest reading is also considered abnormal if it is less than 30 microns thinner than the central reading, again if it is also correlated with an abnormality on another quad map. The fifth item is a difference of greater than 1.00 diopter in the amount of corneal astigmatism between eyes (Figures 5.24 and 5.25). The last item is a localized steep area on the mean power map, especially if correlated with other abnormalities (Figure 5.26).

These guidelines are meant to help alert the clinician to a poor candidate. The example below is an actual patient who preoperatively had a steep posterior difference, a thinnest spot of the cornea greater

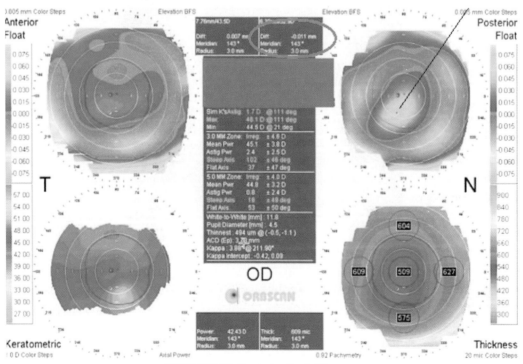

FIGURE 5.21: Posterior float difference

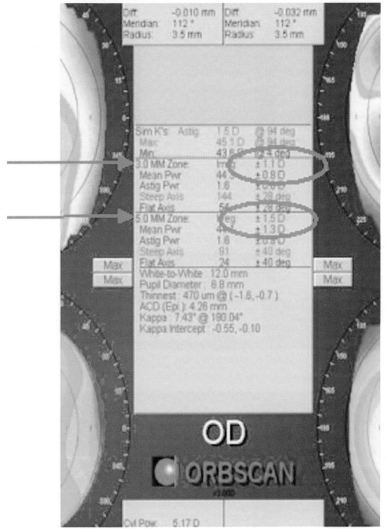

FIGURE 5.22A: 3 mm and 5 mm irregularity

than 30 microns thinner than the central reading, and a higher amount of irregularity in the central 3 and 5 mm zones (Figure 5.27). As you follow this patient's course postoperatively you can see progressive steepening and topographic irregular astigmatism at the 4 month and 17 month visits indicating keratoectasia (Figures 5.28 and 5.29).

CLINICAL EXAMPLES

As with all topographies, an abnormal tear film layer can significantly distort the readings. Below is an example of normal topography on a patient, and then a repeat topography taken after 3 minutes of drying (Figures 5.30 and 5.31). Note the significant change is surface quality and validity of the dry eye reading. The next example is that of a Keratoconus patient (Figure 5.32). Note the larger posterior float difference, the well-correlated steep anterior float, the well correlated steep power reading on the mean power map, the thinnest spot of the cornea not being central and being greater than 30 microns thinner

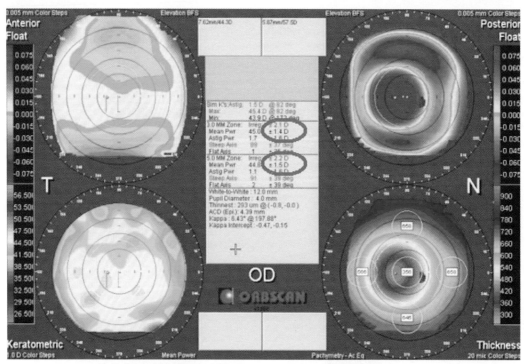

FIGURE 5.22B: 3 mm and 5 mm irregularity

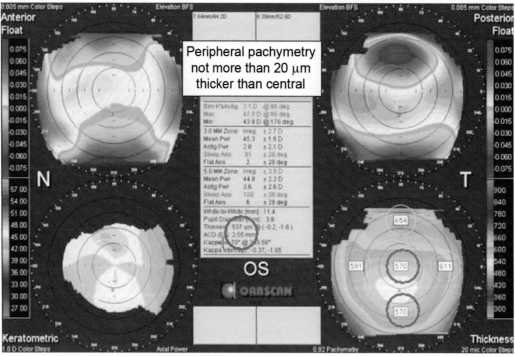

FIGURE 5.23: Peripheral thickness comparison

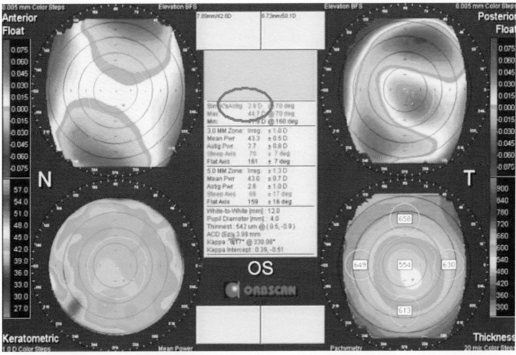

FIGURE 5.24: Astigmatism variance between eyes

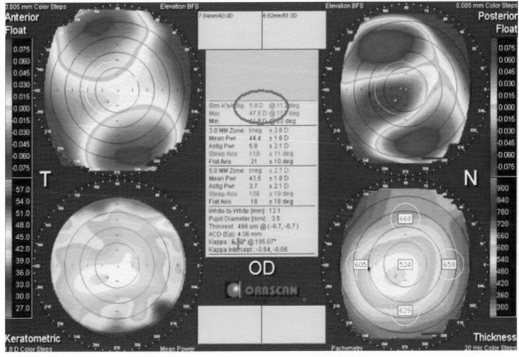

FIGURE 5.25: Astigmatism variance between eyes

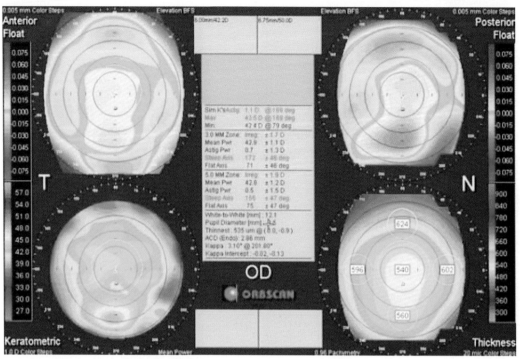

FIGURE 5.26: Steep keratometry on mean power map

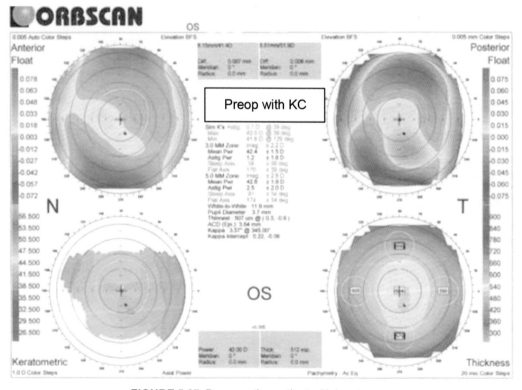

FIGURE 5.27: Preoperative patient with keratoconus

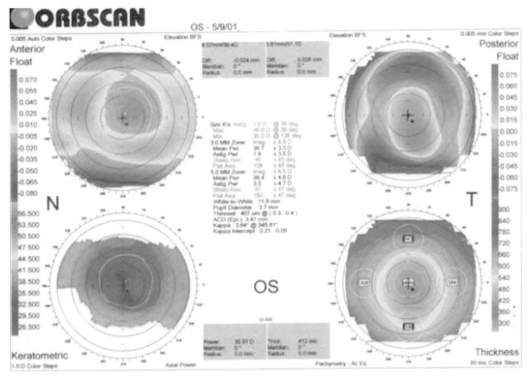

FIGURE 5.28: Four months postoperative LASIK with KC

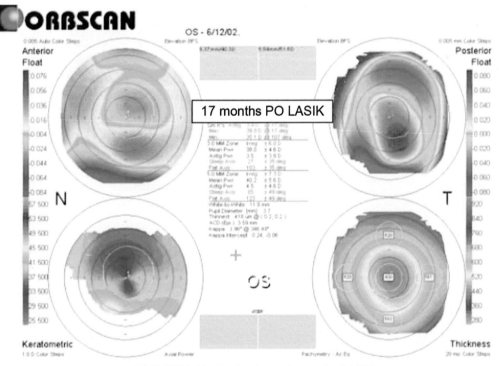

17 months PO LASIK

FIGURE 5.29: 17 Months postoperative LASIK

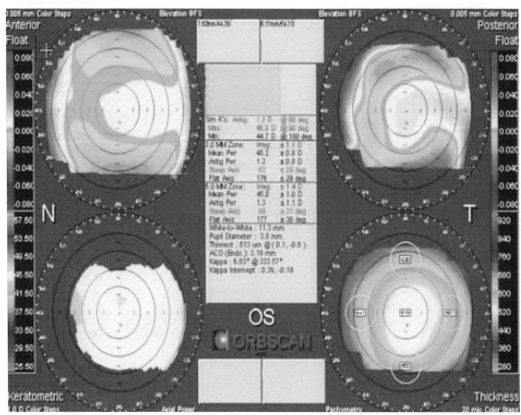

FIGURE 5.30: Normal Orbscan

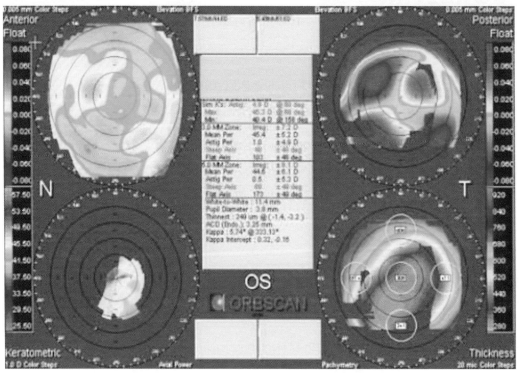

FIGURE 5.31 Orbscan after 3 minutes of desiccation

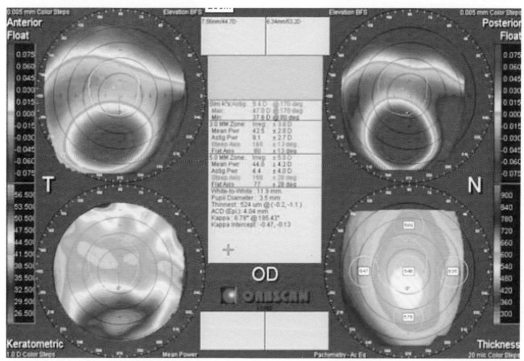

FIGURE 5.32: Keratoconus with normal pachymetry

than the central reading, and the large amounts of irregularity in the central 3 mm and 5 mm zones. The final example is of pellucid marginal degeneration (Figure 5.33). Note the classic large amount of against the rule astigmatism, the large posterior float difference, the well-correlated anterior elevation abnormality, and the large amounts of irregularity in the central 3mm and 5mm zones.

ZYOPTIX

The Zyoptix wavefront diagnostic system version 2.38 is a Hartman-Schack wavefront abberometer developed by Bausch and Lomb. This system is combined with the information obtained from the Orbscan to form the basis for wavefront-guided ablations through the Zylink platform and Technolas 21Z excimer laser.

The first step in any abberometer is data acquisition. In the dual workstation system patient demographics are entered into the Orbscan, including manifest refraction, and this information is simply exported into the Zywave database. The current FDA indications are myopia less than 7.00 diopters and astigmatism less than 3.00 diopters. This information can be entered in plus or minus format and there is a quick conversion button on the Zywave screen. The patient status (i.e. preoperative dilated or undilated, postoperative etc.) is entered and then testing can begin.

It is recommended that an undilated Zywave be taken and then an anterior segment exam is performed. The Zywave will use Hartman-Schack technology and its lenslet array to capture up to 9000 data points. These are then analyzed using Zernike polynomials and the data is displayed up to 5th order Zernike terms. It is crucial that the raw data received at this stage be verified for good quality

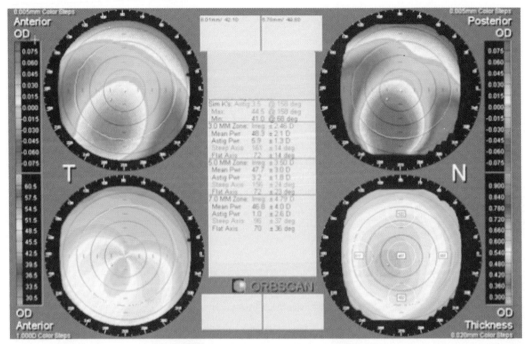

FIGURE 5.33: Pellucid marginal degeneration

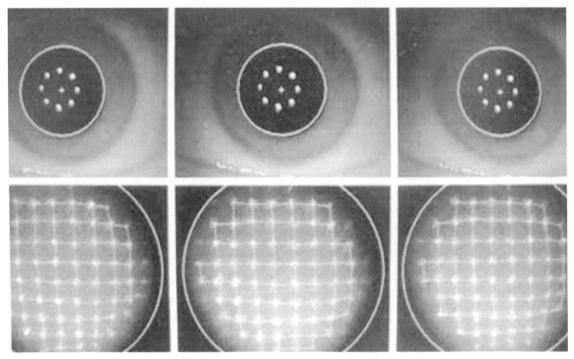

FIGURE 5.34: Zywave raw data

before proceeding. The Zywave will obtain five scans and the best three sets of raw data will be automatically selected for analysis. The examiner needs to verify proper centration of the scans, good quality of the scans, and good accuracy of the scans before proceeding (Figure 5.34). Centration of the

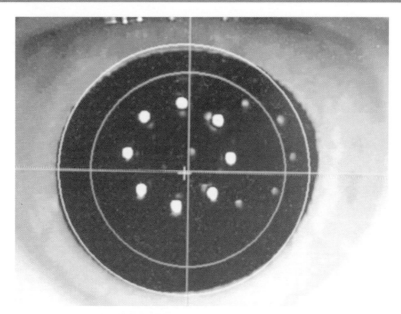

FIGURE 5.35: Well-centered Zywave scan

No.	Dia.[mm]	PPR	OK
1.	5.98	-2.04 / -0.86 / 144°	✓
2.	6.02	-2.27 / -0.72 / 147°	✗
3.	5.98	-2.19 / -0.81 / 145°	✓
4.	5.89	-2.34 / -0.67 / 136°	✗
5.	5.89	-2.13 / -0.90 / 137°	✓

FIGURE 5.36: Predicted phoropter refractions (PPR's)

Zywave scans is verified be looking at the three sets of raw data to see that the central "x" is near pupil center, and that the outer ring around the raw data is green. If it is not centered the outer ring will be yellow and the Zywave needs to be repeated (Figure 5.35). The Zywave system comes with an alignment aid, which greatly improves the ease of acquisition and verification of centration. This aid has color bars and rings that change in size and color until optimally centered and crisp, and then the scan can be taken. The next item is to verify that the raw data is of good quality. The examiner must look at the three sets of raw data and see that all the centroids are sharp, and that the lines from other centroids connect them all. If the lines are broken around the extreme edges it is still ok, but any break in the central areas denotes poor quality and needs to be repeated.

Lastly, the Zywave will display all five sets of Predicted Phoropter Refractions (PPR's). Three will be highlighted and checked as the best three chosen by the computer for analysis (Figure 5.36). It is our practice to not only verify the tight deviations among the chosen three, but to verify that all five PPR's correlate tightly with each other and with the subjective refraction. A range greater than 0.75 diopters

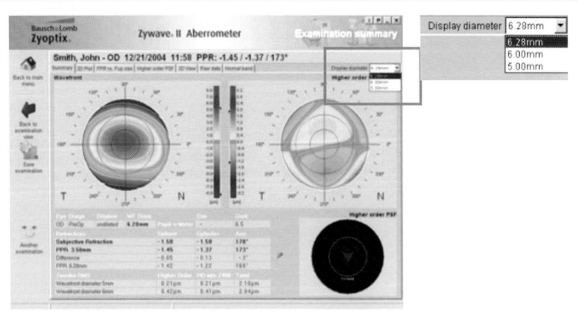

FIGURE 5.37: Examination summary

on sphere, 0.50 diopters on cylinder and 015 degrees on axis is considered unacceptable. An examination summary screen will display the subjective refraction, the PPR at the 3.5 mm zone, and the differences between them. It will highlight in red any deviation larger than the amounts mentioned.

If the undilated pupil size is large enough to allow for the desired optical zone for the individual patient, then no further testing is required. If, however, the pupil size is not large enough, then dilation should be performed with 2.5 percent phenylephrine and 0.5 percent mydriacyl. A full 20 minutes should be allowed for dilation to ensure that there is no asymmetrical shift to the pupil during mid dilation that might then alter the centration of the captured Zywave over the actual physiologic pupil center during treatment.

After successful data capture the surgeon has the ability to review the wavefront data at three different pupil sizes (Figure 5.37). The data can be viewed at a 5 mm zone, a more standard 6 mm zone, or at the size of the captured pupil. This can be view in a higher-order point spread function showing a graphic splay of how light is scattered based on HOA's only. It can be viewed graphically broken down by each individual type of HOA at the 5 mm or 6 mm zones and have the graphs displayed over a normal amount of each of these aberrations for the given zone size. Or it can be displayed as a color map of the HOA's similar to the color topographic maps we are accustom to viewing. One of the most useful features of these displays is the ability to choose a standard viewing zone (not related to treatment zone) for examining the three mentioned displays of HOA's. This allows the surgeon, over time, to be able to use pattern recognition for different types and amount of HOA's similar to how pattern recognition is used in topographic maps today. It would be impossible to do this if all HOA maps were displayed at different zone sizes as opposed to displaying them all at the same zone size. Again as a reminder the 6mm zone chosen to display the HOA data does not then mandate that the treatment be at a 6 mm zone. The surgeon may still choose any zone desired for treatment from 5.5 mm to 7.0 mm.

After capturing and reviewing the Zywave data the surgeon may then comfortably discuss the benefits of wavefront treatment with each patient. Individual markers for custom treatment very from surgeon to surgeon, but generally patients with larger pupil sizes, higher prescriptions, residual bed issues, higher amounts of HOA's to begin with, and higher quality of vision expectations are good candidates for wavefront treatments.

ACKNOWLEDGEMENT

Orbscan Figures, *Courtesy* Andrew L Moyes, MD and Paul M Karpecki, OD.

REFERENCE

1. Rao SN, Raviv T, Majmudar PA, Epstein RJ. Role of Orbscan II in screening keratoconus suspects before refractive corneal surgery. Ophthalmology. 2002 Sep;109(9):1642-6.

Chapter

6

Orbscan Corneal Mapping in Refractive Surgery

Francisco Sánchez León

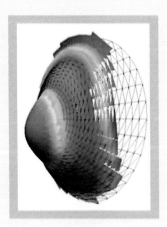

INTRODUCTION

Today corneal topography plays several critical roles in different refractive surgery decisions. Conventional axial and tangential topography maps are not enought to demostrate a healthy cornea and we can not decide either if Lasik surgery, any type of surface laser refractive procedure or intracorneal rings for early keratoconus are suitable procedures indicated for any case based only on surface topographic evaluation.

Maw 1, mentioned that he served as consultant of six cases of postoperative LASIK ectasia ocurred in low to moderate myopia, unfurtunatly none of the eyes he examined had undergone a preoperative evaluation with Orbscan, so he was unable to analize the posterior elevation or the displacement of either the posterior float or cornal thinning. This is unfare for a LASIK patient, in the times when technologies are capable of such analysis.

Bausch & Lomb's Orbscan® IIz is a fully integrated multidimensional diagnostic system that elevates diagnostics beyond mere topography. Unlike current topography systems which scan the surface of the eye at standard points, the Orbscan II acquires over 9000 data points in 1.5 seconds to meticulously map the entire corneal surface (11 mm), and analyze elevation and curvature measurements on both the anterior and posterior surfaces of the cornea.

The Orbscan® system (Bausch & Lomb, Rochester, NY) uses the principle of projection. Forty scanning slit beams (20 from the left and 20 from the right with up to 240 data points per slit) are used to scan the cornea from limbus to limbus and to measure independently the x, y, and z locations of several thousand points on each surface. The images captured are then used to construct the anterior corneal surface, posterior corneal surface, and anterior iris and anterior lens surfaces. Data regarding the cornel pachymetry and anterior chamber depth are also displayed. In the newer version of the Orbscan® system, a placido disk has been mounted to this device in order to improve the accuracy of the curvature measurements.

An advantage of this device is that it measures all surfaces of the anterior segment. Scanning time (1.2-1.5 seconds) is required, this device use a tracking system to track the eye movements in order to minimize the influence of involuntary eye movement.

By providing more comprehensive pre-op diagnostics and planning, exclusionary criteria such as keratoconus, pre-keratoconus, and corneal thinning can be identified to optimize outcomes in both primary treatments and enhancements. The Orbscan II may help explain decreased visual acuity post-op, and is designed to allow the surgeon to more accurately prescribe retreatments, if necessary. This technology is capable of detecting and analyzing posterior corneal abnormalities where corneal anomalies first appear.

ORBSCAN CORNEAL MAPPING FOR REFRACTIVE SURGERY DIAGNOSTICS

The Orbscan II (Figure 6.1), together with other diagnostic tools such as aberrometry , pupillometry and pachymetry, provides us with an unprecedented opportunity to select patients for an appropriate technique (LASIK, LASEK, PRK, Phakik IOL, Intracorneal Rings), minimizing complications such as long-term corneal posterior ectasia.

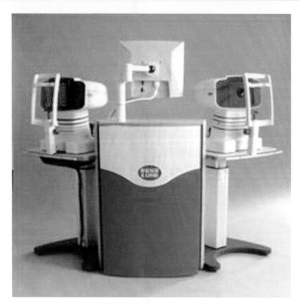

FIGURE 6.1: Orbscan IIz

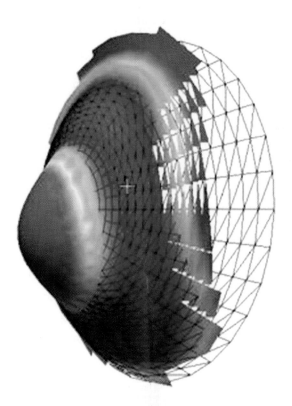

FIGURE 6.2: Ectasia

Posterior ectasia has been identified after refractive surgery techniques such as Lasik, where insufficient corneal tissue has been left behind postoperatively.[2] It has manifested itself as a forward 'bulging' of corneal tissue (Figure 6.2), developing from the posterior corneal surface. Indeed, several researchers indicates that up to 90 percent of kerataconus developing in the untreated eye appear first from the posterior surface. This is thought to be related to leaving the cornea with too little tissue postoperatively; and indeed although this is established, there are other indicators which could also put a patient at risk. **The Orbscan II provide us additional information to predict these risk.**

It has become a universally accepted the standard to leave at least 250 μm residual stromal bed as a safety measure in Lasik, and the Orbscan II has played its part to make it happend. However, the true validity of this limit is in some doubt.[4] The average cornea can range in thickness from 490 to 600 μm, so it is not logical to leave a standard 250 μm in all cases.

A number of surgeons support the view that a percentage thickness of the cornea should remain instead, and/or that a minimum of at least 260 μm to 280 μm is a more realistic standard. To facilitate this, intraoperative pachymetry (corneal thickness measurement) can be performed to provide a more accurate idea of how much tissue will remain after a procedure 5. This in itself has limitations, but gives an additional safety criterion, rather than merely relying on manufacturers' estimations of flap thickness.

In summary, the residual stromal bed is by far from our clinical perspectiver theonly indicator for safe preoperative screening. So, how does the Orbscan II influence decisions on whether or not to treat? It is important to understand that selection criteria for refractive surgery never stands alone, and it is the clinician's responsibility to bring together all the information gathered in the screening process, before deciding whether it is safe to proceed. The Orbscan influences this decision in a number of ways.

Unlike other modern topography systems, the Orbscan is based on slit scanning technology in addition to traditional placido-based techniques (Figure 6.3).

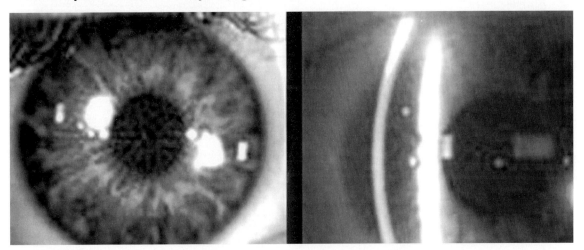

FIGURE 6.3: Slit scanning technology in the Orbscan

The placido image gives us information on axial keratometric readings, by converting distortion of the rings into topographical data. A series of illuminated annular rings are projected onto the cornea. Using the corneal tear film as a mirror, the reflected image of the rings is captured by a digital video camera. The captured image is then subjected to an algorithm to detect and identify the position of the rings in relation to the video keratographic axis. Once these borders are detected, the digital image is 'reconstructed' to show anterior corneal curvature.

Orbscan goes much further than this; slit-beam scanners and triangulation are used to derive the actual spatial location of thousands of points on the surface. Each beam sweep across the cornea gives information on corneal elevation, or height, from the anterior corneal surface, posterior surface and iris. To represent the corneal surface data in a way that is easily understood, the computer calculates a hypothetical sphere that matches as close as possible to the actual corneal shape being measured. This is called the best fit sphere (BFS). It then compares the real surface to the hypothetical sphere, showing areas 'above' the surface of the sphere in warm colours, and areas 'below' the surface in cool colours.

This has many uses, but for the purposes of refractive surgery selection, 'bulges' in both the posterior and anterior surface can indicate patients who may be at risk of ectasia development. This enables the surgeon to screen them out early in the selection process.

A 'quad map' can be produced, which gives four different maps each portraying different information about the cornea (Figure 6.4). The bottom left hand map is the axial keratometry map, based on placido technology. This is similar to maps produced from the majority of commercially available topography systems, and provides detailed keratometric information across the diameter of the cornea.

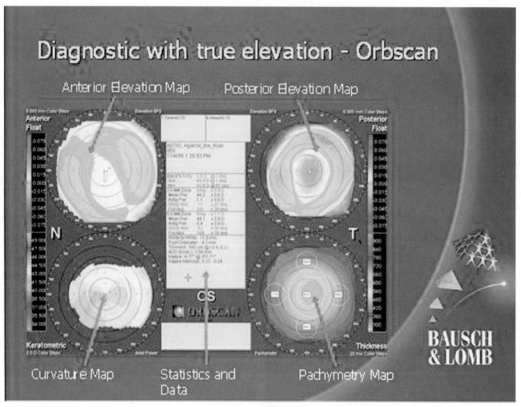

FIGURE 6.4: Quad map

For LASIK selection, this information is important for a number of reasons. The 'K' readings it is important, because limits of K readings are between certain values; the cornea must be neither too steep nor too flat. It is difficult for the microkeratome (blade designed for flap cutting), to create a good quality corneal flap in Lasik if either of these extremes is the case, as this can lead to surgical flap complications.

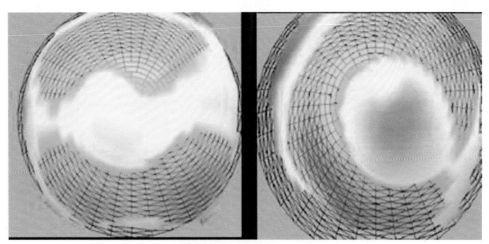

FIGURE 6.5: Elevation map

In addition, K readings of more than 48 D are an indication of potential kerataconus, particularly where this is decentred inferonasally. Details of the K readings can be found in the stats and data information in the centre of the quad map.

The top left hand map of Figure 6.5 is the anterior elevation map, and as with the top right hand posterior elevation map, slit scanning provides the means of creating the information. As mentioned before, slit scanning provides elevation data, and this also can create a 3D interpretation of the cornea. Looking at both elevation maps, if it is imagined that the green tissue is at sea level, then the warmer colours are above sea level, or towards the viewer, and the cooler colours are below, or further away from the viewer.

A 3 D interpretation of both elevation maps can be seen in Figure 6.5. The meshwork affect indicates how the cornea would appear if it were entirely spherical and is referred to as the reference sphere.

This elevation data can be interpreted usefully in a number of ways. First the difference between the highest and lowest points is a potential kerataconus indicator, if over 100 μm; Rousch criteria[6] (Figure 6.6).

In addition, on the posterior map, the highest elevation value can again be interpreted as a kerataconus indicator, or at least as a screen for those patients who may be at risk of developing kerectasia postoperatively. This provides safety criteria to avoid treating patients at risk. From the work of Vukich[7] and Potgeiter,[8] 55D elevation has been recommended as an absolute cut off. As can be seen from Figures 6.5 and 6.6, the elevation on the right hand side (posterior elevation) is more advanced than that on the left (anterior elevation), indicating that 'bulges' develop from the posterior surface of the cornea in the first instance.

From studying the relationship between the two elevation maps, further information can be gleaned. A ratio can be calculated between the posterior and anterior surfaces, which gives an indication of the relative difference in curvature between the two maps.[9] Figure 6.7 shows two corneal cross-sections.

This very simplistic diagram (Figure 6.7) shows us that the same elevation data for the posterior surface can have a different impact on the stability of the cornea. In diagram B where the ratio is high at

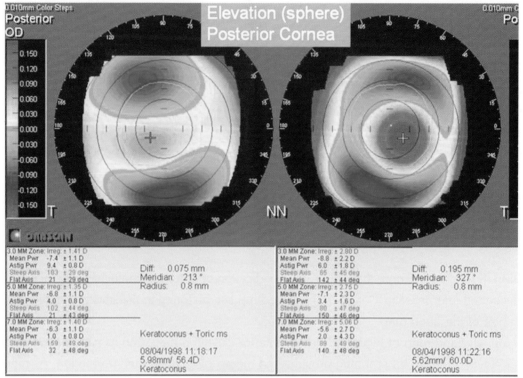

0.010mm Color Steps

Elevation (sphere)
Posterior Cornea

Posterior
OD

0.150
0.120
0.090
0.060
0.030
0.000
-0.030
-0.060
-0.090
-0.120
-0.150

NN

3.0 MM Zone:	Irreg:	± 1.41 D
Mean Pwr	-7.4	± 1.1 D
Astig Pwr	9.4	± 0.8 D
Steep Axis	103	± 29 deg
Flat Axis	21	± 29 deg
5.0 MM Zone:	Irreg:	± 1.35 D
Mean Pwr	-6.8	± 1.1 D
Astig Pwr	4.0	± 0.8 D
Steep Axis	102	± 44 deg
Flat Axis	21	± 43 deg
7.0 MM Zone:	Irreg:	± 1.40 D
Mean Pwr	-6.3	± 1.1 D
Astig Pwr	1.0	± 0.8 D
Steep Axis	159	± 49 deg
Flat Axis	32	± 48 deg

Diff: 0.075 mm
Meridian: 213 °
Radius: 0.8 mm

Keratoconus + Toric ms

08/04/1998 11:18:17
5.98mm/ 56.4D
Keratoconus

3.0 MM Zone:	Irreg:	± 2.80 D
Mean Pwr	-8.8	± 2.2 D
Astig Pwr	6.0	± 1.8 D
Steep Axis	65	± 45 deg
Flat Axis	142	± 44 deg
5.0 MM Zone:	Irreg:	± 2.75 D
Mean Pwr	-7.1	± 2.3 D
Astig Pwr	3.4	± 1.6 D
Steep Axis	80	± 47 deg
Flat Axis	150	± 46 deg
7.0 MM Zone:	Irreg:	± 5.06 D
Mean Pwr	-5.6	± 2.7 D
Astig Pwr	2.0	± 4.3 D
Steep Axis	89	± 49 deg
Flat Axis	140	± 48 deg

Diff: 0.195 mm
Meridian: 327 °
Radius: 0.8 mm

Keratoconus + Toric ms

08/04/1998 11:22:16
5.62mm/ 60.0D
Keratoconus

FIGURE 6.6: Elevation

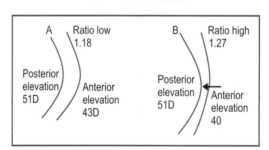

FIGURE 6.7: Corneal cross-sections

1.27, it can be seen that a weak area (indicated by the arrow) develops which is not apparent in A, even though posterior elevation data is the same for both. This information on elevation and ratio would rarely be used as exclusion criteria alone, but by considering these together, more conclusive information can be obtained. For example, a high ratio of say 1.26 would be far more concerning if the posterior elevation was high at 55 D, the cornea was of borderline thickness, and the preoperative prescription high.

The final map to study is the pachymetry map. This is map four of our quad map in Figure 6.4. Traditionally, pachymetry has been measured using ultrasound, which provides a reading of corneal thickness from Bowman's membrane to Descemet's membrane. Through slit scanning technology, Orbscan provides us with a pachymetry reading from the precorneal tear film to the endothelium, therefore slightly thicker readings can be expected.[10] The Orbscan can, however, be calibrated to take this into consideration when comparing readings. The true advantage of the pachymetry map is that it

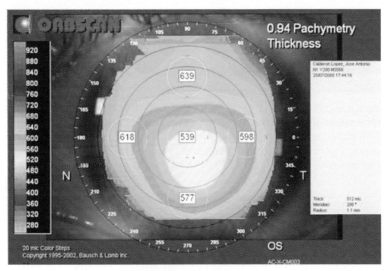

FIGURE 6.8: Pachymetry

provides us with thickness information across the cornea from limbus to limbus, not just in single points as with ultrasound. This once again gives the opportunity to detect areas of weakness, thinning or scarring. Auffarth et al[11] state that the relationship between the highest point on anterior and posterior elevation maps, and the thinnest point (shown by a yellow dot) is an indicator of kerataconus.

The relationship between pachymetry readings can be looked at, and it has been suggested that 100µm should be a cut-off criteria between thickness regions on the map. Figure 6.8 shows the relationship between the central reading in the white circle, and the four peripheral readings, indicated by the arrows. Once again these criteria would be used alongside otherinformation, but alone would not exclude a patient. The readings within the circles are averages of measurements within the area, but the Orbscan also flags the thinnest point, indicated by a yellow dot.

In conclusion, it can be seen that much information can be obtained from analysis of Orbscan maps, and this information does not have the scope to cover it all. The most important message is that the criteria does not stand alone, and by looking at all the maps together along with other information, an informed decision can be made as to whether it is safe to proceed to surgery.

SELECTION CRITERIA

The diagnosis of keratoconus proper, seldom proves to be problematic, and represents the undisputed black end of the spectrum, as would be the case for the patient with simple with the rule astigmatism who would be on the white end of the spectrum. However, in between a large grey area exists, consisting of aginst-the rule astigmatism, asymmetric astigmatism, non-orthogonal astigmatism, irregular astigmatismand forme fruste keratoconus.

Over the past number of years since true elevation corneal topography became available, a set of criteria (Table 6.1 and 6.2)[6,8,9] were developed to distinguish to distinguish among these entities. Altough corneal topography provides us with the most clues for the diagnosis of early keratoconus, other clinical criteria also need to be considered.

TABLE 6.1: Rousch's Orbscan criteria for subclinical keratoconus detection

1. Elevation difference superior of 100 mm at the central optical zone of 7 mm
2. Clinical difference superior of 100 mm at the central optical zone of 7 mm
3. Anterior elevation superior of 40 mm at the central optical zone of 7 mm from BFS
4. Posterior elevation superior of 50 mm at the central optical zone of 7 mm from BFS
5. Posterior BFS reference > 55D

TABLE 6.2: Efkarpides's Orbscan criteria for subclinical keratoconus detection

1. Anterior/Posterior BFS of reference difference in mm superior to 1.25 to 1.27
2. Morphological difference between anterior and posterior face (warpage)
3. Remarkable convergence of points (highest point on anterior elevation, highest point on posterior elevation, thinnest point in pachymetry, steepest curvature on the power map)
4. Infero-temporal displacement of these remarkable points
5. Color code statistical analysis (Normal Band Scale). Elevation values, curvature, pachymetry of more than 2 standard deviations from controls.

These would include the patient's age, a family history of keratoconus, history of systemic or local pathology, asociated with keratoconus, refractive stability, as well as wheter a good and crisp endpoint could be achieved on refractive testing of the subject.

No single cornea topographic sign is in its own right diagnostic of fruste keratoconus, but rather a combination of a set of criteria. One might look at each of these criteria as a "alarm sign" noted, with the porobability for *early keratoconus* propotionate to the number of alarms present.

These criteria can be divide into the following categories:

a. Power map changes
b. Posterior elevation maps
c. Pachymetry
d. Composite/integrated topography information

Power Maps

A. Mean corneal curvature >45 diopters. Mean corneal curvature measuring in excess of 45 diopters is a well established feature of keratoconus.

B. Bow–tie/broken-tie pattern. In addition to steep corneal curvatures, the bow-tie or broken bow-tie appereence of astigmatic pattern might be indicative of early keratoconus, and also a well known criteria.

C. Central corneal asymetry. A change within the central 3 mm optical zone of the cornea of more than 3 diopters from superior or inferior can be correlatedwith the presence of vertical coma. However, this may be merely a sign of asymetrical astigmatism, and is not necesarily an indicator of pathology.

Posterior Elevation

The elevation map displays corneal height or elevation relative to a reference plane, which may be a spherical or aspherical surface depending on the topographer. It is important to note that the elevation display depends on reference surface size, shape, alignment, and fitting zone. This map shows the three-dimensional shape of the cornea and is useful in measuring the amount of tissue removed by a procedure, assessing postoperative visual problems, or planning/monitoring surgical procedures

Many surgeons think the first sign of keratectasia appers on the posterior surface of the cornea, not on the anterior topography map. Considering this, the importance of recognizing a change in the posterior surface deserves special emphasis.[1-3] While one would not perform corneal laser surgery on eyes with keratoconus, keratoconus suspects or posterior ectasia defined by technologies with the capability of posterior corneal float analysis, it might prove useful to look at the criteria for early form of keratoconus in order to define those cases, and distinguish them from eyes that would be suited to laser refractive surgery.

Laser clinics had shown that 5 to 8 percent of patients screened for refractive procedure are not good candidates because ketatoconus detection by simple axial topography, however, a mexican study demostrated that 3.13 percent of population screened for Laser eye surgery had posterior ectasia criteria by Orbscan, despite having axial topography clasified as normal (unpublished data).[3]

We have found four different posterior float pattens in patients screened for Laser eye surgery: complete positive band 71.87 percent, ncomplete postitive band 18.75 percent, butterfly wings cummon in patients with high astigmatism 6.25 percent, and central island 3.13 percent (Figure 6.9). In other words, if we don´t know posterir float features from every case, we have at least 3 percent risk of unstable LASIK result or iatrogenic ectasia in the worst case.[3]

Best fit sphere > 55 diopters. The most common reference surface for viewing elevation maps is the "best fit sphere". This geometric surface is constructed by fitting a spherical spline with the least square of difference values though the three dimensional elevation data from the cornea, whether it be the anterior or posterior profile. The sphere can thus be employed to judge the average profile of the surface in question. A best fit sphere (BFS) with the power of 55 diopters or more on the posterior profile, could be indicative of posterior ectasia. This criterium is not diagnostic as a sign of early keratoconus per sé, as this sign may also be seen in small diameter corneas.

Posterior high point >50 micron above BFS. Early keratoconus is often seen first on the posterior corneal profile. **Whenever a localized elevation above BFS on the posterior surface measures more than 50 micron in elevation, this might be indicative of an early posterior ectasia.**

Many authors have review the posterior surface's response to LASIK, and Orbscan is an unique technology to evaluate this changes.[12-15] Increased forward shift of the posterior corneal surface is common after myopic LASIK and correlates with the residual corneal thickness and ablation percentage per total corneal thikness.[12]

An excessively thin residual cornea bed or a large ablation percentage may increase the risk of iatrogenic complications, such ectasia. Others have considered that even if a residual corneal bed of

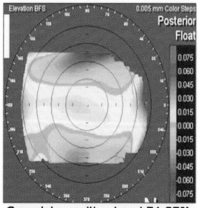

Complete positive band 71.87%

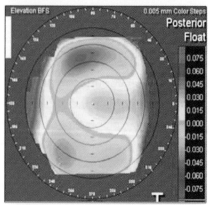

Incomplete positive band 18.75

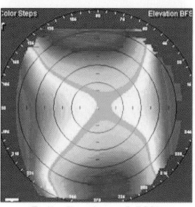

Butterfly wings 6.25%

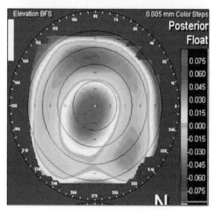

Central island 3.13%

FIGURE 6.9: Posterior float patterns

300mm or thicker is preserved, anterior bulging of the cornea after LASIK can ocurr. Eye with thin corneas and high myopia requiring greater laser ablation are more predisposed to an anterior shift of the posterior central cornea.[13,14]

Roberts 15 with the help of Orbscan proposes a new theory to explain the increased posterior elevation postLASIK, she suggests that the mild ectasia appereance may be due to a backward sweling of the peripheral redistributed cornea rather than a pathological forward bulging of the central corna.

Pachymetry

Thinnest point <470 micron. This constitutes an absolute contra-indication to corneal refractive surgery. In pathological corneas, this thinnest point is often displaced inferotemporal.

Difference of > 100 microns at 7 mm optical zone. A difference of more than 100 microns from the thinnest point to the values at the 7 mm optical zone implies a steep gradient of thinning from the midperiphery towards the thinnest point. These, in conjunction with othe signs, can be indicative of early pathology.[9]

Composite/Integrated Information

As a default, four corneal maps are routinely presented by the Orbscan II (Bausch & Lomb, Orbtek, Salt Lake City, Utha). Elevation topography System. Thes include the anterior elevation profile, posterior elevation profile, power map, and a total pachymetry map. Through integration of the information provide on these maps, one is able to detect subtle, but powerful signs not present on any individual map. These signs include the following:

Bent/warped Cornea

Similarly between anterior and posterior profiles implies a forward bending of those areas shown above the BFS. If these bending is in association with the thinnest point on the cornea. It could related to structural weakness in the cornea, irrespective of wheter the thinnest point still shows and adecuated pachymetry. These sign has to be evaluated within the context other signs above.

Inferotemporal displacement of the highest point. Infero-temporal displacementof the highest point on the anterior as well as the posterior elevation profile can be indicative of early keratoconus, but must also be seen in context (Figure 6.10)

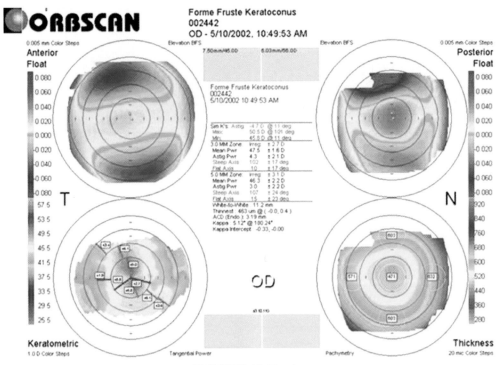

FIGURE 6.10: Keratoconus

Correlation of Signs of the Highest Point on the Posterior Elevation

This is probably the strongest topographic sign indicative of early keratoconus. If the highest point on the posterior elevation coincides with the highst point of anterior elevation, the thinnest point on pachymetry, and the point of steepest curvature on the power map, one has to very carefull regarding your decision

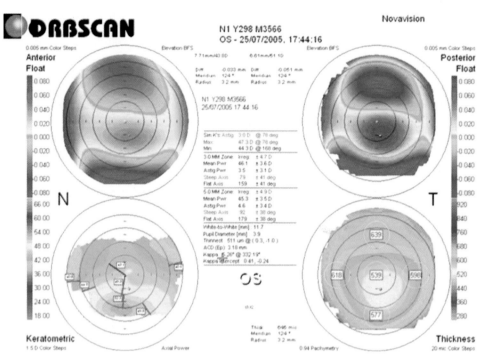

FIGURE 6.11: Keratoconus

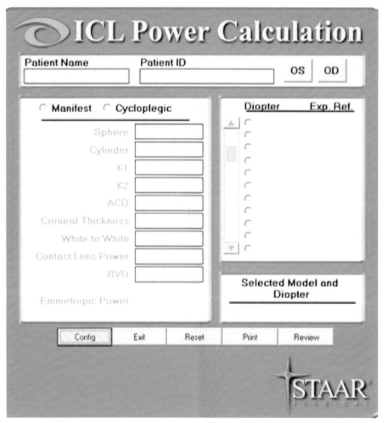

FIGURE 6.12: ICL power calculation for phakic IOL (STAAR)

to operate. This signs implies that the thinnest point represents an structural weakness, wich cause a forward bending of the cornea (as is noted on the posterior and anterior elevation maps), further supported by the curvature change on the power map (Figure 6.11)

Recognizing keratoconus an the other forms of corneal pathology like pellucid marginal degeneration that contra-indicate corneal laser refractive surgery is central to safe clinical practice. As profesionals is our own resposability to keep the prestige of refractive surgery, and LASIK safe desicion must be our mision.

Finally, if some criteria of unhealthy cornea or posterior ectasia have been found, other refractive surgical techniques can be attepted such as phakic IOL in the case of fruste keratoconus or thin cornea for a of high myopia patient (Figure 6.12); or in the scenario of a keratoconus, intracorneal rings can be attempted, orbscan offers us the posibility in helping to take this decision and follow up.

REFERENCES

1. Maw R. Avoiding Postoperative LASIK Ectasia. Cataract and Refractive Surgery Today. Nov-Dec 2003.
2. Seiler T. Koufala K, Richter G. Iatrogenic keratectasia after laser in situ keratomileuisis. J Cataract Refrac Surg 1998; 14: 312-317.
3. Vaca, Oscar. Posterior Float Features in Population Screened for Laser Eye Surgery. Mexican Cornea and Refractive Surgery Society 1999.
4. Ambrosio R, Klyce SD, Wilson SE. Corneal topogrphic and pachymetric screening of keratorefractive patients. J Refractive Surg. 2003; 19:24-29
5. Ou RJ, Shaw EL, Glasgow BJ. Keratectasia after laser in situ keratomileusis (LASIK):evaluation of the calculated residual stromal bed thickness. Am j Ophthalmol. 2002 Nov; 134 (5): 771-3
6. Roush C. Orbscan II Manual (Salt Lake City, Utha. Orbtek)
7. Vukich J et al. Early spatial changes in the posterior corneal surface after laser in situ keratomileusis. J Cataract Refract Surg 2003, 29:778-784
8. Potgeiter F. Custome Lasik Surgical Techniques and Complications. Buranto L., Brint S. Slack. 2004: 435-437
9. Assouline M. Chirugie Ceil-Le Kératocone. De nouveaux critéres de detection de kératocone infraclinique. www.inclo.com/le-keratocone.php
10. Fakhry M, Artola A, Belda J, Alio J. Comparison of corneal pachymetry using ultrasound and Orbscan II . J Cataract Refract Surg 2002; 28:248-252
11. Auffarth GU, Tetz MR, Biazid Y, Volcker HE. Keratoconus evaluation using the Orbscan Topography System. J Cataract Refract Surg 2002, 26:222-228
12. Lee DH,Seo S,Jeong KW,et al. Early spatial changes in the posterior corneal surface after laser in situ keratomileusis. J Cataracy Refract Surg. 2003;29;778-784.
13. Twa MD,Roberts C, Mahmound AM, Chang JS Jr. Response of the posterior corneal surface to laser in situ Keratomileusis for myopia. J Cataract Refract Surg. 2003;31:61-71.
14. Miyata K,Tokunaga T, Nakahara M, et al. Residual bed thickness and corneal foward shifth after laser in situ Keratomileusis. J Cataract Refract Surg. 2004;30:1067-1072.
15. Grzybowski DM, Roberts CJ, Mahmound AM, Chang JS Jr. Model for nonectatic in posterior corneal elevation after ablative procedures. J Cataract Refract Surg. 2005;31:72-81.
16. Cairns G McGhee NJ, Collins MJ,et al. Accuracy of Orbscan II slit scanning elevation topography. J Cataract Refract Surg. 2002;28:2181-2187.

Chapter 7

Nidek OPD Scan in Clinical Practice

Gregg Feinerman
Timothy Peters
Kim Nguyen
Marcus Solorzano
Shiela Scott

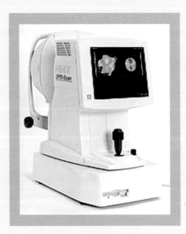

INTRODUCTION

Corneal topography and wavefront analysis are both essential data that provide useful information to the refractive surgeon. Unlike corneal topography, wavefront analysis provides us with information about the overall refractive status of the eye, including the cornea, lens and retina. It also demonstrates aberrations that occur with pupillary dilation.

Over the past five years wavefront technology has been proven to be useful in both custom ablation planning and in screening patients for refractive surgery. Wavefront analysis helps explain visual aberrations when they are not obvious on corneal topography. Patients with visual aberrations following refractive surgery may have unremarkable corneal topography maps, but their symptoms may be explained on wavefront analysis[1]. In such cases, wavefront analysis will commonly show elevated values for vertical coma and trefoil.

NIDEK OPD SCAN

The Nidek OPD Scan is a scanning slit refractometer using skiascopic technology with simultaneous Placido disc corneal topography (Figure 7.1). It is the first diagnostic instrument to combine corneal topography, autorefraction, and wavefront analysis. The Nidek OPD Scan takes the autorefraction, keratometry, and wavefront measurements simultaneously in 0.4 seconds. Compared to other autorefractors, it measures the largest range of spherocylinder refractive error in the industry. It measures between –20 D and +22 D of sphere and 12 D of cylinder. After performing the autorefraction the technician performs the corneal topography (also in less than one second). Unlike Hartmann-Shack

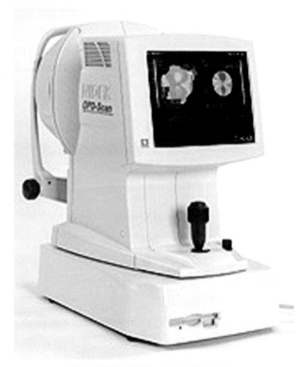

FIGURE 7.1: The Nidek OPD Scan

systems, the Nidek OPD-Scan uses dynamic retinoscopy to measure aberrations through 1,440 data points (highest number of all wavefront machines).[2] These points create refractive power maps with more data than on other systems. Unlike the grid on Hartmann-Shack wavefront systems, there is no mixing of data points with the scanning slit technology.

Guide to Clinical Interpretation with the Nidek OPD Scan

Nidek OPD Scan Six Map Display

Refractive (Snell's Law) map: Look at the color and topography patterns, keratometry, and Sim K values, as you would normally do for corneal topography maps. The scale should be set so that green represents 44 diopters in the scale settings section of the software. The dioptric power steps should be set to either 0.5 diopter or 1 diopter steps.

IROC (Tangential) map: Look at peripheral color patterns to look for peripheral changes beyond the 4 mm zone. The scale should be set so that green represents 44 diopters in the scale settings section of the software. The dioptric power steps should be set to either 0.5 diopter or 1 diopter steps.

OPD (Optical Path Difference to Emmetropia) map: Look at color patterns and overall dioptric power error scale for the 6 mm optical zone. ARK (Sphere/Cylinder/Astigmatism) values are displayed at the 2.5 mm, 3 mm and 5 mm zone. The irregular component of S/C/A at the 3 mm and 5mm ring zone are quantified using RMS values in diopters. RMS diopter values below 0.5 on the OPD map are regular or near normal sphere and cylinder patterns (radially linear and radially symmetric). The components of S/C/A become more irregular at values greater than 0.5 RMS (diopters). Look for irregular patterns associated with double vision (two or three power lobes similar to a three leaf clover pattern) or ghosting (significant variation in central power from nasal to temporal within 4 mm zone). The scale should be set so that green equals "0" diopters in the scale settings section of the software. The dioptric power steps should be set to either 0.5 diopter or 1 diopter steps.

Total order aberration map: This map displays how an emmetropic wavefront deviates through the entire optical system. Both lower and higher order aberrations are displayed in this map. The scale should be set so that green equals "0" microns in 0.5 mm or 1.0 mm steps in the scale settings section of the software.

Higher order aberration map: Determine the Higher Order (HO) wavefront percent by dividing Higher Order RMS wavefront error by Total Order RMS wavefront error (HO WF RMS error/TO WF RMS error = % of HO aberrations). This map displays only the irregular S/C/A or Higher Order aberrations of the optical system. The scale should be set so that green equals "0" microns in 0.5 mm or 1.0 mm steps in the scale settings section of the software.

The percentage of HO aberrations that is significant will vary for preoperative and postoperative patients. Preoperative HO/TO percent aberrations are abnormal after 20%, and postoperative HO/TO percent aberrations are suspect after 50%. However, this is a subjective observation that does not have clinical meaning until one reviews all of the available corneal topography, ARK, and OPD wavefront data.

Zernike graph: Examine the coefficients 6 through 27th and look for values of 0.5 RMS mm or higher for clinical significance. As for Zernike, the irregular (higher order) components of S/C/A can be measured and described optically as coma, trefoil and pentafoil and irregular (higher order) sphere can be described and measured by spherical aberrations (12th and 24th coefficient). RMS mm values below 0.5 mm are considered low and not clinically significant. RMS Values above 0.5 mm generally correlate to subjective visual complaints. This would apply to all higher order Zernike coefficients starting from 6 to 27th as displayed on the Zernike Graph. The Zernike Graph coefficient values are in microns of light (not tissue).

RMS error is the best measure of dispersion around the best-fit sinusoid (Figure 7.2). It expresses a degree of irregularity or reliability of S/C/A values. Emmetropic patients will generally have very uniform topography maps, normal keratometry, low RMS values and low Zernike values. The progression of error increases for conditions such as asymmetrical astigmatism and keratoconus.

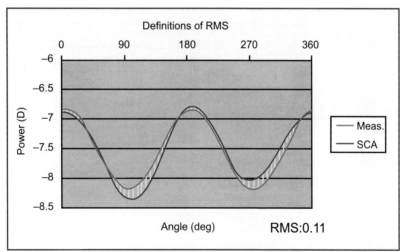

FIGURE 7.2: Definition of RMS

Summary

Examine the simulated keratometry and patterns on the topography maps, the ARK Data and RMS values and patterns on the OPD map, the ratio of HO/TO WF error from the wavefront maps and the HO Zernike RMS coefficients from 6 to 27th to determine:

1. If the visual errors are caused by irregular astigmatism or by irregular spherical error, and to what degree by looking at Zernike coefficients.
2. Compare the RMS OPD values to a known normal range (0.0 to 0.5 diopters) to identify irregular vs. regular profiles.
3. Evaluate whether HO/TO WF error percent aberration value is clinically significant by examining the Zernike RMS coefficient values. A value of 0.0 to 0.5 mm is not clinically significant. Values above

0.5 mm are clinically significant. This would apply to all higher order Zernike coefficients starting from 6 to 27th as displayed on the Zernike Graph.

CLINICAL EXAMPLES

Normal Bowtie Astigmatism (Figure 7.3)

The following patient demonstrates typical bowtie astigmatism on the axial map. The OPD map has RMS values below 0.50 D, which correlates to the clinical picture of regular astigmatism.

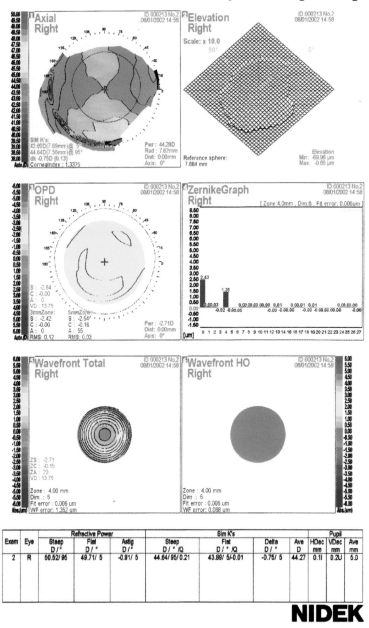

| Exam | Eye | Refractive Power | | | Sim K's | | | | Pupil | | |
		Steep D/°	Flat D/°	Astig D/°	Steep D/°/Q	Flat D/°/Q	Delta D/°	Ave D	HDec mm	VDec mm	Ave mm
2	R	50.52/95	49.71/5	-0.81/5	44.64/95/0.21	43.89/5/-0.01	-0.75/5	44.27	0.1I	0.2U	5.0

NIDEK

FIGURE 7.3: Normal bowtie astigmatism

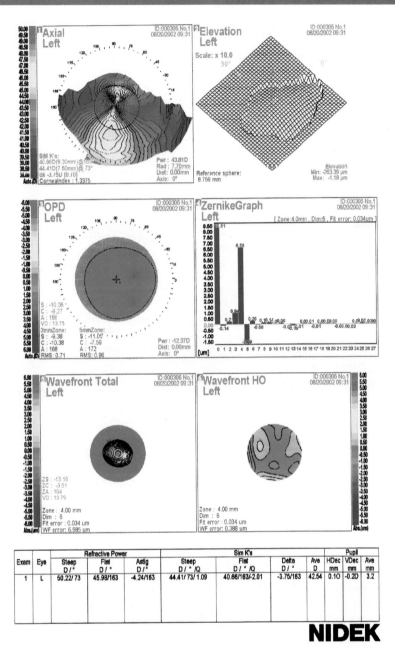

FIGURE 7.4: Keratoconus

Keratoconus (Figure 7.4)

This 20 year-old male presented for refractive surgery. Manifest refraction was –10.00 –8.00 × 165 (20/40). The refractive map revealed high keratometry readings with asymmetric astigmatism. OPD Map readings showed the irregular component of S/C/A at the three and five-millimeter zone using RMS values in diopters. RMS dioptric values measured greater than 0.50 D, which is associated with irregular astigmatism.

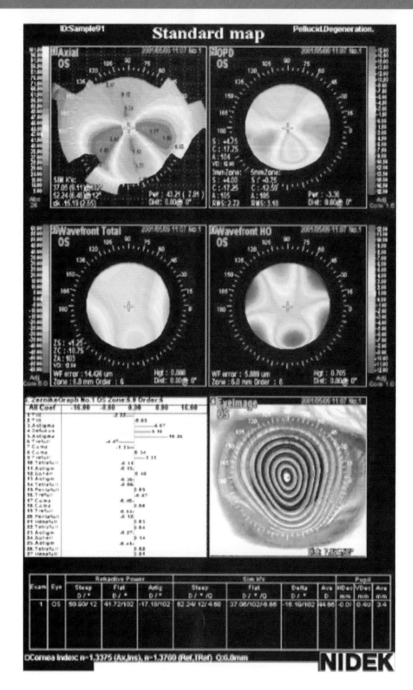

FIGURE 7.5: Pellucid marginal degeneration

Pellucid Marginal Degeneration (Figure 7.5)

This example demonstrates classic loop cylinder on corneal topography which is classic for pellucid marginal degeneration. Wavefront RMS values are elevated (2.72D @ 3 mm and 3.10 @ 5 mm) and consistent with irregular astigmatism.

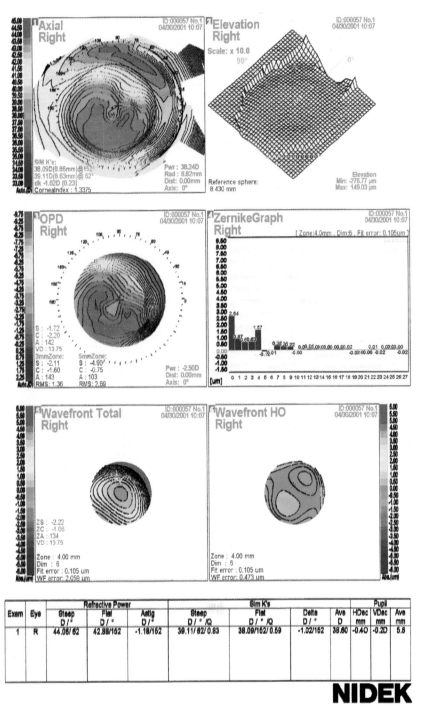

FIGURE 7.6: Decentered LASIK ablation

Decentered LASIK Ablation (Figure 7.6)

This 40-year-old patient was treated at another laser center and presented to the Feinerman Vision Center for correction of her LASIK complication. Her main complaint was decreased best-corrected vision and visual aberrations that worsened at night. BCVA was 20/60 in her right eye.

123

The corneal topography and OPD maps of the right eye demonstrate an inferotemporally decentered ablation. RMS diopter values far exceed 0.5 D, which correlate to the patient's visual complaints.

Significant spherical and coma aberrations are present. Individual Zernike RMS values greater than 0.5 D in either direction correlate with the patient's visual problems.

The OPD Map is the better indicator of what is wrong in diopters. In this case, I would not place much value in the Zernike coefficients, other than the fact that higher values generally correlate with visual complaints. This patient has an off-center power distribution noted on the OPD map. Custom ablation may be an option for cases of decentered ablations.

CONCLUSION

The Nidek OPD Scan is the only diagnostic instrument that incorporates corneal topography, autorefraction, and wavefront analysis in one system. The six map display displays the data in a manner that makes it easy for the surgeon to interpret. In the future, we will be able to utilize Nidek's Final Fit™ software to incorporate this data for custom ablation treatments.

REFERENCES

1. Beyond LASIK - Wavefront Analysis and Customized Ablation. Highlights of Ophthalmology 2001.
2. Nidek OPD Scan Manual, 2002

Chapter

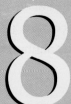

Anterior
Keratoconus

Amar Agarwal
Sunita Agarwal
Athiya Agarwal

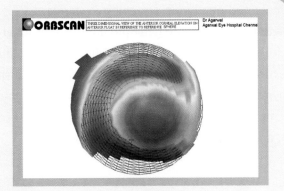

INTRODUCTION

Keratoconus is characterized by non-inflammatory stromal thinning and anterior protrusion of the cornea. Keratoconus is a slowly progressive condition often presenting in the teen or early twenties with decreased vision or visual distortion. Family history of keratoconus is seen occasionally. Patients with this disorder are poor candidates for refractive surgery because of the possibility of exacerbating keratectasia[1]. The development of corneal ectasia is a well recognized complication of LASIK and attributed to unrecognized preoperative forme fruste Keratoconus.

ORBSCAN

The ORBSCAN (BAUSCH and LOMB) corneal topography system uses a scanning optical slit scan that is fundamentally different than the corneal topography that analyses the reflected images from the anterior corneal surface. The high-resolution video camera captures 40 light slits at 45 degrees angle projected through the cornea similarly as seen during slit lamp examination. It has an acquisition time of 4 seconds.[2] The diagnosis of keratoconus is a clinical one and early diagnosis can be difficult on clinical examination alone. ORBSCAN has become a useful tool for evaluating the disease, and with the advent of its use, morphology and any subtle changes in the topography can be detected in early keratoconus. We always use the ORBSCAN system to evaluate our potential LASIK candidates preoperatively to rule out anterior keratoconus.

TECHNIQUE

All eyes to undergo LASIK are examined by ORBSCAN. Eyes are screened using quad maps with the normal band (NB) filter turned on. Four maps included: (a) anterior corneal elevation: NB = ± 25 μ of best-fit sphere, (b) posterior corneal elevation: NB = ± 25 μ of best-fit sphere, (c) keratometric mean curvature: NB = 40 to 48 D, K, and (d) Corneal thickness (pachymetry): NB = 500 to 600 μ. Map features within normal band are colored green. This effectively filters out variation falling within normal band. When abnormalities are seen on the normal band quad map screening, a standard scale quad map is examined. For those cases with anterior keratoconus, we also generate three-dimensional views of anterior and posterior corneal elevation. The following parameters are considered to detect anterior keratoconus: (a) radii of anterior and posterior curvature of the cornea, (b) posterior best-fit sphere, (c) difference between the thickest corneal pachymetry value in 7 mm zone and thinnest pachymetry value of the cornea, (d) normal band (NB) scale map, (e) elevation on the anterior float of the cornea, (f) elevation on the posterior float of the cornea, and (g) location of the cone on the cornea.

ANTERIOR KERATOCONUS

On ORBSCAN analysis in patients with anterior keratoconus the average ratio of radius of the anterior curvature to the posterior curvature of cornea is 1.25 (range 1.21 to 1.38), average posterior best-fit sphere is –56.98 Dsph (range –52.1 Dsph to –64.5), average difference in pachymetry value between thinnest point on the cornea and thickest point in 7 mm zone on the cornea is 172.7 µm (range 117 µm to 282 µm), average elevation of anterior corneal float is 55.25 µm (range 25 µm to 103 µm), average elevation of posterior corneal float is 113.6 µm (range 41 µm to 167 µm). Figures 8.1 to 8.6 show the various topographic features of an eye with anterior keratoconus. In Figure 8.1 (general quad map) upper left corner map is the anterior float, upper right corner map is posterior float, lower left corner is keratometric map while the lower right is the pachymetry map showing a difference of 282 µm between the thickest pachymetry value in 7 mm zone of cornea (597 µm) and thinnest pachymetry value (315 µm). In Figure 8.2, normal band scale map of anterior surface shows significant elevation on the anterior and posterior float with abnormal keratometric and pachymetry maps. Figure 8.3 is three-dimensional representation of the anterior float with reference sphere 64 µm. Figure 8.4 shows three-dimensional representation of posterior float with reference sphere. Figure 8.5 shows amount of elevation (color coded) of the anterior corneal surface in microns (64 µm). Figure 8.6 shows amount of elevation (color coded) of the posterior corneal surface in microns (167 µm).

DISCUSSION

Topography is valuable for preoperative ophthalmic examination of LASIK candidates. Three-dimensional imaging allows surgeons to look at corneal thickness, as well as the corneal anterior and posterior surface and can predict the shape of cornea after LASIK surgery. Topographic analysis using three-dimensional slit scan system allows us to predict which candidates would do well with LASIK and also

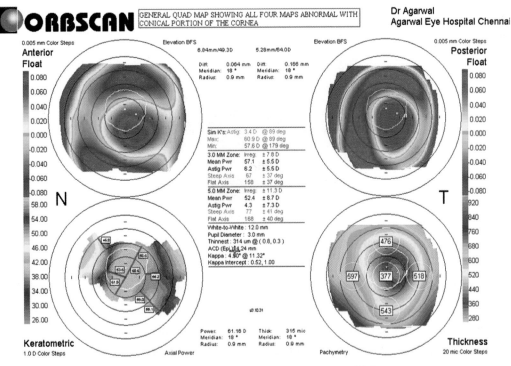

FIGURE 8.1: Showing general quad map of an eye with keratoconus

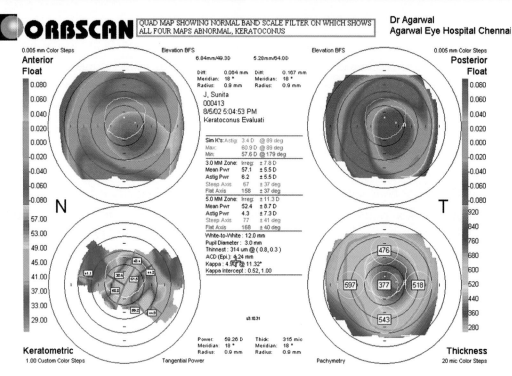

FIGURE 8.2: Showing quad map with normal band scale filter on in the same eye as in Figure 8.1

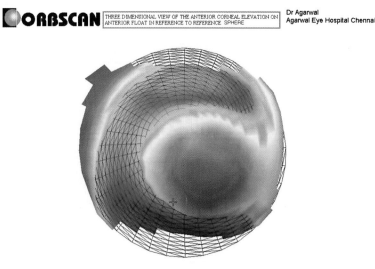

FIGURE 8.3: Showing three-dimensional anterior float

confers the ability to screen for subtle configurations which may be contraindication to LASIK.[3] It is known that corneal ectasias and keratoconus have posterior corneal elevation as the earliest manifestation. In addition Wang et al have shown that the posterior corneal elevation increases after LASIK, and the increase is correlated with residual corneal bed thickness.[4] We found that patients with positive keratoconus have higher posterior and anterior elevation on Orbscan II topography.

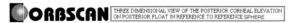

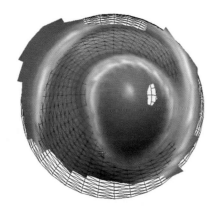

FIGURE 8.4: Showing three-dimensional posterior float

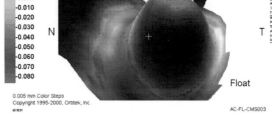

FIGURE 8.5: Showing three-dimensional anterior corneal elevation measured in microns

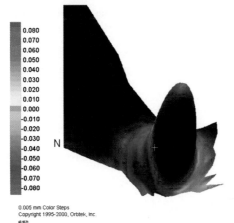

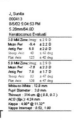

FIGURE 8.6: Showing three-dimensional posterior corneal elevation measured in microns

Elevation is not measured directly by placido-based topographers, but certain assumptions allow the construction of elevation maps. Elevation of a point on the corneal surface displays the height of the point on the corneal surface relative to a spherical reference surface. Reference surface is chosen to be a sphere. Best mathematical approximation of the actual corneal surface called best-fit sphere is calculated. Posterior corneal surface topographic changes after LASIK are known. Increased negative keratometric diopters and oblate asphericity of the PCC are common after LASIK leading to mild keratectasia.[5,6] Lamellar refractive surgery reduces the biomechanical strength of cornea that may lead to mechanical instability and keratectasia. Iatrogenic keratectasia represents a complication after LASIK that may limit the range of myopic correction.[7] Corneal ectasia has also been reported after LASIK in cases of forme fruste keratoconus.[8] Posterior corneal bulge may be correlated with residual corneal bed thickness. The risk of keratectasia may be increased if the residual corneal bed is thinner than 250μm.[9] Age, attempted correction and the optical zone diameter are other parameters that have to be considered to avoid post-LASIK ectasia.[10,11]

CONCLUSION

The ORBSCAN provides reliable, reproducible data of the anterior corneal surface; posterior corneal surface, keratometry, and pachymetry values with three-dimensional presentations and all LASIK candidates must be evaluated by this method preoperatively to detect an " early keratoconus". We suggest that Orbscan II is an important preoperative investigative tool to decide the suitable candidate for LASIK and thus avoiding any complication of LASIK surgery and helping the patient out by contact lens or keratoplasty. The following parameters must be analyzed in all LASIK candidates to rule out keratoconus: (a) ratio of radii of anterior to posterior curvature of cornea: > 1.21 and < 1.27, (b) posterior best fit sphere: > –52.0 Dsph, (c) difference between thickest corneal pachymetry value at 7mm zone and thinnest pachymetry value: > 100 μm, and (d) posterior corneal elevation > 50 μm.

REFERENCES

1. Seiler T, Quurke AW. Iatrogenic keratectasia after LASIK in a case of forme fruste keratoconus. J Cataract Refract Surg 1998;24:1007-9.
2. Fedor P, Kaufman S Corneal topography and imaging. eMedicine Journal, 2001;vol 2, no 6.
3. McDermott G K Topography's benefits for LASIK. Review of Ophthalmology. Editorial, vol no: 9:03 issue.
4. Wang Z, Chen J, Yang B. Posterior corneal surface topographic changes after laser in situ keratomileusis are related to residual corneal bed thickness. Ophthalmology 1999; 106: 406-9; discussion 409-10.
5. Seitz B, Torres F, Langenbucher A, et al. Posterior corneal curvature changes after myopic laser in situ keratomileusis. Ophthalmology 2001 April; 108 (4): 666-72.
6. Geggel H S, Talley A R. Delayed onset keratectasia following laser in situ keratomileusis. J Cataract Refract Surg 1999 Apr; 25(4): 582-6.
7. Seiler T, Koufala K, Richter G. Iatrogenic keratectasia after laser in situ keratomileusis. J Refract Surg 1998 May-June; 14(3): 312-7.
8. Seiler T, Quurke A W. Iatrogenic keratectasia after laser in situ keratomileusis in a case of Forme Fruste keratoconus. J Refract Surg 1998 Jul;24(7): 1007-9.
9. Wang Z, Chen J, Yang B. Posterior corneal surface topographic changes after laser in situ keratomileusis are related to residual corneal bed thickness. Ophthalmology 1999 Feb; 106(2): 406-9.
10. Pallikaris I G, Kymionis G D. Astyrakakis N I. Corneal ectasia induced by laser in situ keratomileusis. J Cataract Refract Surg 2001 Nov; 27(11): 1796-802.
11. Argento C, Cosentino M J, Tytium A et al. Corneal ectasia after laser in situ keratomileusis. J Cataract Refract Surg 2001 Sep; 27(9): 1440-810.

Corneal Topographers and Wavefront Aberrometrers: Complementary Tools

Tracy Schroeder Swartz
Ming Wang
Arun C Gulani

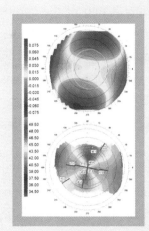

INTRODUCTION

The accessibility of the cornea and the non-intraocular designation of its anatomical status makes it the focus of refractive surgery. The cornea has therewith enjoyed this privilege for decades of refractive surgery. These very advantages also have us refractive surgeons constantly vying to make this delicately transparent yet inherently elastic tissue more predictable.

Thus began our search for that perfect tool which could study and analyze the cornea and also determine our consistency for cornea-based refractive surgery. Corneal topographers have been the gold standard for understanding corneal shape which is the basis of laser refractive surgery. Recently with the advent of aberrometers, the bar has been raised. We have a new technology as well as a new language to address the cornea with and thereby translate the same into effective and accurate surgical outcomes.

This bridge from topography to wavefront technology is actually an adjunct and not about the past or future. These are complimentary technologies as of now and this chapter therewith addresses the application of the two.

With the advent of complex topographic systems and wavefront aberrometers, opthalmologists now benefit from a deeper understanding of the optics of the cornea and their effect on vision.

KERATOMETERS

The first instrument to measure the surface of the cornea was the ophthalmometer. This device measured the curvature of the cornea using reflected rings. It is important to remember the following assumptions related to keratometry:[1]

- The formula used is based on spherical geometry. The cornea, however, is not spherical but is a prolate (flattened) ellipsoid. Thus, the central radius is slightly steeper than actually measured.

- Keratometry is based on four data points within the central 3 mm of the cornea. It provides no insight into the area inside or outside of the 3 mm ring

- Keratometry theory assumes paraxial optics. While the approximation may be clinically acceptable for fitting contacts or estimating corneal astigmatism, it may not be when measuring peripheral curvature

- Keratometers assume alignment of the corneal apex, line of sight and instrument axis. However, this rarely occurs during actual measurement

- The formula used to calculate the radius (r) approximates the distance to the convex focal point, which in the case of the Reichert keratometer, may introduce up to 0.12 D of error. This error may increase, if the instrument is not correctly focused or the operator accommodates during measurement

- Since the indexes may differ between manufacturers, one must be careful comparing the readings in diopters between different instruments.

CORNEAL TOPOGRAPHY

Such assumptions result in significant errors when considering the peripheral cornea, especially in eyes with irregular surfaces such as in keratoconus or S/P keratorefractive surgery. With the growth of computers, came the corneal topography systems widely used today to evaluate the shape characteristics of the cornea.

Early videokeratoscopes used axial power maps to illustrate the information from captured raw data. The power at each point was calculated according to the Javal ophthalmometer convention, and suffered many of keratometry's assumptions.

The axial map is a traditional but poor descriptor of corneal refraction because it does not take into account spherical aberration.[2,3] Despite its limits, the axial map became known as "the corneal topography map". With the development of arc-step algorithms, placido systems could not only approximate axial power, but also measure corneal shape. Elevation maps became available. An example of an axial and elevation map of an eye with with-the-rule astigmatism is shown in Figure 9.1.

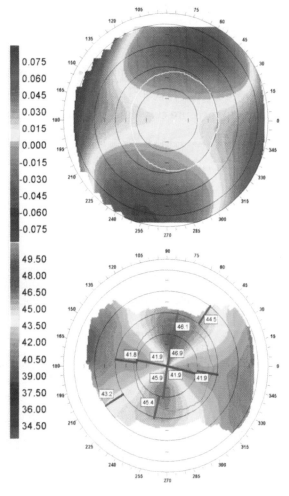

FIGURE 9.1: An axial (bottom) and elevation (top) map of an eye showing with-the-rule astigmatism

133

In the early to the mid-1990s, the explosion of excimer laser refractive surgery necessitated more accurate optical instruments to create more detailed representation of the corneal surface. At this point, the path divided as two parallel paths emerged. Some believed the answers to problems encountered in refractive surgery could be answered using elevation-based topography, while others supported wavefront aberrometry-based platforms.

ELEVATION-BASED TOPOGRAPHY

Placido disk imaging systems are limited to evaluation of the anterior cornea only, and calculate rather than directly measure elevation data. Systems emerged which directly measured corneal elevation, and evaluated anatomy posterior to the anterior cornea. The PAR Corneal topography system (PAR CTS) was the first system to directly measure anterior elevation topography, using principles of triangulation. The distortion of a grid projected on to the cornea was mathematically compared to the true grid in a reference plane. Because the geometry of the reference surface and the grid projection is known, rays can be intersected in three-dimensional space to compute the X, Y and Z coordinates of the surface. [4] This system was generally accepted to be more accurate, when measuring complex bicurve and multicurve test surfaces, but poor reproducibility was reported.

Slit-scanning technology addressed both the need for direct measurement of elevation as well as evaluation of the posterior structures within the eye. The ORBSCAN II (Bausch & Lomb, Roschester, New York) combined a placido disk to measure curvature and slit scanning to measure both surfaces of

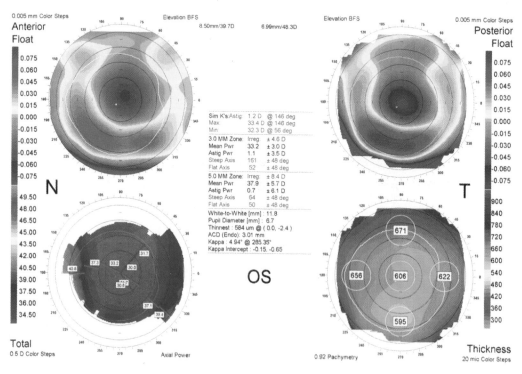

FIGURE 9.2: An example of a Quad map in a patient S/P myopic LASIK

the cornea. The most commonly used display for this system is the Quad map, shown in Figure 9.2. A placido image is captured to evaluate curvature data. Then, over 1.5 seconds, two scanning slit lamps project a total of 40 images each at 45 degrees of the video axis. A proprietary tracking system reduced eye movements. It produced pachymetry and anterior chamber depth information for the first time. This system remains the only type capable of evaluation of the posterior surface. Thus, there is no way to validate the information found in the posterior map.

Another technology was developed to address two problems associated with currently used topographic technology: assumptions inherent to power calculation and paracentral measurement of the cornea. The Pentacam (Oculus) addressed these deficiencies. It is a rotating Scheimpflug camera which provides a complete picture from the anterior surface of the cornea to the posterior surface of the lens, as shown in Figure 9.3.

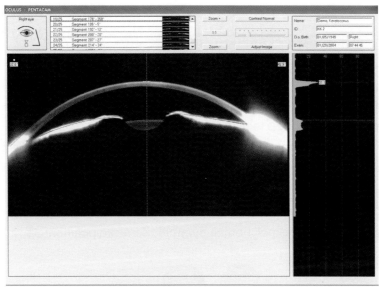

FIGURE 9.3: Scheimpflug image

As topographic systems advanced, understanding of the optics resulting from changes in shape induced by disease or refractive surgery, and the need to correct optical problems grew. Unfortunately, significantly irregular corneas, dry eyes, and scarring may cause topographic systems to fail.

Programs such as the Custom Corneal Ablation Planner (Custom CAP) utilized elevation data and computer analysis to create custom ablation profiles in an attempt to correct decentered ablations and relieve patients of visual distortion. An example is shown in Figure 9.4. Topography-driven programs fail to address the refractive error, however, and refractive changes induced by such treatments were somewhat unpredictable.

WAVEFRONT: ANOTHER VIEW OF CORNEAL OPTICS

Just as topographic analysis was facilitated by computers, so was measurement of optical aberrations. This advance in technology occurred slightly later and parallel to the growth of topography. The most

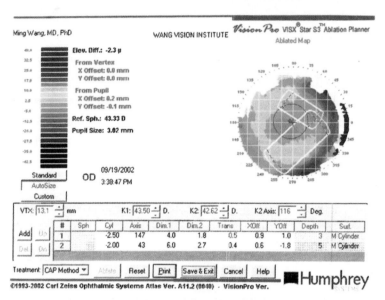

FIGURE 9.4: Custom CAP case

common types of aberrometers are the Hartmann-Shack and the ray tracing models. Hartmann-Shack models utilize several hundred lenslets to measure the wavefront. Ray tracing models utilize individual rays of light to measure the wavefront. Both models measure aberrations as a deviation from the plane wave in microns, and measurements are limited by pupil size. This is problematic in eyes with smaller pupils.

The shape of the wavefront is then mathematically described, most commonly using Zernicke polynomials.[5] Figure 9.5 shows this polynomial pyramid. Zernicke polynomials, are a combination of

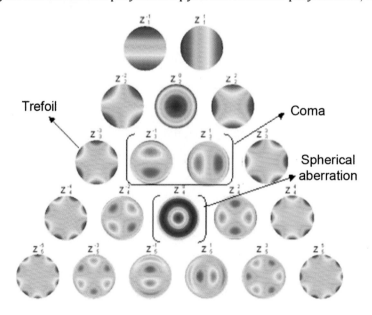

FIGURE 9.5: Zernicke polynomial pyramid

radial trigometric functions which describe the wavefront mathematically. While second order terms of defocus and astigmatism are addressed by the manifest refraction, the irregular astigmatism primarily attributed to the cornea can be described by higher order terms such as coma, spherical aberration, and trefoil.

Just as topographers exhibit difficulty capturing irregular corneal surfaces, aberrometers falter on irregular wavefronts (typically due to irregular astigmatism). This is especially true for diseased eyes and those S/P keratorefractive procedures. Smolek and Klyce studied Zernicke fitting methods for corneal elevation and reported 4th order Zernicke polynomials may not be adequate in their description of corneal aberrations in significantly aberrant eyes.[6]

Because topography failed to address lower order aberrations, and aberrometry failed to address focal topography irregularities, advanced methods were needed. Several case examples later in this chapter demonstrate, how using several systems to gain information about the topography and aberrometry combined in beneficial in determination of the etiology of the visual complaint. It is also beneficial in creating a management plan for surgery.

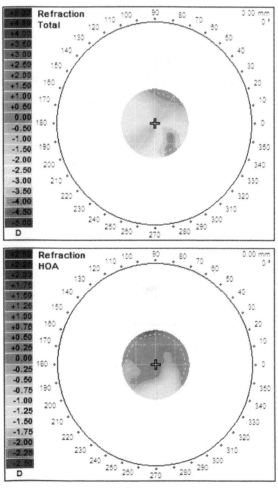

FIGURE 9.6A

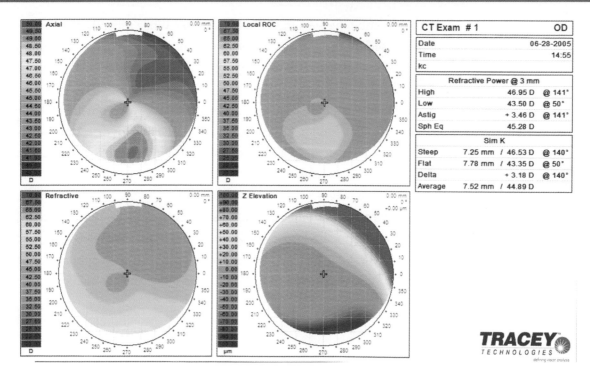

FIGURE 9.6B

FIGURES 9.6A and B: The aberrations found in a keratoconic patient with a 4 mm pupil (A) and the topography (B) of the same eye

As the limitations of wavefront became apparent, interest turned to corneal wavefront measurements— the ability to measure the amount of aberration attributable to the cornea alone. Systems which subtracted the corneal wavefront from the total ocular wavefront emerged. The EyeSys system is capable of using wavefront aberrometry and corneal topography to develop a corneal wavefront map. Figure 9.6 illustrates the aberrations found in a keratoconic patient with a 4 mm pupil (A) as well as the topography (B). Figure 9.7 illustrates the corneal and internal aberrations of the same eye.

It has been suggested that surgeons consider the rule of three when considering corneal surgery: for every 3 microns of distortion from the ideal shape of the corneal, about a +1 micron difference in the OPD map and –1 micron difference in the wavefront error map. It should be noted, however, that the precision of both excimer lasers and wavefront aberrometers far surpasses that of human healing.

CASES

As previously suggested, rather than look at the technologies as separate, it is advantageous to consider them in conjunction with each other. Using both topography and wavefront measurements to determine the etiology of a visual complaint, can be advantageous in the clinical setting. This is illustrated by the following case discussions:

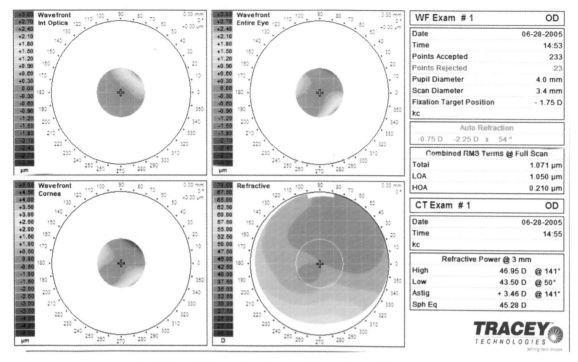

FIGURE 9.7: Corneal and internal aberrations of the same eye

Case I: Double Vision Complaints S/P LASIK

Patient WR presented complaining of "terrible night vision OS after LASIK. Preoperatively, he was significantly nearsighted, and correctable to 20/20. Postoperatively, he refracted to $-2.75+1.75 \times 160$, with a BVA of 20/30. An RGP improved his vision to 20/20 with a significant reduction in monocular diplopia. His preoperative wavescan map is shown in Figure 9.8A, with the preoperative topography in the upper right corner of the difference map shown in Figure 9.8B. Elevation mapping revealed a decentered ablation. Significant coma is evident in the aberrometry map, as expected with decentered ablations. We performed a Custom CAP treatment, which treats the decentered ablation directly without taking the refractive error into account, and the visual distortion improved significantly, indicated by the drop in the RMS value shown in Figure 9.9.

CASE II: Night Vision Complaints S/P LASIK

Patient WR presented with complaints of "terrible night vision, starbursts and halos" after LASIK in 2000. Preoperatively, she was -2.50 DS. Postoperatively, she refracted to $-1.00+0.25 \times 160$, with a BVA of 20/30 OD, her dominant eye. Figure 9.10A shows her topography, revealing central irregularities. Wavescan, found in Figure 9.10B, revealed coma and trefoil. We suspected the central irregularities were exaggerated by her dry eye, and treated her aggressively with punctual occlusion, Restasis BID, and Liqugel nightly. Her symptoms improved slightly, and she is waiting for more advanced custom treatment.

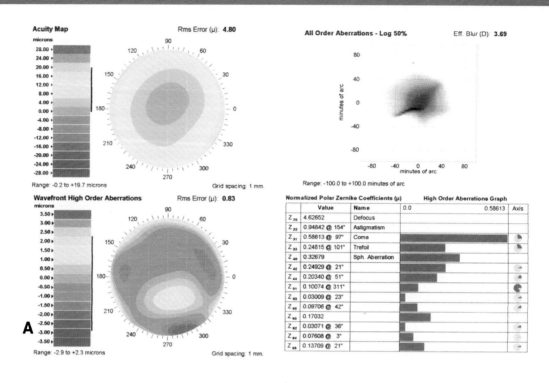

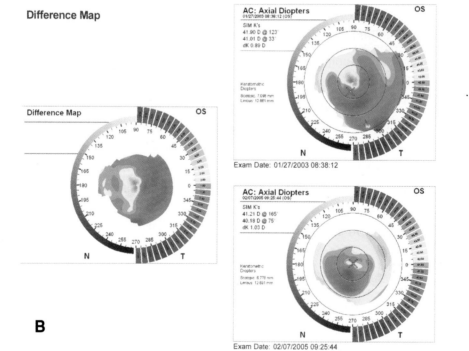

FIGURES 9.8A and B: Preoperative wavescan map (A), and topography difference map (B) showing the change in topography following a Custom CAP treatment

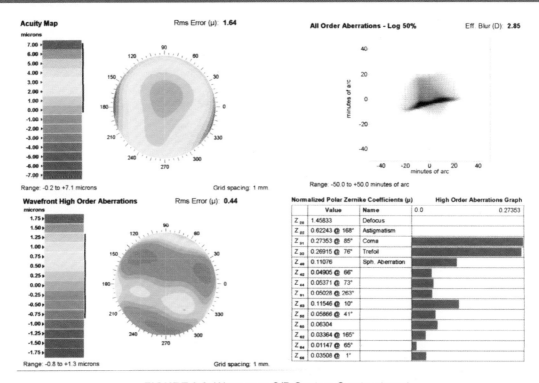

FIGURE 9.9: Wavescan S/P Custom Cap treatment

CASE III: Complaint of Multiple Images after Hyperopic LASIK

Patient TD presented complaining of light sensitivity, ghosting, halos and starbursts at night. Preoperatively she was +4.50D OU. Postoperatively she refracted to PL, 20/25+ OD, +0.25+0.50 × 150, 20/25+ OS. Despite her unaided 20/20- Snellen acuity, she complained bitterly about her quality of vision. Topography found a smaller optical zone OS with greater steepening in the dominant left eye, as shown on the axial map in Figure 9.11A. Wavescan found significant spherical aberration (Figure 9.11B). Note the spherical aberration is negative due to the hyperopic treatment. We have prescribed Alphagan P in an attempt to decrease the pupil size and minimize the night vision issues, and fit the patient with gas perm lenses.

Case IV: Double Vision with Loss of Best Correction S/P LASIK

Patient RD presented for evaluation of double vision S/P LASIK, even with glasses. Preoperatively, he was –4.75+0.75 × 105, with a BVA of 20/20. After his original surgery, he underwent two enhancements and AK in the affected eye, leaving him -2.00 with a best corrected acuity of . He was fit with an RGP, which he reported did not resolve the diplopia, so he rarely wore the lens. Clinical notes from the fitting doctor report BCCLVA of 20/25. The topography was surprisingly regular in the pupillary zone despite the repeated corneal surgery. Wavefront analysis found significant COMA and trefoil, and can be seen in Figure 9.12. We attribute this to early lenticular changes, and elected to monitor rather than proceed with corrective ablation.

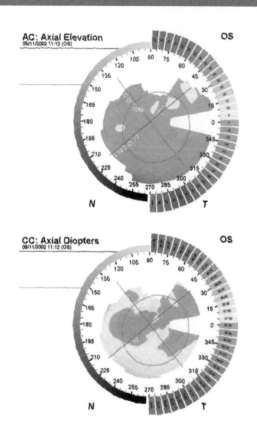

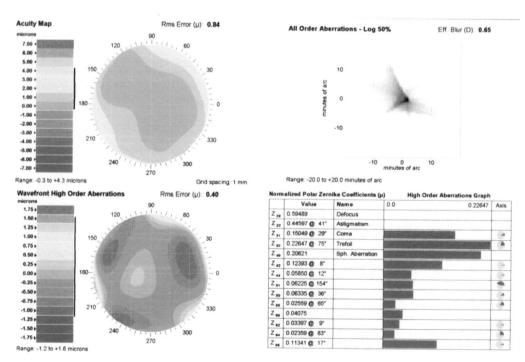

Acuity Map　　　　Rms Error (μ): **0.84**

All Order Aberrations - Log 50%　　Eff. Blur (D): **0.65**

Range: -0.3 to +4.3 microns　　　Grid spacing: 1 mm.

Range: -20.0 to +20.0 minutes of arc

Wavefront High Order Aberrations　　Rms Error (μ): **0.40**

Range: -1.2 to +1.6 microns

Normalized Polar Zernike Coefficients (μ)			High Order Aberrations Graph		
	Value	Name	0.0	0.22647	Axis
Z_{20}	0.59489	Defocus			
Z_{22}	0.44597 @ 41°	Astigmatism			
Z_{31}	0.15049 @ 29°	Coma			
Z_{33}	0.22647 @ 75°	Trefoil			
Z_{40}	0.20621	Sph. Aberration			
Z_{42}	0.12393 @ 8°				
Z_{44}	0.05850 @ 12°				
Z_{51}	0.06225 @ 154°				
Z_{53}	0.06335 @ 36°				
Z_{55}	0.02559 @ 65°				
Z_{60}	0.04075				
Z_{62}	0.03397 @ 9°				
Z_{64}	0.02359 @ 83°				
Z_{66}	0.11341 @ 17°				

FIGURES 9.10A and B: Central irregularities were revealed with topography, (A) while Aberrometry found coma and trefoil. Dry eye treatment only partially resolved this patient's complaints (B)

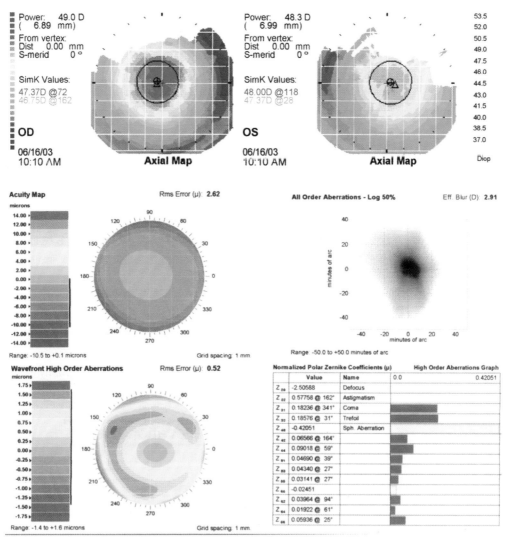

FIGURE 9.11: This patient complained of glare and night vision disturbances secondary to the higher order aberrations caused by the small area of central steepening OS

Case V: Hyperopic Keratorefractive Surgery Results in Steep Cornea

A 19-year-old female presented for LASIK evaluation. Manifest refraction was +1.75+05.0 × 25 OD (20/40) and +0.75 OS (20/25). Cycloplegic found latent hyperopia: +4.25 OD (20/50) and +1.50 (20/40) OS. Her preoperative topography was normal, and is shown in Figure 9.13A. After considerable discussion, she elected to undergo LASIK in both eyes. The latent hyperopia OD was partially addressed, and the goal was a correction of +2.75 OD, +1.00 OS. She underwent bilateral femtosecond laser assisted keratomileusis using a VISX Star 4 laser.

S/P LASIK, the patient complained of blurred vison OD, and the UCVA dropped to 20/50. Manifest refraction found +1.50+1.25 × 180 while the cycloplegic again revealed the latent hyperopia: +3.00+1.25 × 180, yielding a VA of 20/30. Her visual complaint was relieved with simple hyperopic correction, and the patient underwent an enhancement by relift of +1.50+1.25 × 180.

143

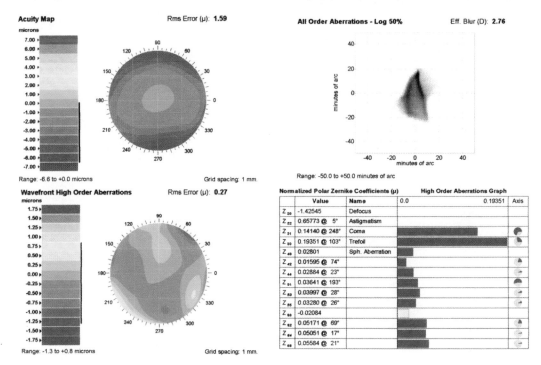

FIGURE 9.12: Aberrometry revealed the cause of the patient's complaint when topography found a relatively normal shape: early cataracts

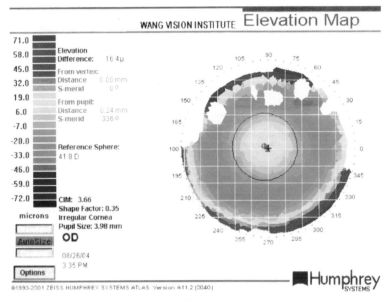

FIGURE 9.13A

At one month, she presented complaining of decreased vision OD, multiple images, and "an unbalanced feeling". Manifest refraction found –1.50+0.75 × 75, and corrected her to only 20/50. Her elevation maps reveal marked central steepening OD as seen on the elevation map in Figure 9.13A. Her wavefront aberrometry measurements revealed coma OD, shown in Figure 9.13B and C.

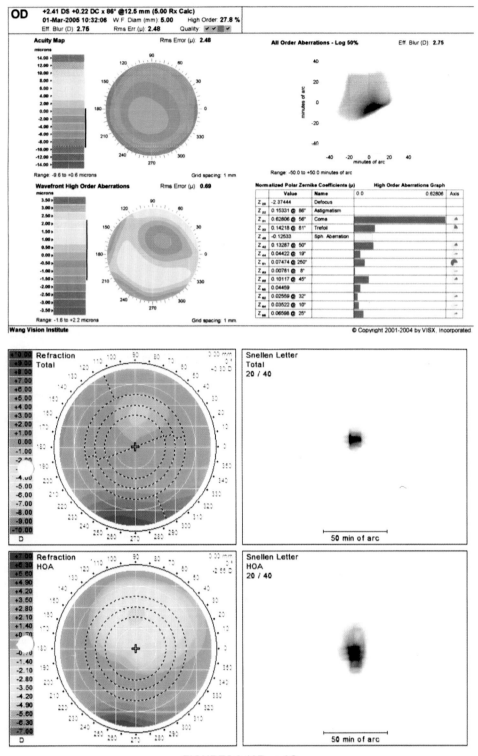

FIGURES 9.13B and C

FIGURES 9.13A to C: Elevation maps reveal marked central steepening OD S/P hyperopic LASIK with hyperopic enhancement, as seen on the elevation map in 9.13A. Her Wavescan map (B) and Itrace map (C) revealed coma, and reported hyperopic refractions despite a manifest of −1.50 DS

Interestingly, the Wavescan and I-Trace both found hyperopic refractions. The coma suggested a decentered apex, and topography revealed a significant steepening just above the geographical center. Neither correction of the manifest refraction with a soft lens nor Alphagan-P to change the pupil size corrected the patient's complaint. While a gas perm lens did restore functional vision, the patient is not able to tolerate the lens. It appears that the patient only uses the tip of the cornea for vision, resulting in the preferred myopia refraction. As time progressed and the naturally smoothing of the cornea occurrs, her symptoms are lessening, and we may perform a custom treatment in the future.

CONCLUSION

While topographers and aberrometers may work well in virgin eyes, for surgeons striving for technology to address irregular astigmatism, current systems fall short. Improved understanding of the relationship between aberrometry, topography and corneal optics must be gained with continued advancement of the current technology.

Several generalizations can be made regarding the relationship between topography and wavefront aberrometry. The loss of the prolate cornea results in an increase in spherical aberration. Irregular astigmatism may be associated with an increase in coma and trefoil. Decentered ablations have been linked to increased coma. The irregular surface associated with dry eyes has been found to be improved with punctual occlusion and accompanied by a secondary reduction in HO aberrations.[7]

For patients with visual complaints S/P keratorefractive surgery, it is advantageous to obtain information from various sources about the etiology of the visual complaint. Using wavefront aberrometry and corneal topography to investigate the source of the patient's problem, and better understand the visual system as a whole, will better enable us to manage our patient's. Systems such as the Advanced Corneal Ablation Pattern (VISX), which combine topographic and wavefront information to create computerized simulations for surgery, may enable correction of irregular surfaces as well as refractive errors.

REFERENCES

1. Horner DG, Salmon TO, Soni PS. Chapter 17, Corneal Topography. In Benjamin WJ Editor: Borish's Clinical Refraction, Philadelphia: WB Saunders Company, 1998.
2. Klein SA. A corneal topography algorithm that produces continuous curvature. Optom Vis Sci 1992; 69: 829-834.
3. Roberts C. The Accuracy of "Power" maps to display curvature data in corneal topography systems. Invest Ophtalmol Vis Sci 1994; 35: 3524-3532.
4. Belin MW, Cambier JL, Nabors JR, Ratliff CD. PAR Corneal Topography System (PAR CTS): the clinical application of close-range photogrammetry. Optom Vis Sci 1995; 72:828-37.
5. Campbell C. A New Method for Describing the Aberrations of the Eye Using Zernike Polynomials, Optometry and Vision Science 80(1): 79-83; Jan 2003.
6. Smolek MK, Kyce SD. Zernicke Polynomial Fitting Fials to Represent All Visuall Signficant Corneal Aberrations. Invest Ophthalmol Vis Sci. 2003; 44: 4676-81.
7. Pepose J, Huang B, Mirza A, Qazi M. Effect of Punctal Occlusion on Wavefront Aberrations in Dry Eyes after LASIK. Invest Ophthalmol Vis Sci 2003 44: E-Abstract 2628.

Section

II

LASIK, LASEK and PRK

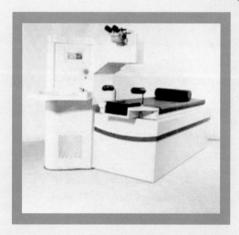

10

The Excimer Laser Beam Profile Topography and Classification

Arun C Gulani

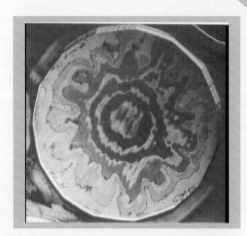

INTRODUCTION

"The Excimer laser is an extension of our own precision at sub-micron tolerance." It is important for us to "*see*" and "*watch*" this invisible laser on a routine and regular basis in achieving the goal of predictable refractive surgery.

EXCIMER LASER ENERGY BEAM PROFILE

The Excimer laser energy beam profile indicates the overall distribution of energy density.[1] This beam profile needs to be homogenous so as to result in a reproducible clinical profile and thus consistent refractive predictability. The refractive outcomes of these highly sensitive lasers are dependent on their accuracy which is believed to be inherent in LASIK (Laser assisted *in situ* keratomileusis). The excimer laser output is basically non-homogenous at the source and a precise combinations of lenses, prisms and mirrors are used to achieve the homogenous beam profile[2-5] output which is directly responsible for homogenous refractive corneal sculpting. The sensitive requirements of these laser systems could result in a dramatic alteration in beam quality and quantity.[6-7] Also there is laser to laser variance.[8-9] Understanding these principles and controllable intricacies of this sub-micron precision cutting tool (The Excimer Laser) will help lay the groundwork for LASIK and decrease the need for repeat surgical enhancements[10-11] in achieving the goal of emmetropia (Gulani AC, Krueger R. LASIK Complication Management: Principles and Techniques LASIK Video GrandRounds Course 433 American Academy of Ophthalmology Conference, California– Nov 2003).

EXCIMER BEAM PROFILE TESTING

We need to produce a homogenous beam profile with repeatable consistency in our quest for safe and predictable refractive surgery. Excimer beam profile testing for prevalent lasers can be classified into direct and indirect techniques. The direct technique analyzes the beam directly and reveals a 3-dimensional top-hat pattern representing the beam profile and homogeneity. The indirect technique uses ablatable testing material with the laser in order to then analyze the obtained pattern and record the beam profile on that particular ablatable testing plate. Examples of indirect testing material include the Chiron plates, PMMA plates, Aluminum foil, ExACT Beam profile film, Wratten gelatin, etc. I have used the CIBA ExACT beam profile tester comprising of a thin micron layer of foil covering a multilayered polymer adherent to a test plastic. The endpoint is a uniformly yellow ablation pattern . What this means is that the laser ablation is begun on this plate and breakthrough (first break in surface layer) achieved at a certain number of pulses, i.e. 50 pulses. The ablation is further continued from this point on till we get a full homogenous coloration in the ablation zone at a certain number of pulses, i.e. 12 pulses. Thus for a total of 62 pulses for a precalibrated laser, we get a homogenous ablation profile denoted by the full yellow discoloration on this testing plate.

EXCIMER BEAM PROFILE TOPOGRAPHY

150

I have been using a different and much more visually informative technique of analyzing excimer beam

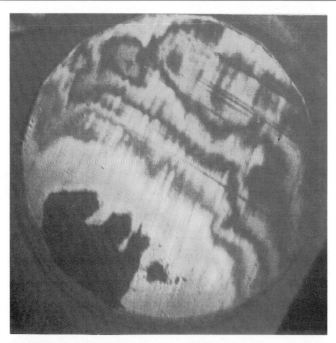

FIGURE 10.1: Excimer beam profile topography on ExACT film showing the impact waves around the breakthrough ablation area (seen as a dark spot). This is a hot spot in a non-homogenous beam

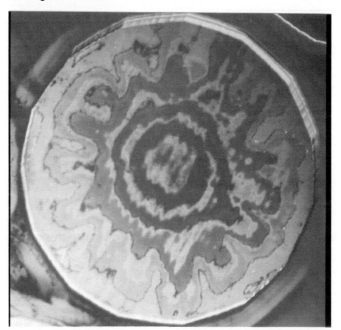

FIGURE 10.2: Excimer beam profile topography on ExACT film showing the impact waves around the breakthrough ablation area (seen in the center). This is a well-centered homogenous beam

homogeneity and profile using the ExACT film. In my technique, I stop at first breakthrough and do not proceed to full ablation testing. This plate is then tilted at an angle and a fiberoptic light incident to it reveals a wave pattern around the area of breakthrough on this plate. These wave patterns represent the profile around the impact zone of the beam and reveal beam profile in its own content, i.e. heterogenous (Figure 10.1) or homogenous (Figure 10.2) as well as beam displacement, i.e. decentration.

I have termed this appearance as Excimer Beam Profile Topography[12] since it represents the negative imprint of the final corneal topography post-LASIK and is a direct correlate of the laser ablation pattern on the patient's cornea. Further, I have classified the excimer laser beam profiles (Figure 10.3) in order to simplify and standardize laser beam profile reporting and discussion (Gulani AC. *See and Watch the Invisible Excimer Laser in Refractive Sugery*. ECLSO meeting. Geneva, Switzerland, Sept.1999).

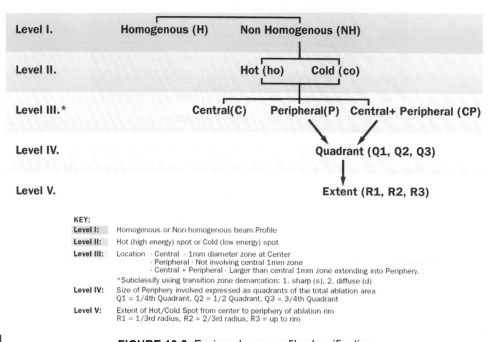

FIGURE 10.3: Excimer beam profile classification

This nomenclature will help exchange of information in a more systematic manner. Presently we report laser beam abnormality in a descriptive way only. Once we use this classification (Excimer Beam Profile Classification) we could record the beam profiles accurately, send accurate beam descriptions by telephone/Fax/e-mail to service personel accross the world as well as among peers on the same standardized language of information exchange.

For example, using the classification system, **NHhoPQ1R1** would imply a nonhomogenous (NH) beam profile with a hot spot (ho) in the periphery (P) involving upto 1/4th Quadrant (Q1) at a distance of 1/3rd the radius of the ablated area. As indicated above the terminology NHhoPQ1R1 is more precise a terminology rather than descriptive explanations of such beam abnormalities. Not only will we be clear as we discuss beam abnormalities but also we or the service personel could get an idea by denoting specifications therein, i.e. if the area between the normal and abnormal ablation pattern is sharp then the cause most likely is the optical system alignment, while if this zone is diffuse, then the causative factor is a contaminant debris. We need to be much more involved with this technology revolution and play our role of serious gatekeepers towards emerging advances as also everyday surgical outcomes.

SUMMARY

The Excimer laser is indeed a remarkable milestone in refractive surgery. It is the most important tool in laser refractive surgery where corneal sculpting is the basis of refractive change. As we forge ahead with advanced in intraocular refractive techniques we need to be more accurate in our understanding and outcomes of what I believe will finally become Laser enhanced fine tuning in refractive surgery. We must gain control and learn to check with dedicated accuracy the workings and management of the same and also to increase our ability to converse with each other using a standardized laser language as we progress symbiotically towards the perfection of laser refractive surgery.

REFERENCES

1. Trokel SL, Srinivasan R, Braren B. Excimer laser surgey of the cornea. Am J of Ophthalmol 1983; 96: 710-5.
2. Machat JJ. Fundamental concepts and principles of the Excimer laser and LASIK. In Machat J (Ed): The Art of LASIK. Slack Inc, 1998; 3: 41-3.
3. Gulani AC, Alio Jorge, Vukich John, Krueger R. Advanced Topography and Wavefront Lasik: Applied and Simplified. Instructive Course. European Society of Cataract and Refractive Surgery-Paris (France), Sept 2004.
4. Gulani AC, Probst L. Cons of presbyopic lasik. In LASIK: Advances, Controversies and Custom. Slack Inc 2004; 32B:367-9.
5. Gulani AC. Hyperopic lasik surgery. In Textbook of Ophthalmology. E-medicine Inc.
6. Neumann AC, Gulani AC. Lamellar surgery: Counterpoint and complications. In Elander R (Eds): Textbook of Refractive Surgery. WB Saunders, 1997;24:291-7.
7. Gimble HV. Early postoperative complications: 24 to 48 hours. In Gimble HV (Ed): LASIK Complications: Prevention and Management. Slack Inc, 1998; 6: 100.
8. Gulani AC, Probst L, Cox I, Veith R. Wavefront in Lasik: The Zyoptix. Platform. Ophthalmol Clin N Am 2004;17: 173-81.
9. Casebeer JC. A systematized approach to LASIK. In Burrato L (Ed): LASIK: Principles and Techniques. Slack Inc, 1998; 18: 228.
10. Gulani AC. New instrument for revision lamellar refractive surgery. J cataract Refract Surg 1998; 24: 595.
11. Gulani AC. Lasik corneal complications: A new stratified classification. Ophthalmology 1999; 106:1457-58.
12. Gulani AC et al. Innovative real-time ilumination system for LASIK surgery: Clinical and surgical ophthalmology. Journal of Canadian Society of Cataract and Refractive Surgery 2003;1/21(6): 244-46.

Chapter

11

Posterior Corneal Changes in Refractive Surgery

Amar Agarwal
Soosan Jacob
Sunita Agarwal
Athiya Agarwal
Nilesh Kanjani

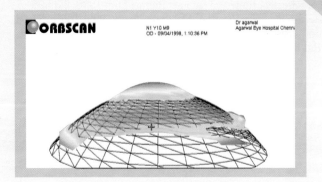

INTRODUCTION

The development of corneal ectasia is a well-recognized complication of LASIK and amongst other contributory factors, unrecognized preoperative forme fruste keratoconus is also an important one. Patients with this disorder are poor candidates for refractive surgery because of the possibility of exacerbating keratectasia. It is known that posterior corneal elevation is an early presenting sign in keratoconus and hence it is imperative to evaluate posterior corneal curvature (PCC) in *every* LASIK candidate.

TOPOGRAPHY

Topography is valuable for preoperative ophthalmic examination of LASIK candidates. Three-dimensional imaging allows surgeons to look at corneal thickness, as well as the corneal anterior and posterior surface and it can also predict the shape of the cornea after LASIK surgery. Topographic analysis using three dimensional slit scan system allows us to predict which candidates would do well with LASIK and also confers the ability to screen for subtle configurations which may be a contraindication to LASIK.

ORBSCAN

The ORBSCAN (Baush & Lamb) corneal topography system uses a scanning optical slit scan which makes it fundamentally different from the corneal topography that analyzes the reflected images from the anterior corneal surface. The high-resolution video camera captures 40 light slits at 45 degrees angle projected through the cornea similarly as seen during slit lamp examination. The slits are projected on to the anterior segment of the eye: the anterior cornea, the posterior cornea, the anterior iris and anterior lens. The data collected from these four surfaces are used to create a topographic map. Each surface point from the diffusely reflected slit beams that overlap in the central 5 mm zone is independently triangulated to x, y, and z coordinates, providing three-dimensional data.

This technique provides more information about the anterior segment of the eye, such as anterior and posterior corneal curvature, elevation maps of the anterior and posterior corneal surface and corneal thickness. It has an acquisition time of 4 seconds.[1] This improves the diagnostic accuracy. It also has passive eye-tracker from frame to frame and 43 frames are taken to ensure accuracy. It is easy to interpret and has good repeatability.

PRIMARY POSTERIOR CORNEAL ELEVATION

The diagnosis of frank keratoconus is a clinical one. Early diagnosis of forme fruste can be difficult on clinical examination alone. ORBSCAN has become a useful tool for evaluating the disease, and with its advent, abnormalities in posterior corneal surface topography have been identified in keratoconus. Posterior corneal surface data are problematic because they are not a direct measure and there are less published information on normal values for each age group. In the patient with increased posterior corneal elevation in the absence of other changes, it is unknown whether this finding represents a manifestation of early keratoconus. The decision to proceed with refractive surgery is therefore more difficult.

Posterior Corneal Topography

One should always use the ORBSCAN system to evaluate potential LASIK candidates preoperatively to rule out primary posterior corneal elevations. Eyes are screened using quad maps with the normal band (NB) filter turned on. Four maps include: (a) anterior corneal elevation: NB = ± 25 μ of best-fit sphere, (b) posterior corneal elvevation: NB = ± 25 μ of best fit sphere, (c) keratometric mean curvature: NB = 40 to 48 D, and (d) corneal thickness (pachymetry): NB = 500 to 600 μ. Map features within normal band are colored green. This effectively filters out variations falling within the normal band. When abnormalities are seen on normal band quad map screening, a standard scale quad map should be examined. For those cases with posterior corneal elevation, three-dimensional views of posterior corneal elevation can also be generated. In all eyes with posterior corneal elevation, the following parameters are generated: (a) radii of anterior and posterior curvature of the cornea, (b) posterior best fit sphere, and (c) difference between the corneal pachymetry value in 7 mm zone and thinnest pachymetry value of the cornea.

Preexisting Posterior Corneal Abnormalities

Figures 11.1 to 11.6 show the various topographic features of an eye with primary posterior corneal elevation detected during pre-LASIK assessment. In Figure 11.1 (general quad map) upper left corner map is the anterior float, upper right corner map is posterior float, lower left corner is keratometric map while the lower right is the pachymetry map showing a difference of 100 μm between the thickest pachymetry value in 7 mm zone of cornea and thinnest pachymetry value. In Figure 11.2, normal band scale map of anterior surface shows "with the rule astigmatism" in an otherwise normal anterior surface (shown in green), the posterior float shows significant elevation inferotemporally. In Figure 11.2 only the abnormal areas are shown in red for ease in detection. Figure 11.3 is three-dimensional representation of the maps in Figure 11.2. Figure 11.4 shows three-dimensional representation of anterior corneal surface with reference sphere. Figure 11.5 shows three-dimensional representation of posterior corneal surface showing a significant posterior corneal elevation. Figure 11.6 shows amount of elevation (color coded) of the posterior corneal surface in microns (50 μm).

In the light of the fact that keratoconus may have posterior corneal elevation as the earliest manifestation, preoperative analysis of posterior corneal curvature to detect a posterior corneal bulge is important to avoid post-LASIK keratectasia. The rate of progression of posterior corneal elevation to frank keratoconus is unknown. It is also difficult to specify that exact amount of posterior corneal elevation beyond which it may be unsafe to carry out LASIK. Atypical elevation in the posterior corneal map more than 45 μm should alert us against a post-LASIK surprise. ORBSCAN provides reliable, reproducible data of the posterior corneal surface and all LASIK candidates must be evaluated by this method preoperatively to detect an "early keratoconus."

Elevation is not measured directly by Placido based topographers, but certain assumptions allow the construction of elevation maps. Elevation of a point on the corneal surface displays the height of the point on the corneal surface relative to a spherical reference surface. Reference surface is chosen to be

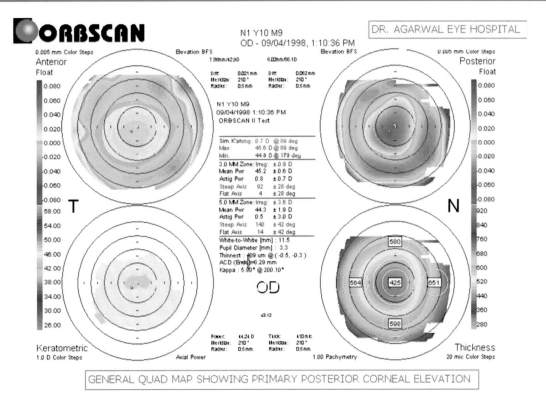

GENERAL QUAD MAP SHOWING PRIMARY POSTERIOR CORNEAL ELEVATION

FIGURE 11.1: Showing general quad map of an eye with primary posterior corneal elevation. Notice the red areas seen in the top right picture showing the primary posterior corneal elevation

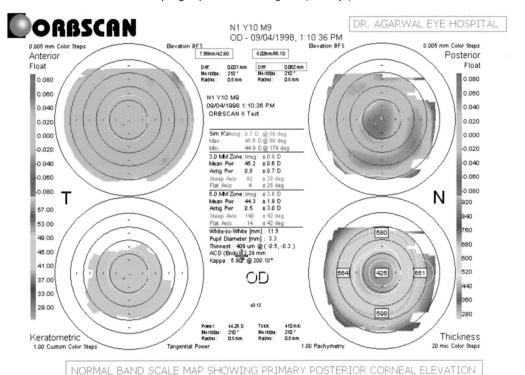

NORMAL BAND SCALE MAP SHOWING PRIMARY POSTERIOR CORNEAL ELEVATION

FIGURE 11.2: Showing quad map with normal band scale filter on in the same eye as in Figure 11.1

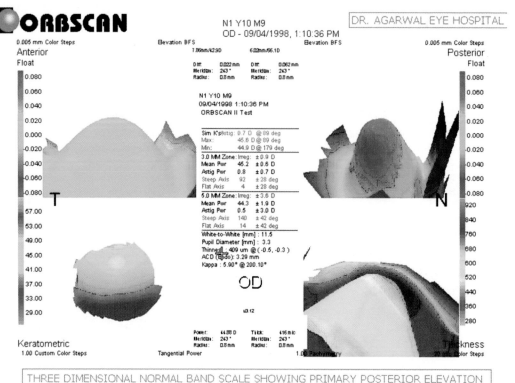

FIGURE 11.3: Showing three-dimensional normal band scale map. In the top right note the red area which shows the elevation on the posterior cornea. The anterior cornea is normal

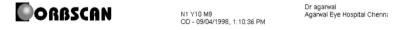

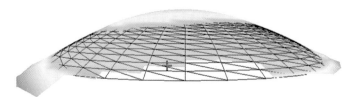

FIGURE 11.4: Showing three-dimensional anterior float. Notice it is normal

a sphere. Best mathematical approximation of the actual corneal surface called best-fit sphere is calculated. One of the criteria for defining forme fruste keratoconus is a posterior best fit sphere of > 55.0 D.

Ratio of radii of anterior to posterior curvature of cornea ≥ 1.21 and ≤ 1.27 has been considered as a keratoconus suspect. Average pachymetry difference between thickest and the thinnest point on the cornea in the 7 mm zone should normally be less than 100 μm.

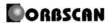

N1 Y10 M9
OD - 09/04/1998, 1:10:36 PM

Dr agarwal
Agarwal Eye Hospital Chenn;

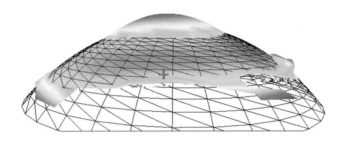

FIGURE 11.5: Showing three-dimensional posterior float. Notice that there is marked elevation as seen in the red areas

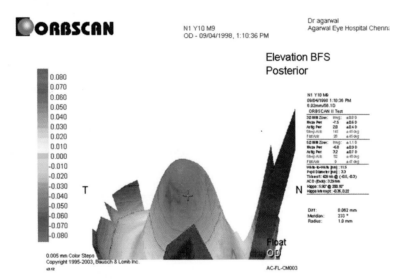

FIGURE 11.6: Showing three-dimensional posterior corneal elevation measured in microns

Agarwal Criteria to Diagnose Primary Posterior Corneal Elevation

1. Ratio of the radii of anterior and posterior curvature of the cornea should be more than 1.2. In Figure 11.2 note the radii of the anterior curvature is 7.86 mm and the radii of the posterior curvature is 6.02 mm. The ratio is 1.3.
2. Posterior best fit sphere should be more than 52 D. In Figure 11.2 note the posterior best fit sphere is 56.1 D.
3. Difference between the thickest and thinnest corneal pachymetry value in the 7 mm zone should be more than 100 microns. The thickest pachymetry value as seen in Figure 11.2 is 651 microns and the thinnest value is 409 microns. The difference is 242 microns.
4. The thinnest point on the cornea should correspond with the highest point of elevation of the posterior corneal surface. The thinnest point as seen in Figure 11.2 bottom right picture is seen as a

159

cross. This point or cursor corresponds to the same cross or cursor in Figure 11.2 top right picture which indicates the highest point of elevation on the posterior cornea.

5. Elevation of the posterior corneal surface should be more than 45 microns above the posterior best fit sphere. In Figure 11.2 you will notice it is 0.062 mm or 62 microns.

IATROGENIC KERATECTASIA

Iatrogenic keratectasia may be seen in some patients following ablative refractive surgery (Figures 11.7 and 11.8). The anterior cornea is composed of alternating collagen fibrils and has a more complicated interwoven structure than the deeper stroma and it acts as the major stress-bearing layer. The flap used for LASIK is made in this layer and thus results in a weakening of that strongest layer of the cornea which contributes maximum to the biomechanical stability of the cornea.

The residual bed thickness (RBT) of the cornea is the crucial factor contributing to the biomechanical stability of the cornea after LASIK. The flap as such does not contribute much after its repositioning to the stromal bed. This is easily seen by the fact that the flap can be easily lifted up even up to 1 year after treatment. The decreased RBT as well as the lamellar cut in the cornea both contribute to the decreased biomechanical stability of the cornea. A reduction in the RBT results in a long-term increase in the surface parallel stress on the cornea. The intraocular pressure (IOP) can cause further forward bowing and thinning of a structurally compromised cornea. Inadvertent excessive eye rubbing, prone position

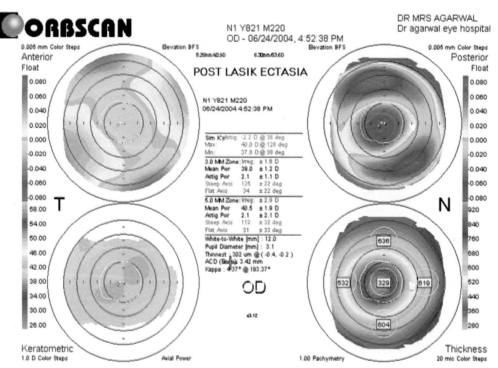

FIGURE 11.7: Shows a patient with iatrogenic keratectasia after lasik. Note the upper right hand corner picture showing the posterior float has thinning and this is also seen in the bottom right picture in which pachymetry reading is 329

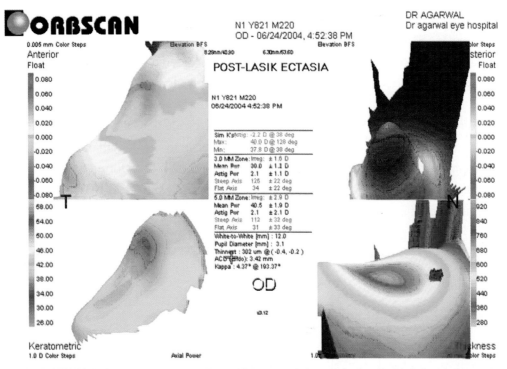

FIGURE 11.8: Shows the same patient with iatrogenic keratectasia after lasik in a 3 D pattern. Notice the ectasia seen clearly in the bottom right picture

sleeping, and the normal wear and tear of the cornea may also play a role. The RBT should not be less than 250 μm to avoid subsequent iatrogenic keratectasias.[2–4] Reoperations should be undertaken very carefully in corneae with RBT less than 300 μm. Increasing myopia after every operation is known as "dandelion keratectasia."

The ablation diameter also plays a very important role in LASIK. Postoperative optical distortions are more common with diameters less than 5.5 mm. Use of larger ablation diameters implies a lesser RBT postoperatively. Considering the formula: Ablation depth (μm) = {(1/3. [diameter (mm)]² × [intended correction diopters (D)]}, [4,5] it becomes clear that to preserve a sufficient bed thickness, the range of myopic correction is limited and the upper limit of possible myopic correction may be around 12 D.[6]

Detection of a mild keratectasia requires knowledge about the posterior curvature of the cornea. Posterior corneal surface topographic changes after LASIK are known. Increased negative keratometric diopters and oblate asphericity of the PCC, which correlate significantly with the intended correction are common after LASIK leading to mild keratectasia.[6,7] This change in posterior power and the risk of keratectasia was more significant with a RBT of 250 μm or less.[8] The difference in the refractive indices results in a 0.2 D difference at the back surface of the cornea becoming equivalent to a 2.0 D change in the front surface of the cornea.[6] Increase in posterior power and asphericity also correlates with the difference between the intended and achieved correction 3 months after LASIK. This is because factors like drying of the stromal bed may result in an ablation depth more than that intended.[6] Reinstein et al predict that the standard deviation of uncertainty in predicting the RBT preoperatively is around 30 μm. [Invest Ophthalmol Vis Sci 40 (Suppl):S403, 1999]. Age, attempted correction, the optical zone diameter and the flap thickness are other parameters that have to be considered to avoid post-LASIK ectasia.[9,10]

The flap thickness may not be uniform throughout its length. In studies by Seitz et al, it has been shown that the Moris model one microkeratome and the Supratome cut deeper towards the hinge, whereas the Automated Corneal Shaper and the Hansatome create flaps that are thinner towards the hinge. Thus, accordingly, the area of corneal ectasia may not be in the center but paracentral, especially if it is also associated with decentered ablation. Flap thickness has also been found to vary considerably, even up to 40 μm, under similar conditions and this may also result in a lesser RBT than intended.[11-17]

It is known that corneal ectasias and keratoconus have posterior corneal elevation as the earliest manifestation.[18] The precise course of progression of posterior corneal elevation to frank keratoconus is not known. Hence it is necessary to study the posterior corneal surface preoperatively in all LASIK candidates.

EFFECT OF POSTERIOR CORNEAL CHANGE ON IOL CALCULATION

The IOL power calculation in post-LASIK eyes is different because of the inaccuracy of keratometry, change in anterior and posterior corneal curvatures, altered relation between the two and change in the standardized index of refraction of the cornea. Irregular astigmatism induced by the procedure, decentered ablations and central islands also add to the problem.

Routine keratometry is not accurate in these patients. Corneal refractive surgery changes the asphericity of the cornea and also produces a wide range of powers in the central 5 mm zone of the cornea. LASIK makes the cornea of a myope more oblate so that keratometry values may be taken from the more peripheral steeper area of the cornea, which results in calculation of a lower than required IOL power resulting in a hyperopic "surprise." Hyperopic LASIK makes the cornea more prolate, thus resulting in a myopic "surprise" post-cataract surgery.

Post-PRK or LASIK, the relation between the anterior and posterior corneal surface changes. The relative thickness of the various corneal layers, each having a different refractive index also changes and there is a change in the curvature of the posterior corneal surface. All these result in the standardized refractive index of 1.3375 no longer being accurate in these eyes.

At present there is no keratometry, which can accurately measure the anterior and posterior curvatures of the cornea. The Orbscan also makes mathematical assumptions of the posterior surface rather than direct measurements. This is important in the LASIK patient because the procedure alters the relation between the anterior and posterior surfaces of the cornea as well as changes the curvature of the posterior cornea.

Thus direct measurements such as manual and automated keratometry and topography are inherently inaccurate in these patients. The corneal power is therefore calculated by the calculation method, the contact lens overrefraction method and by the CVK method. The flattest K reading obtained by any method is taken for IOL power calculation (the steepest K is taken for hyperopes who had undergone

LASIK). One can still aim for 1.00 D of myopia rather than emmetropia to allow for any error, which is almost always in the hyperopic direction in case of pre-LASIK myopes. Also, a third or fourth generation IOL calculating formula should be used for such patients.

REFERENCES

1. Fedor P, Kaufman S. Corneal topography and imaging. Medicine Journal 2001; 2(6).
2. Seiler T, Koufala K, Richter G. Iatrogenic keratectasia after laser in situ keratomileusis. J Refract Surg 1998;14(3):312-7.
3. Seiler T, Quurke A W. Iatrogenic keratectasia after laser in situ keratomileusis in a case of Forme Fruste keratoconus. J Refract Surg 1998;24(7):1007-9.
4. Probost LE, Machat JJ. Mathematics of laser in situ keratomileusis for high myopia. J Cataract refract Surg 1998;24:
5. Mc Donnell PJ. Excimer laser corneal surgery: new strategies and old enemies (review). Invest Ophthalmol Vis Sci 1995;36:4-8.
6. Seitz B, Torres F, Langenbucher A, et al. Posterior corneal curvature changes after myopic laser in situ keratomileusis. Ophthalmology 2001;108 (4): 666-72.
7. Geggel H S, Talley A R. Delayed onset keratectasia following laser in situ keratomileusis. J Cataract Refract Surg 1999;25(4):582-6.
8. Wang Z, Chen J, Yang B. Posterior corneal surface topographic changes after laser in situ keratomileusis are related to residual corneal bed thickness. Ophthalmology 1999;106(2):406-9.
9. Pallikaris IG, Kymionis GD, Astyrakakis NI. Corneal ectasia induced by laser in situ keratomileusis. J Cataract Refract Surg 2001;27(11):1796-802.
10. Argento C, Cosentino M J, Tytium A et al. Corneal ectasia after laser in situ keratomileusis. J Cataract Refract Surg 2001;27(9):1440-8.
11. Binder PS, Moore M, Lambert RW, et al. Comparison of two microkeratome systems. J Refract Surg 1997;13;142-53.
12. Hofmann RF, Bechara SJ. An independent evaluation of second generation suction microkeratomes. Refract Corneal Surg 1992;8:348-54.
13. Schuler A, Jessen K, Hoffmann F. Accuracy of the microkeratome keratectomies in pig eyes. Invest Ophthalmol Vis Sci 1990;31:2022-30.
14. Behrens A, Seitz B, Langenbucher A, et al. Evaluation of corneal flap dimensions and cut quality using a manually guided microkeratome [published erratum appears in J Refract Surg 1999;15:400]. J Refract Surg 1999;15:118-23.
15. Behrens A, Seitz B, Langenbucher A, et al. Evaluation of corneal flap dimensions and cut quality using the Automated Corneal Shaper microkeratome. J Refract Surg 2000;16:83-9.
16. Behrens A, Langenbucher A, Kus MM, et al. Experimental evaluation of two current generation automated microkeratomes: the Hansatomeâ and the Supratomeâ. Am J Ophthalmol. 2000;129:59-67.
17. Jacobs BJ, Deutsch TA, Rubenstein JB. Reproducibility of corneal flap thickness in LASIK. Ophthalmic Surg Lasers 1999;30:350-3.
18. McDermott GK. Topography's benefits for LASIK. Review of Ophthalmology. Editorial 9 (3).

Chapter 12

Topography and Aberrometer-guided Laser

Sunita Agarwal
Athiya Agarwal
Amar Agarwal

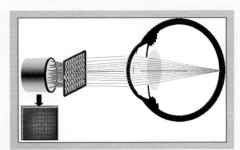

INTRODUCTION

Since as early as middle of 19th century it has been known that the optical quality of human eye suffers from ocular errors (aberrations) besides the commonly known image errors such as myopia, hyperopia and asigmatism.[1] In early 1970's Fyodorov introduced the anterior radial incisions to flatten the central cornea to correct myopia.[2] Astigmatic keratotomy,[3] keratomileusis and keratophakia, epikeratophakia[4] and currently Excimer Laser[5] have been used to manage the various refractive errors. These refractive procedures correct lower order aberrations such as spherical and cylindrical refractive errors however higher order aberrations persist, which affect the quality of vision but may not significantly affect the Snellen visual acuity. Refractive corrective procedures are known to induce aberrations.[6] It is the subtle deviations from the ideal optical system, which can be corrected by wavefront and topography guided (customized ablation) LASIK procedures.[7]

ABERRATIONS

Optical aberration customization can be corneal topography-guided which measures the ocular aberrations detected by corneal topography and treats the irregularities as an integrated part of the laser treatment plan. The second method of optical aberration customization measures the wavefront errors of the entire eye and treats based on these measurements.[7] Wavefront analysis can be done either using Howland's aberroscope[8] or a Hartmann Shack wavefront sensor.[9] These techniques measure all the eye's aberrations including second-order (sphere and cylindrical), third-order (coma–like), fourth-order (spherical), and higher order wavefront aberrations. Based on this information an ideal ablation plan can be formulated which treats lower order as well as higher order aberrations.

ZYOPTIX LASER

Zyoptix™ (Bausch & Lomb) is a system for Personalized Vision Solutions, which incorporates Zywave™ Hartmann Shack aberrometer coupled with Orbscan™ II z multi-dimensional device, which generates the individual ablation profiles to be used with the Technolas® 217 Excimer Laser system. Thus this system utilizes combination of wavefront analysis and corneal topography for optical aberration customization.

ORBSCAN

The Orbscan (Bausch & Lomb) corneal topography system uses a scanning optical slit scan that is fundamentally different than the corneal topography that analyzes the reflected images from the anterior corneal surface. The high-resolution video camera captures 40 light slits at 45 degrees angle projected through the cornea similarly as seen during slit lamp examination. The slits are projected on to the anterior segment of the eye: the anterior cornea, the posterior cornea, the anterior iris and anterior lens. The data collected from these four surfaces are used to create a topographic map. This technique provides more information about anterior segment of the eye, such as anterior and posterior corneal curvature and corneal thickness.[10] It improves the diagnostic accuracy and it has passive eye-tracker from frame to frame, 43 frames are taken to ensure accuracy. It is easy to interpret and has good repeatability. Three different maps are taken, and the one featuring the least eye movements is used. The maximum movements considered acceptable are 200 μ.

ABERROMETER

Zywave™ is based on Hartmann-Shack aberrometry (Figure 12.1) in which a laser diode (780 nm) generates a laser beam that is focused on the retina of the patient's eye (Figure 12.2). An adjustable collimation system compensates for the spherical portion of the refractive error of the eye. Laser diode is turned on for approximately 100 milliseconds. The light reflected from the focal point on the retina (source of wavefront) is directed through an array of small lenses (lenslet) generating a grid like pattern (array) of focal points (Figure 12.3). The position of the focal points are detected by Zywave™. Due to

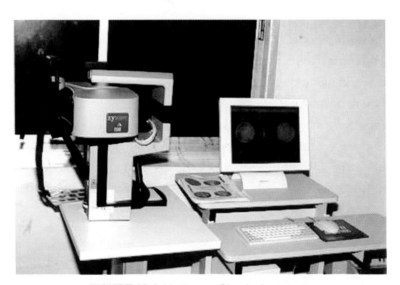

FIGURE 12.1: Hartmann-Shack aberrometer

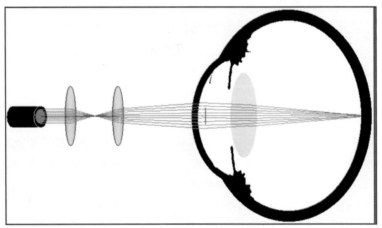

FIGURE 12.2: Zywave projects low-intensity HeNe infrared light into the eye and use the diffuse reflection from the retina

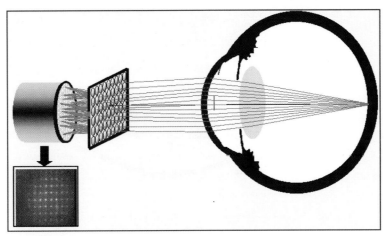

FIGURE 12.3: Schematic illustration of the Bausch & Lomb), Zywave aberrometer. A low-intensity HeNe infrared light is shone into the eye; the reflected light is focused by a number of small lenses (lenslet-array), and pictured by a CCD-camera. The capture image is shown on the bottom left

deviation of the points from their ideal position, the wavefront can be reconstructed. Wavefront display shows: (a) higher order aberrations, (b) predicted phoropter refraction (PPR) calculated for a back vertex correction of 15 mm, and (c) simulated point spread function (PSF). Zywave™ examinations are done with: (a) single examination with undilated pupil, and (b) five examinations with dilated pupil (mydriasis) non-cycloplegic, using 5 percent phenylephrine drops. One of these five measurements, which matched best with the manifest refraction of the undilated pupil, is chosen for the treatment.

ZYLINK

Information gathered from Orbscan and Zywave are then translated into treatment plan using Zylink™ software and copied to a floppy disc. The floppy disc is then inserted into the Technolas 217 system (Figure 12.4), fluence test carried out and a Zyopitx treatment card was inserted. A standard LASIK procedure is then performed with a superiorly hinged flap. A Hansatome™ microkeratome is used to create a flap. Flap thickness varied from 160 μm to 200 μm. A residual stromal bed of 250 μm or more is left in all eyes. Optical zone varied from 6 mm to 7 mm depending upon the pupil size and ablation required. Eye tracker is kept on during laser ablation. Postoperatively all patients are followed up for at least 6 months.

RESULTS

We did a study comprising 150 eyes with myopia and compound myopic astigmatism. Preoperatively, the patients underwent corneal topography with Orbscan II z™ and wavefront analysis with Zywave™ in addition to the routine pre-LASIK work-up. The results were assimilated using Zylink™ and a customized treatment plan was formulated. LASIK was then performed with Technolas® 217 system. All the patients were followed up for at least six months.

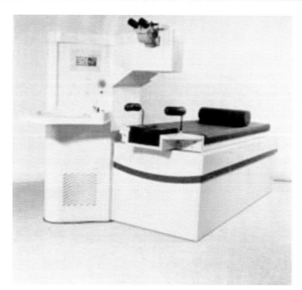

FIGURE 12.4: Technolas 217 Z excimer laser system

Mean preoperative BCVA (in decimal) was 0.83 ± 0.18 (Range 0.33- 1.00). Mean postoperative (6 months) BCVA was 1.00 ± 0.23 (Range 0.33-1.50). Difference was statistically significant (p=0.0003). Out of 150 eyes that underwent customized ablation, 3 eyes (2%) lost two or more lines of best spectacle corrected visual acuity (BSCVA).

Safety Index = Mean postoperative BSCVA/Mean preoperative BSCVA = 1.20 (Figure 12.5). Mean preoperative UCVA was 0.06 ± 0.02 (Range 0.01-0.50). Mean postoperative UCVA was 0.88 ± 0.36 (Range 0.08 – 1.50). Difference was statistically significant (p =0.0001).

Efficacy index = Mean postoperative UCVA/Mean preoperative UCVA = 14.66 (Figure 12.6). Preoperatively, none of the eyes had UCVA of 6/6 or more and one eye (0.66%) had UCVA of 6/12 or more. At 6 months postoperatively, 105 eyes (69.93%) had UCVA of 6/6 or more and 126 eyes (83.91%) had UCVA of 6/12 or more.

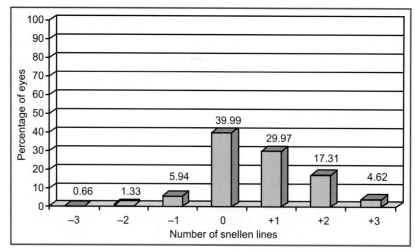

FIGURE 12.5: Shows changes in BSCVA 6 months postoperatively (Safety)

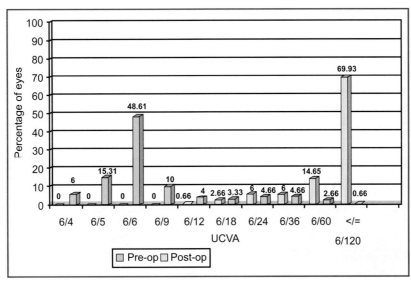

FIGURE 12.6: Compares preoperative and postoperative UCVA (Efficacy)

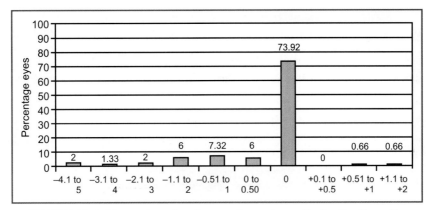

FIGURE 12.7: Shows the refractive results postoperatively after 6 months

Mean preoperative spherical equivalent was –5.25 D ± 1.68 D (Range –0.87 D to –15 D). Mean postoperative spherical equivalent (6 months) was –0.36 D ± 0.931 D (Range –4.25 D to +1.25). Difference between the two was statistically significant ($p < 0.05$) (Figure 12.7). 132 eyes (87.91%) were within ±1.00 D of emmetropia while 120 eyes (79.92%) were within ± 0.05 D of emmetropia. 1 eye (0.66%) was overcorrected by > 0.5 D and 1 eye (0.66%) was overcorrected by >1 D. The mean pupil diameter was 5.1 mm ± 0.62 mm. Preoperatively, 95 eyes (63.27%) had third order aberrations. Forty-two eyes (28%) had second order aberration alone, while 13 eyes (8.65%) had fourth and fifth order aberrations. Postoperatively, 60 eyes (40%) had third-order aberration. Seventy-five eyes (50%) had second order alone while 15 eyes (10%) had higher order aberrations.

DISCUSSION

Hartmann–Shack wavefront sensor was first used by Liang and colleagues to detect ocular aberrations.[11] They applied an adaptive optics deformable mirror to correct the lower and higher-order aberrations of

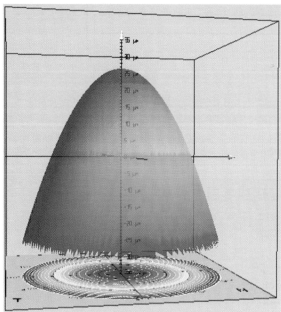

FIGURE 12.8: Second-order sphere

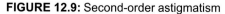

FIGURE 12.9: Second-order astigmatism

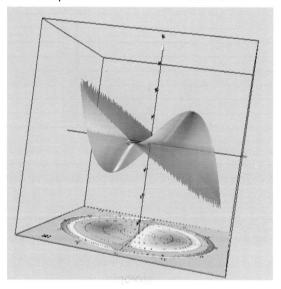

FIGURE 12.10: Third-order coma

the eye. They reported a 6 times increase in contrast sensitivity to high spatial frequency when the pupil was large. This study demonstrated that correction of higher-order aberrations could lead to supernormal vision in normal eyes. Figures 12.8 to 12.10 show various aberrations.

In our series, using Zyoptix and Technolas 217 system, which is wavefront and corneal topography guided, we yielded results that are comparable to standard LASIK procedure.[12] In a series of 347 eyes, McDonald et al[12] reported a postoperative refraction of –0.29 ± 0.45 D (–0.36 ± 0.93 D in our series) with standard LASIK. Fifty-seven percent of the eyes in their series had postoperative UCVA of ≥ 6/6. In our study, 70 percent of the eyes had UCVA of ≥6/6, six months postoperatively.

Higher order aberrations were reduced postoperatively in our study. Third-order aberration (coma) was most common in our series, followed by second-order (defocus and astigmatism) and fourth-order (spherical aberration). Postoperatively, after 6 months, there was considerable decrease in third-order and fourth-order aberrations. While most of the eyes had only defocus and astigmatism (i.e. second - order aberration). A slight increase in fourth-order aberration (spherical) was noted. Spherical aberration is known to increase after LASIK.[13-15] Roberts has reported that cornea changes its shape in response to ablation and this change, along with wound healing effects have to be taken into account before customized correction can nullify higher-order aberrations. Roberts and coworkers suggest that increase in spherical aberrations following LASIK may be caused by a biomechanically-induced steepening and thickening that may occur in midperiphery of the cornea.[13] MacRae and coworkers have reported that simply creating a LASIK flap increases higher-order aberrations in unpredictable manner.[14] They suggest that improved results can be obtained using a surface ablation such as PRK or LASEK, or by doing a two-stage LASIK, with the second stage adjusting for the aberration created by the flap and initial ablation.

Scotopic visual complaints have been the bugbear of LASIK procedures, ranging from mild annoyance to server optical disability.[16,17] Nighttime starbursts, reduced contrast sensitivity and haloes are the most common complaints. [16,17] Spherical aberration that is induced during LASIK may account for this scotopic complaints.[14] Pupil diameter is another factor that is important. When pupil diameter is large, as in young patients, dim light vision is improved after customized correction.[18,19] In our series, 11 percent of the patients complained of haloes around light at night and difficult night driving. In dim light, the mean pupil diameter in these patients was 4.2 mm while it was 5.9 mm in other patients. Smaller pupil diameter and induced higher-order aberration may account for these scotopic visual complaints.

Twenty-five percent of the patients in our series reported improvement in bright light vision, while 40 percent showed improvement in dim light vision. A similar improvement was noted by Cox and co-workers (presentation by Cox IG at Zyoptix Alliance meeting, 2002 reported in *Ocular Surgery News*, July 2002 volume 13, number 7). In our series, treatment optical zone ranged from 6 mm to 7 mm. Treatment with larger optical zones and transition zones as compared to conventional LASIK may be possible since entire corneal topography and not just the central cornea overlying pupil along with wavefront ablation in dilated pupil are considered during treatment. This may induce lesser spherical aberration post-LASIK and account for improved scotopic vision.

Though we did not measure contrast sensitivity and glare acuity postoperatively, our results suggest improved quality of vision and fewer glare problems with Zyoptix treatment. A more temporal appraisal of the procedure has to be carried out with comparison to standard LASIK. Short-term results suggest wavefront and topography-guided LASIK may be a safe and effective procedure which improves the visual performance.

CONCLUSION

Wavefront and topography-guided LASIK procedure leads to better visual performance by decreasing higher order aberration. Scotopic visual complaints may be reduced with this method.

REFERENCES

1. Helmholtz H. Handbuch der physiologischen optik. Leipzig: Leopold Voss.1867; 137-47.
2. Fyodorov SN, Durnev VV. Operation of dosaged dissection of corneal circular ligament.
3. Binder PS, Waring GO III: Keratotomy for astigmatism. In Waring GO III (Eds): Refractive Keratotomy for Myopia and Astigmatism. Mosby Year Book 1992; 1085–1198. In cases of myopia of mild degree. Ann Ophthalmol II: 1979; 1885–90.
4. Kaufmann HE. Correction of aphakia. Am J Ophthalmol 1980;89: 1.
5. McGhee CNJ, Taylor HR, Garty DS, et al. Excimer Lasers in Ophthalmology: Principles and Practice. Martin Duntz: London, 1997.
6. MacRae S, Porter J, Cox IG, et al. Higher-order aberrations after conventional LASIK. ISRS: Dallas, Texas, 2000.
7. MacRae SM: Supernormal vision, hypervision, and customized corneal ablation. Guest Editorial J Cat Refract Surg 2000; 26 (2).
8. Howland HC, Howland B. A subjective method for the measurement of monochromatic aberrations of the eye. J Opt Soc Am 1977; 67:1508-18.
9. Liang J, Williams DR, Miller DT. Supernormal vision and high-resolution retinal imaging through adaptive optics. J Opt Soc Am 1997; 2884-92.
10. Fedor P, Kaufman S. Corneal topography and imaging. eMedicine Journal, 2001; 2(6).
11. Liang J, Williams D. Aberrations and retinal image quality of the normal human eye. J Opt Soc AM A 1997;14:2884-92.
12. McDonald MB, Carr JD, Frantz JM, et al. Laser in situ keratomilieusis for myopia up to –11 diopters with up to –5 diopters of astigmatism with summit autonomous LADARVision excimer laser system. Ophthalmology 2001; 108:309-16.
13. Roberts C. The cornea is not a piece of plastic. J Refract Surg 2000; 16:407-13.
14. MacRae SM, Roberts C, Porter J, et al. The biomechanics of a LASIK flap. ISRS Mid-Summer Meeting: Orlando, Florida, 2001.
15. Applegate RA, Howland HC, Klyce SD. Corneal aberration and refractive surgery. In MacRae S (Ed): Customized Corneal Ablation. Thorofare NJ: Slack, Inc., 2001.
16. Holladay JT, Dudeja DR, Chang J. Functional vision and corneal changes after laser in situ keratomileusis determined by contrast sensitivity, glare testing, and corneal topography. J Cataract Refract Surg 1999; 25: 663-9.
17. Perez-Santonja JJ, Sakla HF, Alio JL. Contrast sensitivity after laser in situ keratomileusis. J Cataract Refract Surg 1998; 24: 183-9.
18. Applegate R, Howland H, Sharp R, et al. Corneal aberrations and visual performance after refractive keratectomy. J Refract Surg 1998; 14: 397-407.
19. Oshika T, Klyce S, Applegate R, et al. Comparison of corneal wavefront aberrations after photorefractive keratectomy and laser in situ keratomileusis. Am J Ophthal 1999; 127:1-7.

Chapter

13

Aberropia:
A New
Refractive
Entity

Sunita Agarwal
Athiya Agarwal
Amar Agarwal

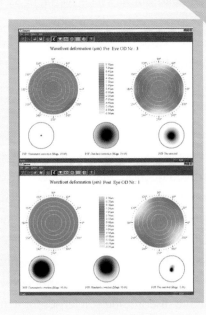

INTRODUCTION

The next evolution to come on to the visual science scene in refractive ocular imaging is the aberrometer, the Orbscan and wavefront analysis. This technology is based on astrophysical principles, which astronomers use to perfect the images impinging on their telescopes. Dr Bille, the Director of the Institute of Applied Physics at the University of Heidelberg first began work in this field while developing this specific technology for astronomy applications in the mid-1970's. For perfect imaging, astrophysicists have to be able to measure and correct the imperfect higher-order aberrations or wavefront distortions that enter their telescopic lens system from the galaxy. To achieve this purpose, adaptive optics are used wherein deformable mirrors reform the distorted wavefront to allow clear visualization of celestial objects. Extrapolating these same principles to the human eye, it was thought that removal of the wavefront aberrations of the eye might finally yield the long awaited and much desired ultimate goal of "super vision."

So far, the only parameters that could be modified to obtain the optical correction for a given patients refractive error were the sphere, cylinder and axis even though this does not give the ideal optical correction many a times. This is because the current modes for correcting the optical aberrations of the eye do not reduce the higher order aberrations. The ideal optical system should be able to correct the optical aberrations in such a way that the spatial resolving ability of the eye is limited only by the limits imposed by the neural retina, i.e. receptor diameter and receptor packing.

Thus, there may be a large group of patients whose best corrected visual acuity (BCVA) may actually improve significantly on removal of the optical aberrations. These optical aberrations are contributed to by the eye's entire optical system, i.e. the cornea, the lens, the vitreous and the retina. This study was conducted to determine the existence of a hitherto unidentified entity which we label as **aberropia** wherein patients with best corrected visual acuity of ≤ 6/9 (0.63), corneal topography not accounting for the lack of improvement in BCVA and with no other known cause for decreased vision improved by ≥ two Snellen lines after refractive correction of their wavefront aberration.

MATERIALS AND METHODS

Sixteen eyes of 10 patients were included in this retrospective study carried out at the Dr Agarwal's Eye Institute, India between May to December 2002. Only patients who had visual acuity less than 6/9 (0.63) prior to the procedure and whose visual acuity improved by more than or equal to two lines after the procedure were included in the study. None of these patients had any other known cause for decreased vision and their corneal topography did not account for the lack of improvement in BCVA. The routine patient evaluation including uncorrected (UCVA) and best corrected (BCVA), slit lamp examination, applanation tonometry, manifest and cycloplegic refractions, Orbscan, aberrometry, corneal pachymetry, corneal diameter, Schirmer test and indirect ophthalmoscopy had been performed for all the patients. Patients wearing contact lenses had been asked to discontinue soft lenses for a minimum of 1 week and rigid gas permeable lenses for a minimum of 2 weeks before the preoperative examination

174

and surgery. Informed consent was obtained form all patients after a thorough explanation of the procedure and its potential benefits and risks.

The Zyoptix procedure was then performed using the Bausch & Lomb) Technolas 217 z machine. The parameters used were: wavelength 193 nm, fluence 130 mJ/cm^2 and ablation zone diameters between 4.8 mm and 6 mm. The Hansatome (Bausch & Lomb)) was used in all the eyes. Either the 180 μm or the 160 μm plate was used in all the eyes. The aberrometer and the Orbscan, which checks the corneal topography, are linked and a zylink created. An appropriate software file is created which is then used to generate the laser treatment file.

Postoperatively, the patients underwent complete examination including UCVA, BCVA, slit lamp examination, Orbscan and aberrometry. The mean follow-up was 37.5 days.

For statistical analysis, the Snellen acuity was converted to the decimal notation. Continuous variables were described with mean, standard deviation, minimum and maximum values.

RESULTS

Sixteen eyes of 10 patients satisfied the inclusion criteria. The mean age of the patients was 29.43 years (range 22 to 35 years). Six patients were females and 4 were males. The mean preoperative pupil diameter measured on aberrometer was 4.69 mm and mean postoperative pupil diameter measured on aberrometer was 4.53 mm.

The mean pre-operative spherical equivalent was – 4.94 D (range –12.50 to –1.5 D). The mean spherical equivalent at 1 month postoperative period was –0.16 ± 0.68 D (range –1.0 to 1.5). Mean preoperative sphere was –4.95 D (range –12.50 to –0.75 D) and the mean postoperative sphere was –0.13 ± 0.68 D (range-1 to 1.5) at 1 month. The mean preoperative cylinder was –1.34 D (range 0 to –3.50). The mean postoperative cylinder was –0.08 ± 0.24 D (range 0 to –0.75 D) at one month. Postoperatively, at the end of first month, 70 percent of the patients were within ± 0.5D and 90 percent were within ± 1D of emmetropia (Figure 13.1). Preoperatively mean RMS (Root Mean square) values (Figure 13.2) were: Z 200 Defocus –9.22, Z 221 Astigmatism 0.12, Z 220 Astigmatism 1.02, Z 311 Coma –0.041, Z 310 Coma –0.04, Z 331 Trefoil 0.23, Z 330 Trefoil 0.016, Z 400 Spherical aberration –0.054, Z 420 Secondary astigmatism 0.103, Z 421 Secondary astigmatism 0.029, Z 440 Quadrafoil – 0.103, Z 441 Quadrafoil –0.021, Z 510 Secondary coma 0.025, Z 511 Secondary coma –0.015, Z 530 Secondary trefoil 0.0049, Z 531 Secondary trefoil -0.00219, Z 550 Pentafoil 0.023, Z 551 Pentafoil 0.046. Postoperative mean RMS values were : Z 200 Defocus –0.429, Z 221 Astigmatism 0.07, Z 220 Astigmatism –0.07, Z 311 Coma 0.149, Z 310 Coma –0.079, Z 331 Trefoil –0.102, Z 330 Trefoil – 0.004, Z 400 Spherical aberration -0.179, Z 420 Secondary astigmatism 0.015, Z 421 Secondary astigmatism 0.031, Z 440 Quadrafoil 0.019, Z 441 Quadrafoil –0.069, Z 510 Secondary coma –0.008, Z 511 Secondary coma 0.008, Z 530 Secondary Trefoil -0.002, Z 531 Secondary Trefoil –0.014, Z 550 Pentafoil 0.006, Z 551 Pentafoil 0.026.

RMS pre- and post-laser showed a reduction in the higher order aberrations (Tables 13.1 and 13.2). 6.25 percent patients achieved 6/9, 31.25 percent patients achieved ≥ 6/6 (1.00), 37.50 percent achieved

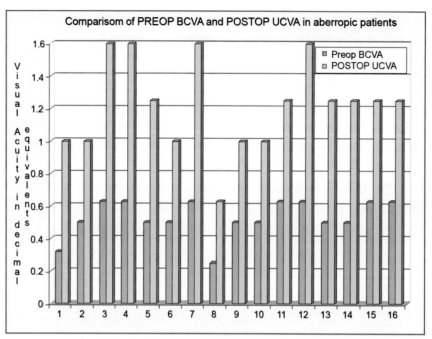

FIGURE 13.1: Preoperative BCVA versus postoperative UCVA

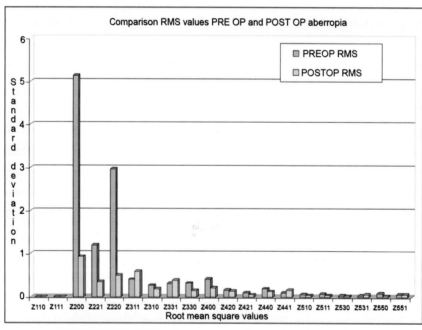

FIGURE 13.2: RMS values preoperative and postoperative

a BCVA of 6/5 (1.25) and 25 percent achieved a BCVA of 6/4 (1.6) (Figure 13.3). Figure 13.4 shows the preoperative Orbscan picture of a patient showing no abnormality. Figures 13.5 and 13.6 show the aberrometer maps of the right eye and left eye of a patient in which we can see the aberrations reduced post-laser.

TABLE 13.1: RMS preoperative of 16 eyes

RMS VALUES PRE LASER

Patient no	Z 110	Z 111	Z 200	Z 221	Z 220	Z 311	Z 310	Z 331	Z 330	Z 400	Z 420	Z 421	Z 440	Z 441	Z 510	Z 511	Z 530	Z 531	Z 550	Z 551	Z 6
1	0	0	-5.77	4.055.	-6.131	0.299	-0.113	0.725	-0.44	0.009	-0.03	0.102	-0.233	0.109	0.131	0.027	-0.048	-0.041	0.052	0.039	-999
2	0	0	-4.323	-1.719	6.005	-0.273	0.022	-0.353	0.275	0.092	0.092	-0.145	0.199	-0.013	-0.006	0.011	0.034	-0.039	0.042	0.042	-9999
3	0	0	-11.8	-0.088	0.116	0.435	-0.658	-0.444	-0.567	-0.779	-0.089	0.043	-0.202	-0.053	-0.052	-0.057	-0.04	-0.001	0.13	0.111	-9999
4	0	0	-12.46	0.514	-0.155	0.29	-0.006	0.016	0.529	-0.91	0.124	0.124	-0.431	-0.222	0.074	-0.04	0.001	-0.063	-0.141	0.119	-9999
5	0	0	-6.535	-0.123	-0.886	0.156	-0.09	0.094	-0.128	-0.084	-0.072	0.035	-0.009	-0.044	0.001	-0.031	0.01	-0.005	0.001	-0.041	-9999
6	0	0	-7.867	0.185	1.704	-0.02	0.414	0.441	0.197	0.365	0.197	0.107	-0.155	-0.002	0.123	0.026	-0.001	0.049	0.048	0.032	-9999
7	0	0	-4.28	0.167	2.571	0.007	-0.089	0.356	0.125	0.585	0.101	-0.002	-0.17	-0.062	-0.077	0.198	0.001	-0.104	-0.022	0.029	-9999
8	0	0	-10.4	0.502	-0.587	-0.007	-0.331	0.165	-0.126	-0.054	-0.071	0.036	-0.118	-0.128	0.009	0.017	-0.007	-0.026	0.063	-0.052	-9999
9	0	0	-17.15	-0.414	-1.217	0.093	-0.106	0.343	-0.18	-0.254	0.009	0.002	0.001	-0.025	0.007	-0.022	-0.007	-0.042	0.037	0.04	-9999
10	0	0	-16.78	-0.162	-0.637	0.122	-0.159	0.279	0.2	-0.181	0.115	0.007	-0.002	0.042	-0.034	-0.028	0.021	-0.043	-0.006	-0.017	-9999
11	0	0	-4.513	2.916	4.661	-0.634	-0.205	0.477	0.44	0.094	0.377	0.058	-0.201	0.101	0.133	-0.147	0.009	0.011	-0.055	0.118	-9999
12	0	0	-5.736	-1.501	5.195	-1.126	0.32	0.665	-0.254	0.218	0.479	0.122	-0.253	-0.045	0.099	-0.025	0.012	-0.006	-0.05	0.11	-9999
13	0	0	-15.46	1.605	2.754	0.378	0.443	0.208	0.458	0.643	-0.083	0.09	0.407	-0.006	-0.021	0.09	0.033	0.032	0.239	0.149	-9999
14	0	0	-15.26	-0.557	2.865	-0.26	-0.059	0.107	0.122	0.168	0.025	-0.256	-0.003	0.257	0.007	0.051	0.136	-0.061	-0.114	0.124	-9999
15	0	0	-4.955	0.735	0.383	-0.401	0.003	0.62	-0.494	-0.676	0.391	0.163	-0.421	-0.264	0.039	-0.261	-0.079	0.241	0.103	-0.067	-9999
16	0	0	-4.367	-0.195	-0.238	0.28	-0.04	0.021	0.11	-0.112	0.084	-0.022	-0.061	0.013	-0.018	-0.063	0.004	0.063	0.044	0	-9999

177

TABLE 13.2: RMS postoperative of 16 eyes

RMS VALUES POST LASER

Pat.no.	Z 110	Z 111	Z 200	Z 221	Z 220	Z 311	Z 310	Z 331	Z 330	Z 400	Z 420	Z 421	Z 440	Z 441	Z 510	Z 511	Z 530	Z 531	Z 550	Z 551	Z 6
1	0	0	-0.022	0.74	-1.294	0.117	-0.067	0.141	0.052	-0.063	-0.076	0.1	0.054	-0.037	-0.028	0.001	0.008	0.007	0.013	0.006	-9999
2	0	0	-0.508	0.12	0.194	-0.085	0.039	-0.12	-0.018	-9999	-9999	-9999	-9999	-9999	-9999	-9999	-9999	-9999	-9999	-9999	-9999
3	0	0	-1.398	-0.606	0.697	-0.558	-0.351	0.841	0.345	-0.39	0.392	0.038	-0.303	-0.038	-0.001	0.103	-0.066	-0.105	-0.021	0.137	-9999
4	0	0	-2.05	-0.499	-0.375	-0.027	-0.269	-0.534	-0.289	-0.58	0.114	0.058	0.236	-0.161	0.034	-0.083	0.004	0.039	0.01	-0.077	-9999
5	0	0	0.229	0.1	-0.123	-9999	-9999	-9999	-9999	-9999	-9999	-9999	-9999	-9999	-9999	-9999	-9999	-9999	-9999	-9999	-9999
6	0	0	-0.036	-0.17	0.425	-0.002	0.069	-0.045	-0.042	-0.342	-0.032	0.094	0.075	-0.05	0.068	0.03	0.064	-0.014	0.012	0.002	-9999
7	0	0	0.687	0.128	-0.028	-0.117	-0.043	0.062	0.088	-0.178	0.179	0.024	-0.045	0.055	0.013	0.016	-0.034	-0.013	-0.013	0.059	-9999
8	0	0	-2.164	0.279	-0.696	-0.25	-0.398	-0.147	-0.128	-0.581	-0.238	0.02	0.032	-0.088	-0.129	0.028	-0.029	0.007	0.089	0.059	-9999
9	0	0	-0.298	0.002	-0.311	0.158	-0.206	0.129	-0.116	-0.105	-0.045	-0.043	-0.1	-0.1	-9999	-9999	-9999	-9999	-9999	-9999	-9999
10	0	0	0.109	0.241	-0.503	0.233	-0.119	-0.16	-0.204	-9999	-9999	-9999	-9999	-9999	-9999	-9999	-9999	-9999	-9999	-9999	-9999
11	0	0	0.034	-0.092	0.076	0.013	-0.03	-0.067	0.003	-9999	-9999	-9999	-9999	-9999	-9999	-9999	-9999	-9999	-9999	-9999	-9999
12	0	0	0.187	0.061	0.004	-0.097	0.015	0.067	0.035	-9999	-9999	-9999	-9999	-9999	-9999	-9999	-9999	-9999	-9999	-9999	-9999
13	0	0	-0.701	0.291	0.598	2.161	0.349	-1.062	-0.201	-0.428	-0.013	0.204	0.258	-0.636	-0.082	0.113	0.069	-0.239	0.062	-9999	-9999
14	0	0	-0.638	0.094	0.391	0.517	-0.328	-0.336	0.188	-0.118	-0.077	0.003	0.157	0.034	-0.006	-0.025	0.004	0.018	-0.066	-9999	-9999
15	0	0	-0.148	0.493	0.017	0.261	0.017	-0.354	0.302	-0.111	0.053	0.07	-0.019	-0.084	-0.007	-0.051	-0.052	0.063	0.011	-9999	-9999
16	0	0	-0.161	-0.038	-0.331	0.072	0.049	-0.05	-0.086	0.025	-0.008	-0.059	-0.028	-9999	-9999	-9999	-9999	-9999	-9999	-9999	-9999

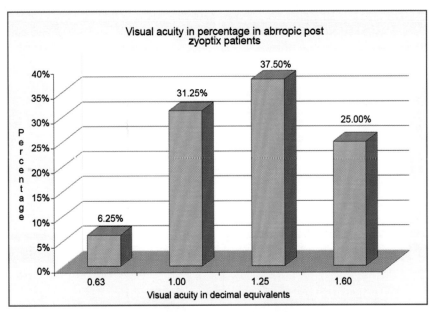

FIGURE 13.3: Percentage values of visual acuity

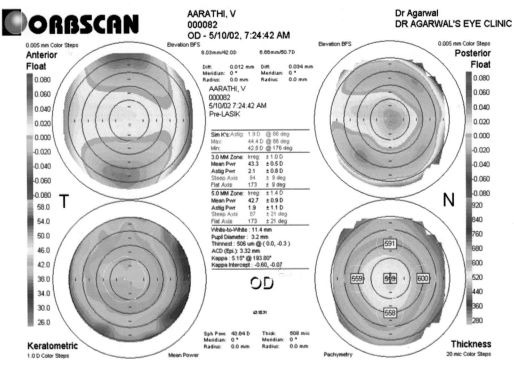

FIGURE 13.4: Preoperative Orbscan

DISCUSSION

Zyoptix is the new generation of excimer laser used for the treatment of refractive disorders. Until recently, refractive disorders were treated with standard techniques, which took into consideration only the subjective refraction. Zyoptix technique, on the other hand, takes into account the patient's subjective

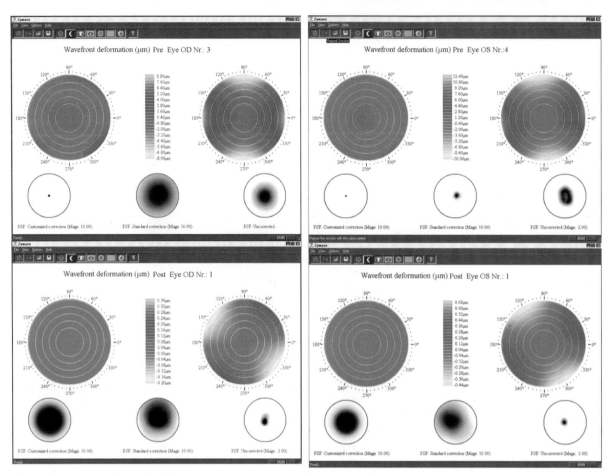

FIGURES 13.5 and 13.6: Pre- and postoperative aberrometry of the right and left eye of the same patient showing removal of higher order aberrations

refraction, ocular optical aberrations and corneal topography, with the latter not only for the diagnosis, but also for the therapeutic treatment, in order to design a personalized treatment based on the total structure of the eye. The wavefront technology in Zyoptix uses the Hartmann-Shack aberrometer based on the Hartmann-Shack principle[1] demonstrated by Liang et al[2] to measure the eye's wave aberration. This wavefront sensor has been improved by increasing the density of samples taken of the wavefront slope in the pupil.[3] All Hartmann-Shack devices are outgoing testing devices in that they evaluate the light being bounced back out through the optical system. A narrow laser beam is focused onto the retina to generate a point source. The out coming light rays which experience all the aberrations of the eye pass through an array of lenses which detects their deviation. The wavefront deformation is calculated by analyzing the direction of the light rays using this lenslet array. Parallel light beams indicate a good wavefront and non-parallel light beams indicate a wavefront with aberrations, which does not give equidistant focal points. This image is then captured onto a CCD camera and the wavefront is reconstructed. The data is explained mathematically in three dimensions with polynomial functions. Most investigators have chosen the Zernike method for this analysis although Taylor series can also be used for the same purpose.[4] Data from the wavefront map is presented as a sum of Zernike polynomials each describing a certain deformation. At any point in the pupil, the wavefront aberration is the optical path difference between the actual image wavefront and the ideal spherical wavefront centered at the image point.[5]

Any refractive error which cannot be corrected by spherocylindrical lens combinations is referred to by physicists as higher-order aberrations, i.e. comma, spherical aberration, chromatic aberration. The Zernike Polynomials, which describe ray points, are used to obtain a best fit toric to correct for the refractive error of the eye. The points are described in the x and y coordinates and the third dimension, height, is described in the z-axis. The local refractive correction of each area of the entrance pupil can be determined by calculating from the wavefront polynomial the corresponding local radii of curvature and hence the required spherocylindrical correction.[6] Thus each small region of the entrance pupil has its own three parameters that characterize the local refractive correction: sphere, cylinder and axis.[6] The global aberrations of the entire optical system including the cornea, lens, vitreous and the retina are thus measured. The great advantage of wavefront analysis is that it can describe these other aberrations.

The first order polynomial describes the spherical error or power of the eye. The second order polynomial describes the regular astigmatic component and its orientation or axis. Third order aberrations are considered to be coma and fourth order aberrations are considered to be spherical aberration. Zernike polynomial descriptions for wavefront analysis typically go up to the tenth order of expression. The first and second orders describe the morphology of a normal straight curve. More local maximum and minimum points require higher orders of the polynomial series to describe the surface. Normal eyes exhibit spherical[7,8] and comma[9,10] aberrations in addition to exhibiting defocus and astigmatism.

Ideally, the difference in the magnitude of the local refractive correction of each area of the entrance pupil should not exceed 0.25 D. Lower spherocylindrical corrections are generally associated with lower wavefront aberrations.[6] These observations regarding variation in local ocular refraction along different meridians are also confirmed by Ivanoff[11] and Jenkins.[12] Van den Brink[13] also commented on the change in refraction across the pupil. Clinically significant changes of at least 0.25 D in one or both components of the spherocylindrical correction might normally be expected for decentrations of about 1 mm. Rayleigh's quarter wavelength rule states that if the wavefront aberration exceeds a quarter of a wavelength, the quality of the retinal image will be impaired significantly.[14] Thus the aberration in eyes starts to become significant when the pupil diameter exceeds 1-2 mm.[6] Thus it is not possible to correct the entire wavefront aberration with a single spherocylindrical lens. As conventional refractive procedures such as Lasik also reduce only the second order aberrations, the visual acuity will still be limited by aberrations of third and higher order aberrations. These patients are likely to undergo tremendous improvement in their BCVA after correction of their aberrations by Zyoptix.

In the Zyoptix system, the aberrometer and the orbscan, which checks the corneal topography, are linked and a zylink created. An appropriate software file is created which is then used to generate the laser treatment file. The truncated gaussian beam shape used in Zyoptix combines the advantages of the common beam shapes, i.e. flat top beam and the gaussian beam, creating a maximized smoothness and minimized thermal effect. Thus Zyoptix gives a smoother corneal surface, reducing glare and increasing visual acuity. The larger optical zones reduce haloes. Zyoptix also causes a reduction of the ablation depth by 15 to 20 percent and a reduced enhancement rate

In a patient with higher order aberrations, lasik does not remove the higher order aberrations and the point-spread function is a large blur. Zyoptix on the other hand, performs customized ablation and removes the higher order aberrations thus minimizing the wavefront deformation. The point-spread function is therefore a small spot of light.

In our study, the mean preoperative spherical equivalent improved from –4.78 D to –0.16 D ± 0.68 and the mean preoperative cylinder improved from –1.34 D to –0.08 D ± 0.24. The aberrations were reduced drastically in all the eyes and the BCVA improved in all cases by ≥ two lines. Reduction of the aberrations of the eye can thus result in an improved BCVA postoperatively.

Improving the optics of the eye by removing aberrations increases the contrast and spatial detail of the retinal image. Reduction of higher order aberrations may not improve high contrast acuity much more in eyes where spherocylindrical lenses alone improve the BCVA to 6/3 (2.00) or better. In contrast, in otherwise normal eyes where the BCVA is limited to 6/9 (0.50) or 6/6 (1.00) due to optical aberrations, reduction of higher order aberrations should improve visual acuity.

Realization of the best possible unaided visual acuity may be limited at the cortical, retinal and the spectacle, corneal, or implant level. All maculae may not be able to support 6/3 (2.00) vision. Insufficient cone density or sub-optimal orientation of cone receptors or a sub-optimal Stiles-Crawford profile of the macula may make 6/3 (2.00) vision impossible. Clinical or sub-clinical amblyopia may make achievement of super vision impossible. But, in spite of this, there may be a certain patient population who have the potential for an improved BCVA on removal of their wavefront aberrations. The corneal topography does not account for the decreased preoperative visual acuity in these patients, neither do they have any other identifiable cause for the decrease in acuity except for an abnormal wavefront. It is important that this subgroup of patients are identified and their optical aberrations neutralized so that they are not deprived of the opportunity to gain in their BCVA.

Wavefront sensing technology, at present, does not in most cases define the exact locale of the pathology causing the aberration. Hence, clinical examination and other refractive tools, such as corneal topographic mapping, along with sound clinical judgment is required for proper understanding of the eye and its individual refractive status. Also, wavefront aberrations may not remain static. Numerous authors[15-18] have shown that ocular optical aberrations probably remain constant between 20 and 40 years of age but increase after that. Aberrations also change during accommodation [19,20] and may be affected by mydriatics.[21] Thus, the patient should be informed about these possibilities while taking the consent for the procedure. Long term studies are required to determine the stability of the post-operative refraction, residual aberrations and changes in BCVA if any.

The question of magnification factor improving visual acuity does not arise as these patients pre-operatively did not improve with contact lenses. Further the refractive error in some of these patients was not very large.

CONCLUSION

In conclusion, removal of the wavefront aberration may extend the benefit of an improved BCVA to patients with an abnormal wavefront. The subgroup of patients with higher order aberrations, normal corneal topography and no other known cause for decreased vision may thus benefit immensely with wavefront guided refractive surgery. Customized refractive surgery tailor-made for these individual patients, aimed at neutralizing the wavefront aberrations of the eye is safer, more predictable, provides better visual acuities and reduces the incidence of unsatisfactory outcomes. Further studies are required to assess the long-term outcomes.

Till now, when we discuss refractive errors we discuss about spherical and a cylindrical correction. But in todays world we have to think of a third parameter which is the aberrations present in the eye which can be anywhere in the optical media. These can be corrected in the corneal level by the laser treatment.

REFERENCES

1. B Platt, RV Shack. Lenticular Hartmann screen. Opt Sci Center News (University of Arizona)1971;5:15-16.
2. J Liang, B Grimm, S Goelz, J Bille. Objective measurement of the wave aberrations of the human eye with the use of a Hartmann-Shack wavefront sensor. J Opt Soc Am 1994;11:1949-57.
3. J Liang, Williams DR, et al. Aberrations and retinal image quality of the normal human eye. J Opt Soc Am A 1997; 14(11): 2873-83.
4. Oshika T, Klyce SD, Applegate RA, et al. Comparison of corneal wavefront aberrations after photorefractive keratectomy and laser in situ keratomileusis. Am J Ophthalmol 1999; 127:1-7.
5. Fincham WHA, Freeman MH. Optics (9th edn). London: Butterworths, 1980. Born M, Wolf E. Principles of Optics (2nd edn). New York: Macmillan, 1964:203-32.
6. WN Charman, G Walsh. Variations in the local refractive correction of the eye across its entrance pupil. Optometry and Vision Science 1989; 66(1):34-40.
7. WM Rosenblum, JL Christensen. Objective and subjective spherical aberration measurement of the human eye. In E Wolf (Ed). Progress in Optics. North-Holland, Amsterdam 1976;13;69-91.
8. MC Campbell, EM Harrison, Simonet P. Psychophysical measurement of the blur on the retina due to optical aberrations of the eye. Vision Res 1990;30:1587-1602.
9. HC Howland, Howland B. A subjective method for the measurement of monochromatic aberrations of the eye. J Opt Soc Am 1977;67:1508-18.
10. G Walsh, WN Charman, Howland HC. Objective technique for the determination of monochromatic aberrations of the human eye. J Opt Soc Am 1984;A1: 987-992.
11. Ivanoff A. About the spherical aberration of the eye. J Opt Soc Am 1956;46: 901-3.
12. Jenkins TCA. Aberrations of the eye and their effects on vision. Part 1. Br J Physiol Opt 1963; 20: 59-91.
13. Van den Brink G. Measurements of the geometric aberrations of the eye. Vision Res. 1962; 2: 233-44.
14. Born M, Wolf E. Principles of Optics (2nd edn). New York: Macmillan, 1964:203-32.
15. Kaemmerer M, Mrochen M, Mierdel P, et al. Optical aberrations of the human eye. Nature Medicine (in press).
16. Oshika T, Klyce SD, Applegate RA, et al. Changes in corneal wavefront aberration with aging. Invest Ophthalmol Vis Sci 1999; 40: 1351-55.
17. Calver RI, Cox MJ, Elliot DB. Effect of aging on the monochromatic aberrations of the human eye. J Opt Soc Am A 1999;16: 2069-78.
18. Guirao A, Gonzalez C, Redondo M, et al. Average optical performance of the human eye as a function of age in a normal population. Invest Ophthalmol Vis Sci 1999; 40 203-13.
19. Krueger R, Kaemerrer M, Mrochen M, et al. Understanding refraction and accommodation through "ingoing optics" aberrometry: A case report. Ophthalmology (in press).
20. He JC, Burns SA, Marcos S. Monochromatic aberrations in the accommodated human eye. Vis Res 2000; 40:41-48.
21. Fankhauser F, Kaemerrer M, Mrochen M, et al. The effect of accommodation, mydriasis, and cycloplegia on aberrometry. ARVO abstract 2248. Invest Ophthalmol Vis Sci 2000; 41; S461.

14

Irregular Astigmatism: LASIK as a Correcting Tool

Jorge L Alió
José I Belda Sanchis
Ahmad MM Shalaby

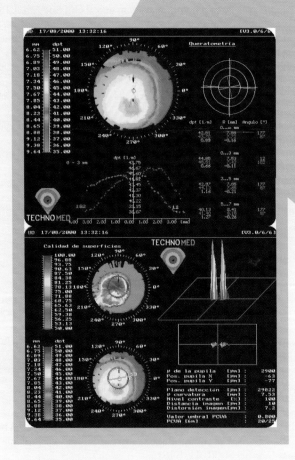

INTRODUCTION

Irregular astigmatism represents one of the problems that are very difficult to manage and frustrating in results to refractive surgeons. It is also one of the worst sequelae of corneal injuries. It can also complicate certain corneal diseases as keratoconus. With the recent evolution of refractive surgery techniques and diagnostic tools, new types of irregular astigmatism are being observed.[1,2]

Astigmatism is defined as irregular if the principal meridians are not 90 degrees apart, usually because of an irregularity of the corneal curvature. It cannot be completely corrected with a spherocylindrical lens.[3] Duke-Elder defines irregular astigmatism as a refractive state in which the refraction in different meridians conforms to no geometric plan and the refracted rays have no planes of symmetry.[4]

The alternatives for correction of irregular astigmatism are very scarce and with very limited expectations. Spectacle correction is usually not useful in the correction of corneal irregular astigmatism as it is difficult to define principle meridians. Hard contact lenses represent a good alternative in which the tear fluid layer under the contact lens evens out the irregularity. We should consider that adaptation and stability of contact lenses is limited by irregularity of the corneal surface and the patient's comfort.

Lamellar and full-thickness corneal grafting are surgical alternatives. The limited availability of corneal donor as well as the biological and refractive complications of allografic corneal graft limit the clinical applicability of these procedures.

Many surgeons have made great efforts in finding a solution to this problem.[5-7] To this date, we believe there should be safe, efficient and predictable methods to resolve this problem. Accordingly, the approach to new surgical methods for the correction of irregular astigmatism is one of the greatest expectations in today's refractive surgery, especially when the very near future is supposed to bring generalization of corneal refractive surgical techniques.

ETIOLOGY OF IRREGULAR ASTIGMATISM

Primary Idiopathic

There is a general prevalence of low levels of irregular astigmatism of unknown cause within the population. This might explain the mildly reduced best-corrected visual acuity (BCVA) in patients presenting for laser vision correction.[1]

Secondary

Dystrophic

In the cornea, keratoconus, which, in optical terms, is primarily an irregularity of the anterior corneal surface, is the best example. Pelucid degeneration and keratoglobus may also be associated with posterior corneal surface irregularity causing irregular astigmatism. In the lens, lenticonus may cause irregular astigmatism; and in the retina, posterior staphyloma.[1]

185

Traumatic

Corneal irregularity is caused commonly by corneal wounds (incision or excision) or burns (chemical, thermal or electrical).[1]

Postinfective

Postherpetic keratitits is the most common form of postkeratitic healing and scarring that may lead to an irregular surface.[1]

Postsurgical

Irregular corneal astigmatism can complicate any of the following refractive surgical procedures: keratoplasty, photorefractive keratectomy (PRK), laser *in situ* keratomileusis (LASIK), radial keratotomy (RK), arcuate keratotomy (AK), and cataract incisions. Scleral encirclement or external plombage may also contribute.[1]

DIAGNOSIS OF IRREGULAR ASTIGMATISM

Clinically, irregular astigmatism will present with one of those typical **retinoscopy** patterns, the most common being spinning and scissoring of the red reflex. On attempting **keratometry,** the mires will appear distorted. **Corneal topography** shows certain patterns for irregular astigmatism that will be discussed in detail later. The most recent and sophisticated technique is the application of **wavefront analysis (aberrometers)**.[8] This emerging method measures the refractive status of the whole internal ocular light path at selected corneal intercepts of incident light pencils. By comparing the wavefront of a pattern of several small beams of coherent light projected through to the retina with the emerging reflected light wavefront, it is possible to measure the refractive path taken by each beam and to infer the specific spatial correction required on each path.

CLINICAL CLASSIFICATION OF IRREGULAR ASTIGMATISM FOLLOWING CORNEAL REFRACTIVE SURGERY

In corneal refractive surgery using laser *in situ* keratomileusis (LASIK), the surgeon uses a microkeratome, whether automated or manual, to fashion a corneal flap and a stromal bed. Once the flap is fashioned and lifted, the excimer laser is used to ablate tissue from the bed for the planned correction, depending on the capabilities of the laser.

In this clinical prespective, irregular astigmatism induced by LASIK can be classified according to its location as:
1. **Superficial:** due to flap irregularities.
2. **Stromal:** induced by bed irregularities.
3. **Mixed:** due to irregularities in both flap and stroma.

CORNEAL TOPOGRAPHY PATTERNS OF IRREGULAR ASTIGMATISM

Topographic classification of irregular astigmatism patterns is very important in the following aspects:

1. To unify terms and concepts when referring to corneal topography images.
2. To determine the cause of the subjective symptoms referred by the patient (haloes, glare, monocular diplopia, etc.).
3. Reaching a topographic basis for retreatment. The topographic approach for treatment patients with a previous unsuccessful excimer laser surgery should allow reshaping the cornea in the pattern appropriate for the specific patient.

Based on the topography, we proposed the following classification for irregular astigmatism:[7]

- **Irregular astigmatism with defined pattern,** and
- **Irregular astigmatism with undefined pattern.**

Irregular Astigmatism with Defined Pattern

We define irregular astigmatism with defined pattern when there is a steep or flat area of at least 2 mm of diameter, at any location of the corneal topography, which is the main cause of the irregular astigmatism. It is divided into five groups:

A. **Decentered Ablation:** Shows a corneal topographic pattern with decentered myopic ablation in more than 1.5 mm in relation to the center of the cornea. The flattening area is not centered in the center of the cornea; the optical zone of the cornea has one flat and one steep area (Figure 14.1A).

B. **Decentered Steep:** Shows a corneal hyperopic treatment decentered in more than 1.5 mm in relation to the center of the cornea (Figure 14.1B).

C. **Central island:** Shows an image with an increase in the central power of the ablation zone for myopic treatment ablation at least 3.00 D and 1.5 mm in diameter, surrounded by areas of lesser curvature (Figure 14.1C).

D. **Central irregularity:** Shows an irregular pattern with more than one area not larger than 1.0mm and no more than 1.50 D in relationship with the flattest radius, located into the area of the myopic ablation treatment (Figure 14.1D).

E. **Peripheral irregularity:** It is a corneal topographic pattern, similar to central island, extending to the periphery. The myopic ablation is not homogeneous, there is a central zone measuring 1.5 mm in diameter and 3.00 D in relation to the flattest radius, connected with the periphery of the ablation zone in one meridian (Figure 14.1E).

Irregular Astigmatism with Undefined Pattern

We consider irregular astigmatism with undefined pattern when the image shows a surface with multiple irregularities; big and small steep and flat areas, defined as more than one area measuring more than 3 mm in diameter in the central 6 mm (Figure 14.1F). The differential between flat and steep areas were not possible to calculate in the Profile Map and Dk showed an irregular line or a plane line. Normally, Dk is the difference between the steep k and the flat k, given in diopters at the cross of the profile map. A

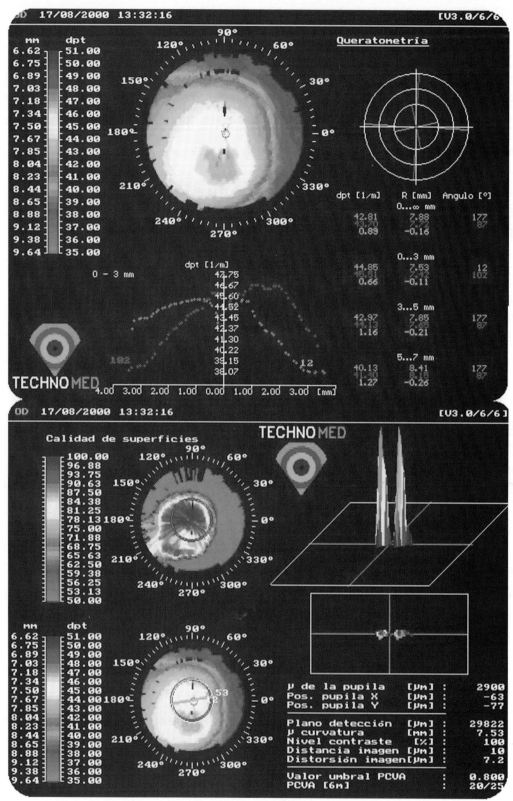

FIGURE 14.1A

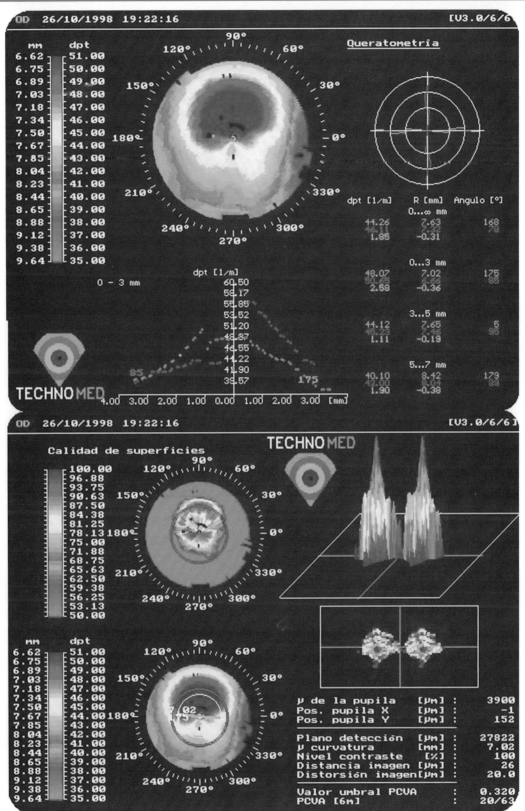

FIGURE 14.1B

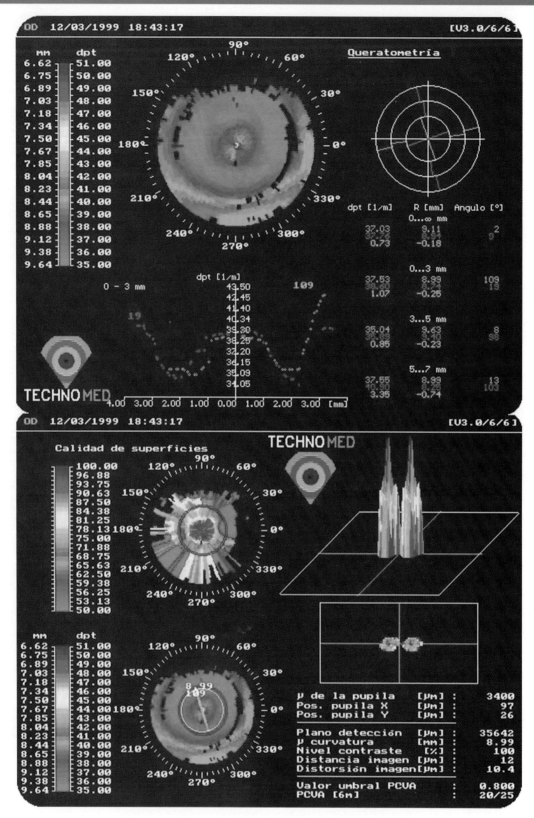

FIGURE 14.1C

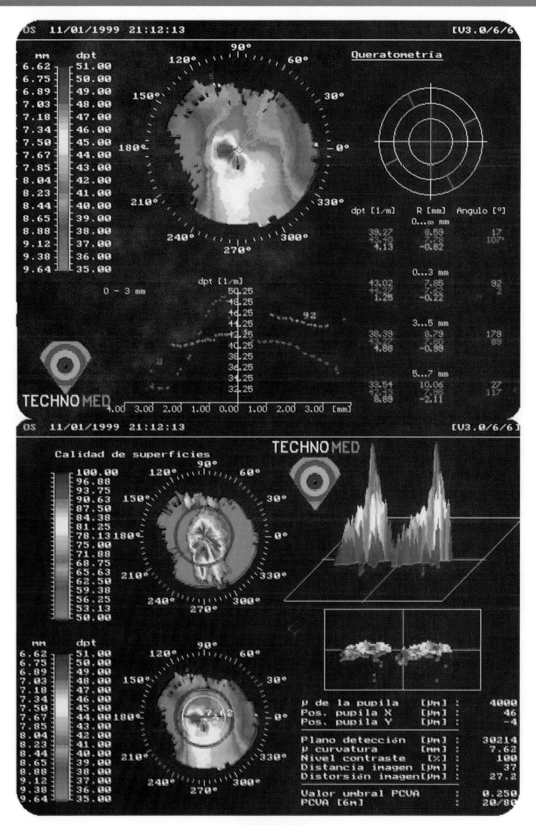

FIGURE 14.1D

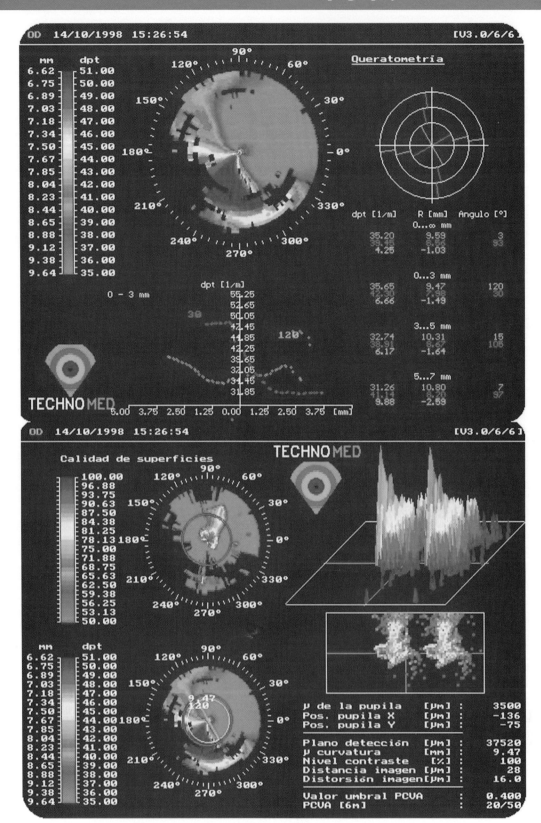

FIGURE 14.1E

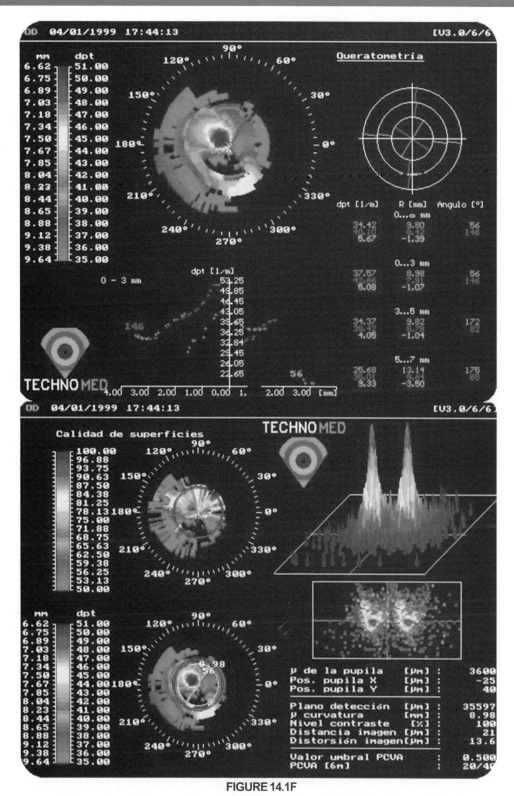

FIGURE 14.1F

FIGURES 14.1A to F: Topographic patterns of irregular astigmatism (with ray tracing study):
A. Decentered ablation, **B.** Decentered steep, **C.** Central Island, **D.** Central irregularity,
E. Peripheral irregularity, **F.** Irregular astigmatism with undefined pattern

plane line is produced when the Dk cannot recognize the difference between the steep k and the flat k in severe corneal surface irregularities.

EVALUATION OF IRREGULAR ASTIGMATISM

In managing irregular astigmatism patients, a meticulous preoperative evaluation is necessary. We perform a complete preoperative ocular examination, including previous medical reports and complete ocular examination: uncorrected and best-corrected visual acuity, pinhole visual acuity and cycloplegic refraction, keratometry, contact ultrasonic pachymetry (Ophthasonic Pachymeter Teknar Inc. St. Louis, USA) and computerized corneal topography.

We perform the corneal topography with Eye Sys 2000 Corneal Analysis System (Eye Sys Co., Houston, Texas, USA). We also use the Ray Tracing mode of the C-SCAN Color-Ellipsoid-Topometer (Technomed GmbH, Germany) to determine the Superficial Corneal Surface Quality (SCSQ) and the Predicted Corneal Visual Acuity (PCVA), in addition to the topography. Recently, we have incorporated the elevation topography of the Orbscan system (Orbtek, Bausch & Lomb, Surgical, Orbscan II Corneal Topography, Salt Lake City, Utah, USA) in our evaluation tools.

Follow-up examinations after surgery were performed at 48 hours, and then at one, three and six months. Postoperative follow-up included: uncorrected and best-corrected visual acuity, pinhole visual acuity and cycloplegic refraction, biomicroscopy with slit-lamp and complete corneal topography screening with the previously mentioned instrumentation.

During the preoperative and postoperative, period the surface quality of the cornea was studied using the Ray Tracing module of the C-SCAN 3.0 (Technomed GmbH, Germany). This device determines the Predicted Corneal Visual Acuity from the videokeratography map, by simulating the propagation of rays emanating from 2 light dots, which impinge on the best-fit image plane after projection via the maximum of 10,800 previously determined corneal surface power values. Refraction and reflection of the rays at the optical interfaces, the pupil diameter, and the anterior chamber depth are taken into account according to laws of geometric optics. The Ray Tracing module calculates the pupil size by the captured image of the pupil during videokeratography. This is measured under the luminance of the videokeratography rings (25.5 cd/m^2) and is automatically integrated into the Ray Tracing analysis with the videokeratography map. Hence, the projection of objects onto a detection plane can be determined. The Ray Tracing module calculates the optical function of the eye by means of optical Ray Tracing, using the cornea as the refractive element of the system. It measured and analyzed the interaction between the corneal shape, the functional optical zone, and the pupil diameter, providing valuable additional information by the resulting diagram. The image points on the detection plane are represented by two intensity peaks that must be spatially resolved to discriminate them separately and individually. The peak distance (distance between the functional maxima) and the distortion index (basic diameter of the point cloud in the detection plane) are parameters defined to help understanding when these two peaks are spatially resolved. They help to objectively quantify the individual retinal image in each subject. We found it very useful to evaluate the corneal surface and corneal healing. It is very useful also to explain visual phenomena referred by the patients, and that cannot be explained by older versions of corneal topographers. We do not consider it a substitution of the EyeSys 2000 Corneal Analysis System (Houston, Texas, USA), but it showed to be a very useful tool.[9]

Subjective symptoms from the pre- and postoperative periods should be noted in the medical report such as haloes, glare, dazzling, corneal and conjunctival dryness, dark-light adaptation and visual satisfaction reported by the patient.

TREATMENT OF IRREGULAR ASTIGMATISM

Treatment options for irregular astigmatism have expanded greatly during recent years. Excimer laser is gaining priority with the advent of finely controlled corneal ablation. Before that, limited alteration of corneal topography was possible by, for instance, selective incision placement, placement and removal of sutures, or penetrating and lamellar keratoplasty. Other "treatment" options for irregular corneal astigmatism include optical correction with hard contact lenses in which the tear fluid layer under the contact lens "evens out"' the irregularity,[1] but the patient's aim to get rid of glasses as well as contact lenses still limits their use. Intracorneal ring segments, originally used for myopia treatment,[10] represent another option that is under investigation.

SURGICAL TECHNIQUES WITH EXCIMER LASER

These represent the main subject of discussion in this chapter. The ultimate goal excimer laser treatment is to correct the refractive error while reducing corneal astigmatism and topographic disparity but not increasing aberrations within the eye. With the advent of the excimer laser, it may be possible to correct directly some forms of corneal irregularity. Before considering any treatment option, the relationship between the topographical irregularity and the refraction must be considered; a therapeutic balance between refractive and corneal astigmatism must be reached so that overall visual function is optimal. In other words, an optimal treatment should include both topographic and refractive values, rather than excluding one.[1]

We have used different methods for the surgical correction of irregular astigmatism. At this moment, we consider three surgical procedures with excimer laser for correction of the irregular astigmatism:

1. **Selective Zonal Ablation (SELZA):** Designed to improve the irregular astigmatism with defined pattern.[7]

2. **Excimer Laser Assisted by Sodium Hyaluronate (ELASHY):** Designed mainly to improve the irregular astigmatism with undefined pattern.[11]

3. **Topographic Linked excimer laser ablation (TOPOLINK):** Combines data of the topography and patient refraction in as software to improve the irregular astigmatism with defined pattern and the refractive error, with the same procedure.[12]

The three surgical procedures were performed under topical anesthesia of Oxibuprocaine 0.2% (Prescaina 0,2%; Laboratorios Llorens, Barcelona, Spain) drops; no patient required sedation. The postoperative treatment consisted of instillation of topical tobramycin 0.3% and dexamethasone 0.1%

drops (Tobradex, Alcon-Cusi, Barcelona, Spain) three times daily for the five days of the follow-up and then discontinued. When the ablation was performed onto the cornea (surface ELASHY, some patients of SELZA), a bandage contact lens (Actifresh 400, power +0.5, diameter 14.3 mm, radius of curvature 8.8 mm – Hydron Ltd., Hampshire, UK) was used during the first three days of the post-operative and the patient was examined daily. It was removed when complete re-epithelialization was observed. Then treatment with topical fluorometholone (FML forte, Alcon-Cusi, Barcelona, Spain) was used three times daily for the three months of follow-up and then stopped.[13]

Non-preserved artificial tears (Sodium Hyaluronate 0.18%, Vislubeâ, CHEMEDICA, Ophthalmic line, München, Germany) were used up to three months in every case. Supplementation with oral pain management medications was also used as necessary.

Statistical Analysis. Statistical Analysis was performed with the SPSS/Pc+4.0 for Windows (SPSS Inc, Madrid, 1996). Measurements typically are reported as the mean $\pm$ 1 standard deviation [using $(n-1)^{1/2}$ in the denominator of the definition for standard deviation, where n is the number of observations for each measurement] and as the range of all measurements at each follow-up visit. Patients' data samples were fitting the normal distribution curves. Statistically significant differences between data sample means were determined by the "t Student's" test; p values less than 0.05 were considered significant. Data concerning the standards for reporting the outcome of refractive surgery procedures, as the safety, efficacy and predictability, was analyzed as previously defined.[14]

Selective Zonal Ablation (SELZA)

In this study, we report the results of a prospective clinically controlled study performed on 31 eyes of 26 patients with irregular astigmatism induced by refractive surgery. All cases were treated with SELZA using an excimer laser of broad circular beam (Visx Twenty/Tweenty, 4.02, Visx, Inc. Sunnyvale, California, USA). The surgical planning was applied using the Munnerlyn formula,[15] modified by Buzard,[16] to calculate the depth of the ablation depending on the amount of correction desired and the ablation zone. In this formula, the resection depth is equal to the dioptric correction, divided by 3, and multiplied by the ablation zone (mm) squared. We used a correction factor of 1.5 times, to avoid undercorrection:

$$\text{Ablation depth} = \frac{(\text{Dioptric correction}) \times 1.5}{3} \times (\text{ablation zone})^2$$

Methods

In general, we use ablation zone of 2.5 to 3.0 mm, depending on the steep area of the corneal topography to be modified. The ablation zone was determined by observing the color map. The form of videokeratoscope provides additional information about the irregular zones, and the profile map gave the values for performed ablation. In cases of irregular corneal surface, treatment was performed on the center of irregularity, which was located using the color map of the corneal topography. First we located the center of the cornea, then we located the exact center of irregularity. Here, we use the dotted boxes in the map (each dot represents 1 mm^2) to detect the exact center of irregularity in relation to the center of the cornea. The amount of ablation is determined using the cross section of the profile map (vertical line corresponding to diopters and horizontal line corresponding to corneal diameter). When the patient had LASIK previously, we lift the flap or we do a new LASIK cut and after we perform excimer laser using PTK mode.

The technique is based on subtraction of tissues to eliminate the induced irregular astigmatism and to achieve a uniform corneal surface using excimer laser; we center the effect of laser on zones where the corneal surface is steeper.

Results

In patients with *irregular astigmatism with a defined pattern*, the visual acuity improved significantly, reaching in many cases near the BCVA before the initial refractive procedure. The difference between the BCVA before the therapeutic procedure was highly statistically significant ($p < 0.001$). The mean BCVA after 3 months of surgery it was 20/25 ± 20/100 (range 20/50–20/20), which was as good as the initial BCVA 20/29 ± 20/100 (range 20/50–20/20). The BCVA before selective ablation improved from 20/40 ± 20/100 (range 20/100–20/25) to 20/25 ± 20/100 (range 20/50–20/20). We did not have any patients with one or more lines lost of BCVA. The **Corneal Uniformity Index** (CUI) before versus after selective zonal ablation with excimer laser improved from 55.65 ± 15.90% (range 20–80%) to 87.83 ± 10.43 percent (range 70–100), a change that was also statistically significant ($p < 0.005$). The **safety index** (the ratio of mean postoperative BCVA over mean preoperative BCVA) was equal to 1.55. The **efficacy** of the procedure in percent UCVA 20/40 was 85 percent.

The **predictability** (astigmatic correction) using CUI was expressed as a percentage. The various relationships between the preoperative CUI and the surgically induced postoperative CUI provided the information about the magnitude of irregular astigmatism correction and the corneal surface uniformity. Correction index, which is the ratio of mean postoperative CUI (87.83 ± 10.43%; range, 70–100%) over the mean preoperative CUI (55.65 ± 15.90%; range, 20–80%), was equal to 1.58.

The results observed in all cases of *irregular astigmatism without a defined pattern* were poor. **Efficacy** in percentage of eyes with UCVA of 20/40 was 6 percent, and **predictability** (astigmatic correction) was 0.58. In some cases, visual acuity became worse: the refraction error and corneal topography were considerably modified.

Discussion

The results of the selective zonal ablations technique were satisfactory as regards the correction of irregular astigmatism with a defined topographic pattern. Visual acuity improved in the postoperative period, achieving values near the initial BCVA of the patients (before the initial surgical procedure). The corneal uniformity index was used to evaluate the central 3 mm zone of the cornea. It started to improve in the early postoperative period and stabilized after 3 months, just as the issues of visual acuity ($p<0.005$). Normally, this refractive procedure requires a stable corneal topography (6 months after the last corneal procedure) and its adequate interpretation.[17] However, our results have proven that it is not suitable for correcting all patterns of irregular astigmatism.

Excimer LASER Associated by Sodium Hyaluronate (ELASHY)

This can be considered as one of the ablatable masking techniques. We report the results of a prospective clinically controlled study performed on 32 eyes of 32 patients with irregular astigmatism.[11] All the patients had been subjected previously to one or more of the following procedures: LASIK, incisional keratotomy, photorefractive keratotomy, phototherapeutic keratotomy, laser thermokeratoplasty, and corneal trauma. Irregular astigmatism was induced thereafter.

Six months after the last corneal procedure, for the aim of stability, the cases were selected for ELASHY.

Methods

The correction of irregular astigmatism was made with a Plano Scan Technolas 217 C-LASIK Scanning-spot Excimer laser (Bausch & Lomb), CHIRON Technolas GmbH, Doranch, Germany) in PTK mode, assisted by viscous masking sodium hyaluronate 0.25% solution (LASERVIS® CHEMEDICA, Ophthalmic line, München, Germany). The physical characteristics of sodium hyaluronate confer important rheological properties to the product. The photoablation rate is similar to that of corneal tissue, forming a stable and uniform coating on the surface of the eye, filling depressions on the cornea and effectively masking tissues to be protected against ablation by the laser pulses.[18,19]

In cases where the irregular astigmatism was induced by a flap irregularity or superficial corneal scarring, ELASHY ablations were performed onto the corneal surface. The epithelium was removed also using the excimer laser assisted by viscous masking. When the irregularity was inside the stroma, at the previous stromal bed, the previous flap was lifted up whenever possible or a new cut was done. Then ELASHY was performed at the stroma and after the procedure the flap was repositioned.

We centered the ablation area at the corneal center and fixed it with the eye-tracking device in the center of the pupillary area. After this, one drop of the viscous masking and fluorescein was scattered on the cornea that should be ablated and spread out with the 23-G cannula (Alcon laboratories, USA) used for the viscous substance instillation. With fluorescein, it was also possible to observe the spot and the effect of laser. Because fluorescent light is emitted during ablation of corneal tissue, cessation of the fluorescence signifies complete removal of the viscous masking solution, i.e. tissue ablation. The laser was prepared for ablation at 15 microns intervals. After each of the intervals, a new drop of the viscous substance was added at the center of the ablation area and again spread out with the same maneuvers with the 23-G cannula. Total treatment was calculated to ablate the prominent areas to the calculated K-value at the 4 to 6 mm optical zone or calculated from the tangential map of the Technomed topographer. Assuming a decrease in the ablative effect of the laser due to the use of the viscous agent, we target at a 50 percent more ablation than the one that corresponds to the real ablation depth necessary for the smoothing procedure.

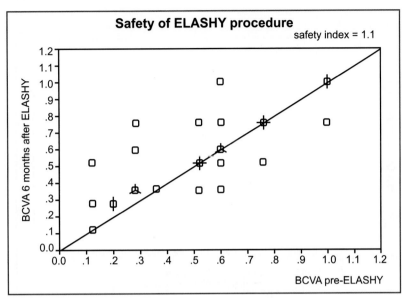

FIGURE 14.2: Safety of ELASHY procedure

Results

Corneal topography corresponded to our established classification of irregular astigmatism: pattern irregular corneal astigmatism was identified in 23 eyes (71.9%) and irregularly irregular corneal astigmatism was identified in the other 9 eyes (28.1%).

The mean preoperative BCVA improved from 20/40 ± 20/80 (range 20/200 to 20/20) to 20/32 ± 20/100 (range 20/200 to 20/20) ($p = 0.013$, Student t test), six months after surgery. There were only 2 eyes losing 2 lines of BCVA (6.3%) and 3 eyes (9.4%) losing 1 line. The procedure was safe with a **safety index** equal to 1.1 (Figure 14.2).

We had 28.1 percent of eyes at 6 months with postoperative UCVA of 20/40 or better with 3.1 percent reaching 20/20. The **efficacy index** of the procedure [*the ratio (mean postoperative UCVA) / (mean preoperative BCVA)*], was equal to 0.74.

As ELASHY is based on the subtraction of tissues to achieve a smoother corneal surface, we expected improvement in the patients' BCVA and subjective symptoms as glare, haloes, etc. rather than changes in the spherical equivalent. The astigmatic correction was evaluated in respect to the improvement of the corneal surface, using the data of the SCSQ provided by the Ray Tracing study (C-SCAN Color-Ellipsoid-Topometer, Technomed GmbH, Germany). The SCSQ (Figure 14.3) pre- vs. post-therapeutic procedure, evaluated by the Ray Tracing study, improved from a mean of 69.38 percent ± 9.48 preoperatively to 73.13 percent ± 8.87, 6 months postoperative ($p = 0.002$, Student t test). Other parameters of the Ray Tracing study also improved. The PCVA improved from a mean of 20/40 ± 20/80 (range 20/100 to 20/16) preoperatively to 20/32 ± 20/80 (range 20/125 to 20/16) ($p = 0.11$, Student t test) postoperatively. Also, the image distortion significantly improved from a mean of 14.39 ± 3.78 (range 8 to 23.2) preoperatively to 13.29 ± 3.87 (range 7.2 to 26) at 6 months ($p = 0.05$, Student t test).

199

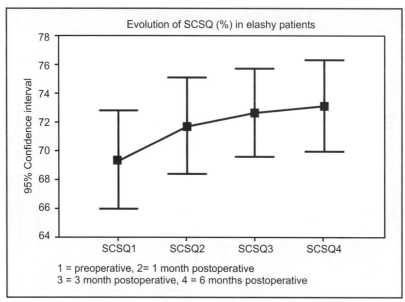

FIGURE 14.3: Evolution of superficial corneal surface quality (SCSQ)

The corneal surface was left smooth. Almost all patients (89.3%) subjectively noted improvement of the visual acuity and disappearance of the visual aberrations that previously impaired their quality of vision. This coincided with the improvement in the peak distortion and the Ray Tracing (Figure 14.4).

Discussion

The results of this study could add the excimer laser plano Scan surgery assisted by sodium hyaluronate 0.25% (LASERVIS® CHEMEDICA, Ophthalmic line, München, Germany) (ELASHY) to the tools useful for the treatment of irregular astigmatism, both with and without defined pattern. The clinical indications include irregular astigmatism caused by irregularity in flap or irregularity on stromal base induced by laser *in situ* keratomileusis (LASIK).

Excimer laser application in PTK mode may be undertaken to improve various visual symptoms through improving the corneal surface.[20, 21] PTK also can help in cases of irregularities and opacities on corneal surface or anterior stroma, induced by LASIK. In 1994, Gibralter and Trokel applied excimer laser in PTK mode to treat a surgically induced irregular astigmatism in two patients. They used the corneal topographic maps to plan focal treatment areas with good results.[5] The correction of irregular astigmatism should be considered in one of these therapeutic indications.

The use of a viscous masking agent should increase the efficiency of the procedure, through protection of the valleys between the irregular corneal peaks, leaving these peaks of pathology exposed to laser treatment. In this study, we used the sodium hyaluronate 0.25% (LASERVIS® CHEMEDICA, Ophthalmic line, München, Germany) for this purpose. When the treatment is performed on corneal surface, Bowman's membrane is removed. However, the new epithelium was able to grow and adhere well to the residual stroma. Interestingly, none of our patients developed significant postoperative haze (grade II–III)—normally seen after PRK—even those subjected to surface treatment. We suggest this effect

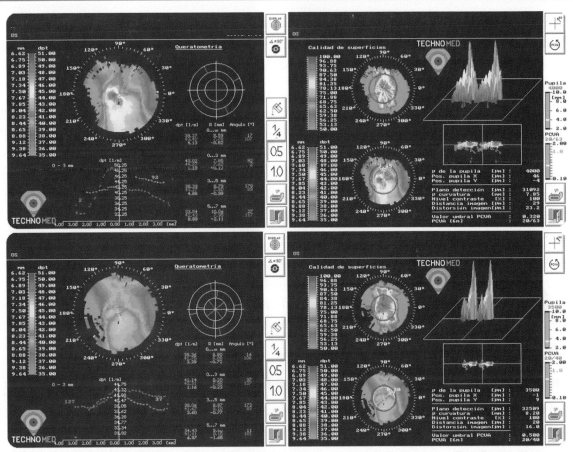

FIGURE 14.4: ELASHY: Preoperative (a) and postoperative (b) corneal topography with Raytracing; note the improvement of the Raytracing.

could be due to the protective properties of the viscoelastic agent, sodium hyaluronate 0.25% (LASERVIS® CHEMEDICA, Ophthalmic line, München, Germany), against the oxidative free radical tissue damage.[22]

Many authors have evaluated different masking agents.[18,19] Methylcellulose is the most commonly used agent and is available in different concentrations. Some properties of the methylcellulose, such as to turn white during ablation due to its low boiling point, make this substance not ideal for the purpose of this study.

We found sodium hyaluronate 0.25% (LASERVIS® CHEMEDICA, Ophthalmic line, München, Germany) the most suitable for our purpose. It has a photoablation rate similar to that of the corneal tissue. Its stability on the corneal surface forms a uniform coating that fills the depressions on the cornea, protecting them against ablation by the laser pulses.[18] Adding fluorescein to the viscous masking solution is very useful to observe the excimer laser action during corneal ablation at the corneal surface. With experience, it is very easy to distinguish between the ablated areas (in dark) and the marked areas (in green) while the laser radiation is ablating the cornea during the treatment.

The actual corneal ablation is equal to 63 percent of the ablation depth programmed in the software of the excimer laser.[23] If the corneal surface has a masking agent, the initial effect of the laser will be ablating the viscous masking.

The viscous masking solution functions to shield the tissues partially. Multiple applications of viscous masking solution often are required, and a familiarity with the ablation characteristics will be learned with experience. When the laser ablation is performed on corneal surface, we increase the ablation by 50 mm, necessary for the epithelium ablation.[24]

ELASHY was originally designed for the correction of those irregular astigmatism cases that did not show a pattern and were not available to SELZA correction, yet it proved to be as effective in cases with pattern irregular astigmatism.

Ray Tracing improved considerably, coinciding with the improvement of the visual subjective symptoms. The superficial corneal surface quality and image distortion were improved, achieving values significantly better than the preoperative values. This demonstrates that a relationship exists between the quality of the corneal surface and the quality of the vision. When the corneal surface is smoothened, the haloes, glare and refractive symptoms improve.[25]

From our results, we can also conclude that the procedure achieves more stability with time, improving from the 3rd to the 6th months. Further follow-up of these cases should be carried on to obtain better judgment of the biomechanical response of these special corneas to the procedure and to decide a proper timing for a re-intervention if necessary.

Topographic Linked Excimer Laser Ablation (TOPOLINK)

About forty percent of human corneas show some irregularities that cannot be taken into account in a standard basis treatment with excimer laser.[26] For these patients, and for those suffering an irregular astigmatism after trauma or refractive surgery, a custom-tailored, topography-based ablation, which has been adapted to the corneal irregularity, would be the best approach to improve not only their refractive problem but also to improve their quality of vision.

This treatment was the first step in customized ablation depending mainly on the corneal topography as well as the refraction for calculating the treatment. It aimed at obtaining the best-corrected visual acuity that can be attained by wearing hard contact lenses. Its requirements were an excimer laser with spot scanning technology, in which a small laser spot delivers a multitude of single shots fired in diverse positions to fashion the desired ablation profile. The laser spot is programmable, thus any profile could be obtained. A videokeratography system that provides an elevation map at high resolution is needed, and specific software is used to create a customized ablation program for the spot scanner laser.

Methods

The aim of this study was to fashion a regular corneal surface in 41 eyes of 41 patients with irregular astigmatism induced by LASIK: 27 eyes (51.9%) had irregular astigmatism with a defined pattern; 14 eyes (48.1%) had irregular astigmatism without a defined pattern.

All cases were treated with a Plano Scan Technolas 217 C-LASIK Scanning-spot Excimer laser (Bausch & Lomb), Chiron Technolas GmbH, Doranch, Germany) assisted by a C-SCAN Color-Ellipsoid-Topometer (Technomed GmbH, Germany). We performed several corneal topographies from same eye; the software of the automated corneal topographer selected the four exactly equal. These corneal maps, the refractive error, the pachymetry value and desired K-readings calculated for each patient were sent to Technolas by modem. The information was analyzed and a special software program for each patient was created, including it in the Technolas 217 C-LASIK excimer laser by system modem.

The basis for the topography-assisted procedure was the preoperative topography.[12,27] This data was transferred into true height data and the treatment for correcting the refractive values in sphere and astigmatism, taking into account the corneal irregularities, was calculated. After that, a postoperative topography was simulated. With this technique, real customized treatment should become a reality, not only treating the refractive error but also improving the patient's visual acuity.

Results

After 3 months of the surgery: The mean preoperative UCVA improved from 20/80 ±0.25 (range 20/400–20/60) to 20/40±0.54 (range 20/100–20/32); mean preoperative BCVA improved from 20/60±0.20 (range 20/200–20/32) to 20/32±0.15 (range 20/60–20/25). This proved to be statistically significant (p<0.001).

Even though emmetropia was our goal, it was considered more important to achieve a regular corneal surface. The spherical equivalent of the individual refraction was taken into account in determining the corneal K-value. Preoperatively, mean sphere was –0.26 ±4.50 D (range –5.75 to +3.70 D) and mean cylinder was –1.71±3.08 D (range –6.00 to +2.56 D). Three months after surgery, the mean sphere was 0.70±1.25 D (range –1.75 to +1.50 D) and the mean cylinder was –0.89±1.00 D (range –1.92 to +1.00).

Corneal topography improved significantly in those cases that presented an irregular astigmatism with a defined pattern. The mean corneal surface quality improved from 45 percent (range 35–60%) to 76.6 percent (range 60.06–96.43%). The corneal surface is left smooth and the Ray Tracing improved in the peak distortion, coinciding with the improvement of the visual acuity (Figure 14.5). In 60.29 percent patients, the visual aberrations disappeared.

At 3 months of follow-up, the **safety** of the procedure was 74.31%, the **efficacy** (Figure 14.6) in percent UCVA 20/40 was 63.68 percent and the **predictability** for the spherical equivalent within the ± 1 D zone was 68.23 percent.

Discussion

Using the corneal topographic map as a guide, excimer laser ablation can be used to create a more regular surface with improved visual acuity. In a program consisting of a combination of phototherapeutic and photorefractive ablation patterns, the amount of tissue to be removed is calculated on the basis of the diameter and steepness of the irregular areas of the corneal surface. At present, customized ablation based on topography can improve spectacle-corrected visual acuity.

Limitations for this technique exist. With this procedure, some irregular astigmatisms cannot be corrected. Some patients could not be selected as candidates for Topolink because any of the following criteria were present:

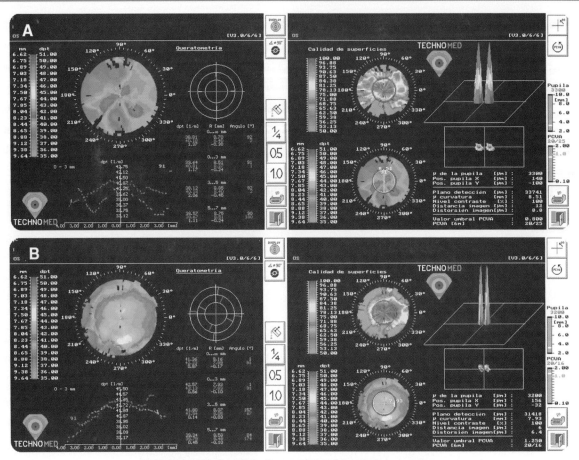

FIGURE 14.5: Topolink: Preoperative **A** and postoperative
B corneal topography with ray tracing

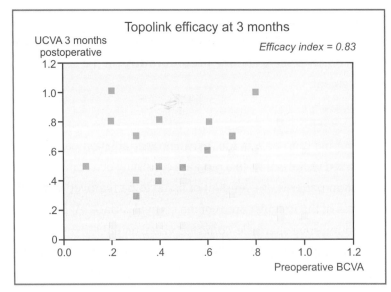

FIGURE 14.6: Safety of the Topolink procedure at 3 months

1. Different between steep and flat meridians more than 10 D at the 6.0 mm treatment area.
2. Corneal pachymetry was not thick enough (< 400 mm).
3. Diameter of the corneal topography more than 5.0 mm.
4. Corneal topography showing an irregular astigmatism with undefined pattern (irregularly irregular).

This preliminary study showed that topographic-assisted LASIK (Topolink) could be a useful tool to treat irregular astigmatism. This technique was, as aforementioned, the early stage of developing customized ablation. The surgeon depends only on the Placido topographic images, their precision and their reproducibility. To the moment, this cannot provide us with the actual customization and we are still left with some patients waiting for a solution.

THE FUTURE

A new view of customization could be achieved with more reliable instruments (elevation topography, aberrometer, etc.). As aforementioned, wavefront analysis (aberrometry, Figure 14.7) can measure the refractive state of the entire internal ocular light path.[8] Using this technology, it has been shown that using only the refractive error of the eye to treat the ammetropia can greatly increase optical aberrations within the eye.[28] Increases in wavefront aberrations are evident after both PRK and LASIK,[29] and increased spherical aberration has been shown to occur in cases of increased corneal astigmatism.[30] This increase in spherical aberration and coma will interfere with visual function, particularly in low-light conditions where the pupil size increases, increasing the effect of aberrations within the eye, a condition that is diminished in the day light where the pupil constricts.[31]

We are now conducting the second phase of a study incorporating the data of the wafefront analysis using the ZyWave aberrometer (Bausch & Lomb, CHIRON Technolas GmbH, Doranch, Germany) together with the elevation topography of the Orbscan II (Orbtek, Bausch & Lomb, Surgical, Orbscan II corneal topography, Salt Lake City, Utah, USA) to correct ametropia.

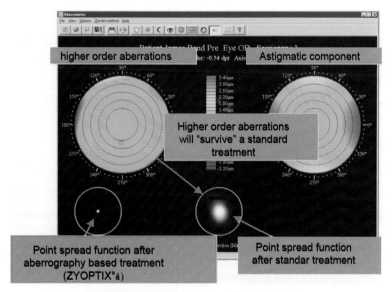

FIGURE 14.7: Aberrometry, clinical example

To the moment, the system is under trial, and is only applicable to regular virgin corneas. With the proper development of the technique, we think that it would provide us with the real customized ablation necessary not only for our desperate irregular astigmatism patients but also for obtaining a super-vision for ametropes who are to be treated for the first time.

OTHER PROCEDURES

Automated Anterior Lamellar Keratoplasty

This technique was originally designed to treat superficial stromal disorders, but it has also been used for the treatment of difficult cases of irregular astigmatism, with very poor results.[32] The surgeon performs phototherapeutic keratectomy or a microkeratome lamellar resection to 250 to 400 mm stromal depth, followed by trasplantation of a donor lamella of the same dimension on to the recipient bed.[33] We have limited experience with this subject. We think it is a good option for patients with thin corneas, and with the preservation of the Descemet's membrane, the complications of rejection should be extremely minimized if not eliminated. However, the subject is out of the scope of discussion in this chapter.

Intracorneal Ring Segments (Intacs)

These segments were originally designed to correct low-to-moderate myopia by inducing flattening of the central cornea through intralamellar insertion of 2 PMMA ring segments in the corneal midperiphery.[34] Studies indicated that the range of corneal asphericity before and after surgery, provided good visual acuity and normal contrast sensitivity.[10, 35] These segments could be used to modify the corneal surface in patients with irregular astigmatism whether natural as in keratoconous or surgically induced.

Contact Lens Management

Contact lenses are sometimes needed in the postoperative management of refractive surgery. This need arises as it has become evident to the refractive surgeon that an undesirable result has occurred. The decision of contact lens fitting has to be based on the impossibility of performing new surgeries, or the willing of the patient.[36]

SUMMARY

It is clear from the previous discussions that the subject of irregular astigmatism is still under investigation. In spite of the availability of various methods attempting to solve this problem, we are left with patients who are not satisfied with their vision and are in need for intervention. Penetrating keratoplasty is an ultimate solution that has to be undertaken only when the patient has no other alternative. More effort should be done to try to help these patients improving their corneal surface quality and BCVA. The evolution of newer techniques and the experience gained by refractive surgeons day after day represent a hope for irregular astigmatism patients.

REFERENCES

1. Goggin M, Alpins N, Schmid LM. Management of irregular astigmatism. Curr Opin Ophthalmol 2000; 11: 260-266

2. Alió JL, Artola A, Claramonte PJ, et al. Complications of photorefractive keratectomy for myopia: two year follow-up of 3000 cases. J Cataract Refract Surg 1998, 24: 619-26.

3. Azar DT, Strauss I. Principles of applied optics. In: Albert DM, Jakobiec FA (Eds): Principles and Practice of Ophthalmology, Philadelphia, WB Saunders Co, 1994; 5: 3603-3621.

4. Duke-Elder S (Ed). Pathological refractive errors. In System of Ophthalmology. London: Publisher; 1970: 363.

5. Gibralter R, Trokel SL. Correction of irregular astigmatism with the excimer laser. Ophthalmology 1994; 101: 1310-1315.

6. Alpins NA. Treatment of irregular astigmatism. J Cataract Refract Surg 1998; 24: 634-646.

7. Alió JL, Artola A, Rodríguez-Mier FA. Selective Zonal Ablations with excimer laser for correction of irregular astigmatism induced by refractive surgery. Ophthalmology 2000; 107: 662-73.

8. Harris WF. Wavefronts and their propagation in astigmatic optical systems. Optom Vis Sci 1996,73:606–12.

9. Dick HB, Krummenauer F, Schwenn O, et al. Objective and subjective evaluation of photic phenomena after monofocal and multifocal intraocular lens implantation. Ophthalmology 1999; 106: 1878-86

10. Holmes-Higgin DK, Burris TE, and The INTACS Study Group. Corneal surface topography and associated visual performance with INTACS for myopia. Phase III clinical trial results. Ophthalmology 2000; 107: 2061-71.

11. Alio JL, Belda JI, Shalaby AMM. Excimer laser assisted by sodium hyaluronate for correction of irregular astigmatism (ELASHY). Accepted for publication to Ophthalmology, September 2000.

12. Wiesinger-Jendritza B, Knorz M, Hugger P, Liermann A. Laser in situ keratomileusis assisted by corneal topography. J Cataract Surg 1998; 24:166-174

13. Sher NA, Kreuger RR, Teal P, et al. Role of topical corticoids and nonsteroidal anti-inflammatory drugs in the etiology of stromal infiltrates after photorefractive keratectomy. J Refract Corneal Surg 1994; 10:587-588.

14. Koch DD, Kohnen T, Obstbaum SA, Rosen ES. Format for reporting refractive surgical data. [letter]. J Cataract Refract Surg 1998; 24:285-287.

15. Munnerlyn C, Koons S, Marshall J. Photorefractive keratectomy: a technique for laser refractive surgery. J Cataract Refract Surg 1988; 14:46-52.

16. Buzard K, Fundingsland B. Treament of irregular astigmatism with a broad beam excimer laser. J Refract Surg 1997; 13:624-636.

17. Seitz B, Behrens A, Langenbucher A. Corneal topography. Curr Opin Ophthalmol 1997; 8: 8-24.

18. Kornmehl EW, Steiner RF, Puliafito CA. A comparative study of masking fluids for excimer laser phototherapeutic keratectomy. Arch Ophthalmol 1991;109:860-863.

19. Kornmehl EW, Steinert RF, Puliafito CA, Reidy W. Morphology of an irregular corneal surface following 193 nm ArF excimer laser large area ablation with 0.3% hydroxypropyl methylcellulose 2910 and 0.1% dextran 70.1% carboxy-methylcellulose sodium or 0.9% saline (ARVO abstracts). Invest Ophthalmol Vis Sci 1990; 31:245.

20. Trokel S.L, Srinivasan R, Braren B. Excimer laser surgery of the cornea. Am J Ophthalmol 1983; 96:705-710.

21. Orndahl M, Fagerholm P, Fitzsimmons T, Tengroth B. Treatment of corneal dystrophies with excimer laser. Acta Ophthalmol 1994; 72: 235-240.

22. Artola A, Alió JL, Bellot JL, Ruiz JM. Protective properties of viscoelastic substances (sodium hyaluronate and 2% hydroxymethyl cellulose) against experimental free radical damage to the corneal endothelium. Cornea 1993; 12: 109-114.

23. Kreuger RR, Trokel SL. Quantification of corneal ablation by ultraviolet light. Arch Ophthalmol 1986; 103:1741-1742.

24. Seiler T, Bendee T, Wollensak J. Ablation rate of human corneal epithelium and Bowman's layer with the excimer laser (193 nm). J Refract Corneal Surg 1990; 6: 99-102.

25. Klyce SD, Smolek MK. Corneal topography of excimer laser photorefractive keratectomy. J Cataract Refract Surg 1993;19:122-130.

26. Bogan SJ, Waring GO III, Ibrahim O, et al. Classification of normal corneal topography based on computer-assisted videokeratography. Arch Ophthalmol 1990; 108: 945-949.

27. Dausch D, Schröder E, Dausch S. Topography-controlled excimer laser photorefractive keratectomy. J Refract Surg 2000; 16: 13-22.

28. Mierdel P, Kaemmerer M, Krinke H-E, Seiler T. Effects of photorefractive keratectomy and cataract surgery on ocular optical errors of higher order. Graefe's Arch Clin Exp Ophthalmol 1999,237:725–729.

29. Oshika T, Klyce SD, Applegate RA, et al. Comparison of corneal wavefront aberrations after photrefractive keratectomy and laser in situ keratomieusis. Am J Ophthalmol 1999,127:1–7.

30. Seiler T, Reckmann W, Maloney RK. Effective spherical aberration of the cornea as a quantitative descriptor in corneal topography. J Cataract Refract Surg 1993,19(Suppl):155–165.

31. Applegate RA, Howard HC. Refractive surgery, optical aberrations and visual performance. J Refract Surg 1997,13:295–299.

32. Sugita J, Kondo J. Deep lamellar keratoplasty with complete removal of pathological stroma for vision improvement. Br J Ophthalmol 1997; 81: 184-8.

33. Melles GRJ, Remeijer L, Geerards AJM, Beekhuis WH. The future of lamellar keratoplasty. Curr Opin Ophthalmol 1999; 10: 253-259.

34. Ruckhofer J, Stoiber J, Alzner E, Grabner G. Intrastromal corneal ring segments (ICRS, KeraVision Ring, Intacs): clinical outcome after 2 years. Klin Monatsbl Augenheilkd 2000; 216:133-42 (abstract).

35. Holmes-Higgin DK, Baker PC, Burris TE, Silvestrini TA. Characterization of the aspheric corneal surface with intrastromal corneal ring segments. J Refract Surg 1999; 15: 520-8.

36. Zadnik K. Contact lens management of patients who have had unsuccessful refractive surgery. Curr Opin Ophthalmol 1999; 10: 260-263.

Chapter

15

Corneal Ectasia Post-LASIK The Orbscan Advantage

Erik L Mertens
Arun C Gulani
Paul Karpecki

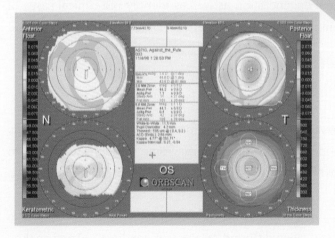

INTRODUCTION

With the advent of corneal topography and its increasing application in practice, our knowledge about the shape of the cornea has rapidly accumulated.[1] Determination of the ability of the cornea to undergo laser refractive surgery is of the utmost importance. The purpose is to avoid corneal ectasia and visual impairment in otherwise healthy eyes. First reported by Prof Theo Seiler[2] this condition is characterized by progressive protuberance and steepening, increasing myopia and or astigmatism with distorted and decreased best corrected vision in the involved eye. Some of the reported cases can be traced back to the preoperative evaluations and lack of recognition for risk factors (Gulani AC: Corneal Topography and Wavefront Instructional Course, ASCRS San Diego, May 2004).

CORNEAL ECTASIA

Postrefractive surgical ectasia was a planned event in automated lamellar keratomileusis for hyperopia where the corneal flap was created at 70% depth to allow for a controlled steepening. This phenomenon has been seen not only with LASIK surgery where the creation of the corneal flap is an additional contributing factor but also with surface photorefractive keratectomy wherein the depth of ablation and repetitive or multiple ablative patterns add to the risk. The most important diagnosis in this direction is that of forme fruste keratoconus.

Over several years data collected in retrospective analysis of post-LASIK ectasias underscores the importance of this diagnosis. These thoughts have been repeatedly addressed but not solved (Gulani AC and Nordan LT—Personal Corresspondence). We shall need to strive to introduce newer and effective measurement criterias and combination technologies to further assist us in this field of obscure clinical findings but drastic postoperative outcomes. Through the years the Orbscan II and orbscan IIZ (Bausch & Lomb) Orbtek, Salt Lake City, Utah) became more and more the standard for preoperative screening amongst refractive surgeons. It is an important diagnostic tool to help separate cases of corneal ectatic disorders like keratoconus and pellucid marginal degeneration as well as identify pre-clinical cases of corneal instability and forme fruste keratoconus (Gulani AC: Advanced Diagnostics Course-B and L-AAO, Washington DC, April 2005).

SELECTION CRITERIA

A lot of these criteria are published throughout the years. Most of the parameters were empirically established by studying the unexpected post-operative ectasia patients. Some surgeons were able to find correlations with preoperative corneal maps and could even quantify abnormal preoperative corneal map findings.[3]

Besides the topographical parameters never forget to look at the clinical signs (fluctuation of subjective refraction, younger patients, history of keratoconus, steep/distorted keratometry readings,…) and analyze the Orbscan maps on the Orbscan IIZ system, NOT ON THE PRINTOUT!!!

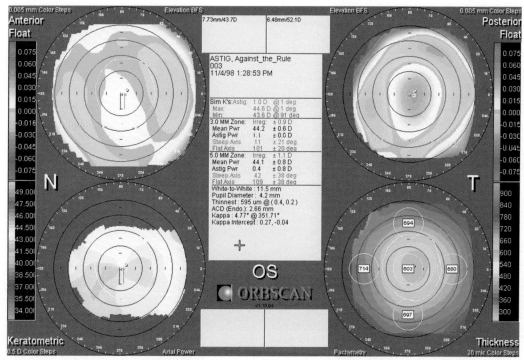

FIGURE 15.1: Typical Quad Map (Orbscan II)

The decision to continue with refractive laser surgery is not based on a single clue, but rather on a combination of a set of criteria. When looking at the Orbscan's Quad Map you can find so called 'red flags' or 'yellow flags'. A 'red flag' definitely means a no-go situation and a 'yellow flag' is suspicious and will drive our attention to look very closely into the other corneal maps. On a typical Quad Map four corneal maps are routinely presented by the Orbscan II (Bausch & Lomb) Orbtek, Salt Lake City, Utah). You will find the anterior elevation map in the upper left quadrant and the posterior elevation map in the upper right quadrant. The keratometric curvature map (power map) is located in the lower left quadrant and the pachymetry[4] map in the lower right quadrant (Figure 15.1). In the center of these four maps a lot of statistics and useful data are displayed.

PACHYMETRY[5]

An absolute contraindication for lamellar corneal laser surgery is a thinnest point of < 470 microns. When pathological, this point is often displaced inferotemporal (Figure 15.2). A difference of <30 microns (yellow flag) or <20 microns (red flag) between the central pachymetry and the peripheral thickness indicators can be seen in abnormal corneas (Figure 15.3). A difference of > 100 microns from the thinnest point to the values at the 7 mm optical zone implies a steep gradient of thinning from the midperiphery towards the thinnest point (yellow flag) (Figure 15.3).

POSTERIOR ELEVATION MAP (FIGURE 15.4)

1. The most common reference surface for viewing elevation maps is the "best fit sphere" (BFS).

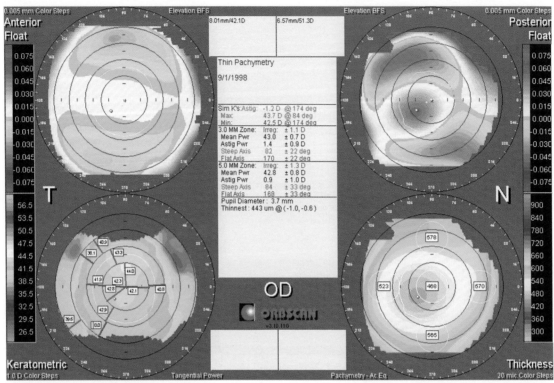

FIGURE 15.2: Thinnest point (443 micron) displaced inferotemporal and a difference of >100 microns from the thinnest point to the values at the 7 mm zone

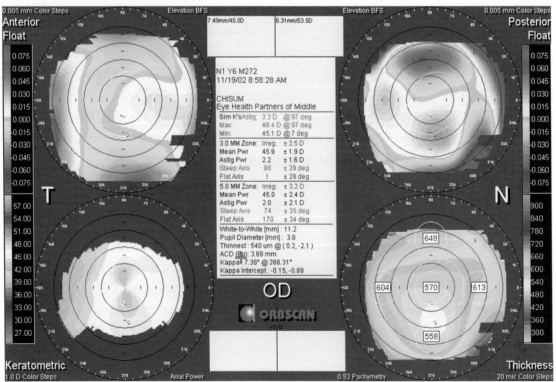

FIGURE 15.3: Abnormal cornea: Less than 20 microns between central pachymetry and peripheral inferior thickness

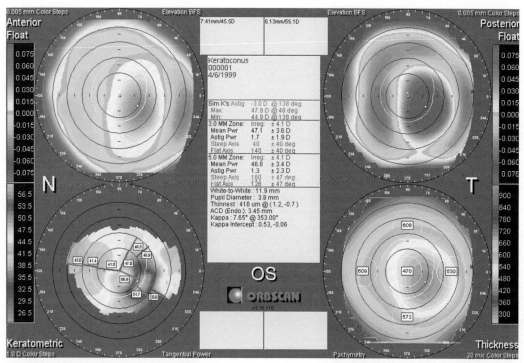

FIGURE 15.4: The posterior elevation map shows multiple red flags. The highest point on the posterior elevation coincides with the highest point on the anterior elevation, the thinnest point on pachymetry, and the point of steepest curvature on the power map

A posterior high point > 50 microns above BFS might be indicative of an early posterior ectasia. However in cylindrical corneas with an astigmatism > 2.5 D this elevation can be induced by the astigmatism and needs to be checked with the other corneal maps (Figure 15.5).

A posterior high point > 35 microns above BFS with corresponding thinning on the pachymetry map is a red flag for LASIK, but not for PRK, LASEK or epi-LASIK.

2. The power of the posterior best fit sphere (BFS) is in normal corneas around 51D. A BFS with a power of more than 55 diopters (Figure 15.4) on the posterior profile, could be indicative of early keratoconus. This criterium is not diagnostic as a sign of early ectasia[6] per se, as this may also be seen in small corneas (WTW<11 mm), very steep corneas or in Asian eyes.

A power between 53 and 54 diopters can be suspicious, and needs to be correlated with other signs and/or symptoms.

3. *Roush criterion*: indicative of early keratoconus is a relative difference > 100 microns between the highest and lowest point on the posterior elevation map (Figure 15.4). A relative difference >70 microns is a yellow flag, except when the cornea is very symmetrical and when it is caused by a regular astigmatism.

POWER MAP

1. Steep corneal curvatures are always suspicious. Keratometric mean power map > 46 diopters or total mean power map > 45 diopters are definitely red flags (Figure 15.6).

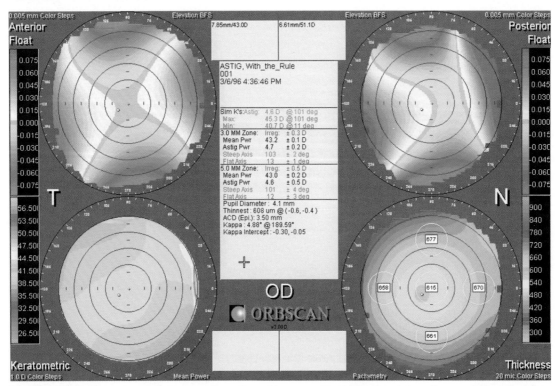

FIGURE 15.5: Normal with-the-rule astigmatism. However, the highest point on the posterior elevation map is > 50 microns

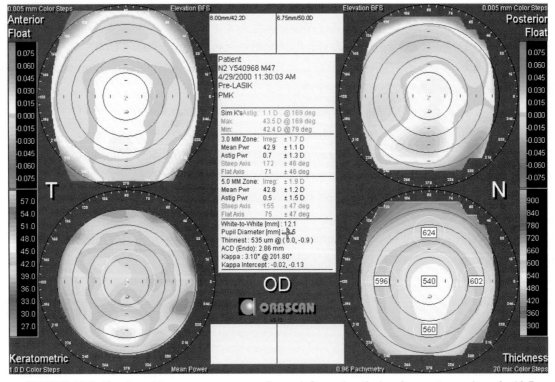

FIGURE 15.6: Keratometric mean power map (lower left quadrant) showing a steepening of >46 D

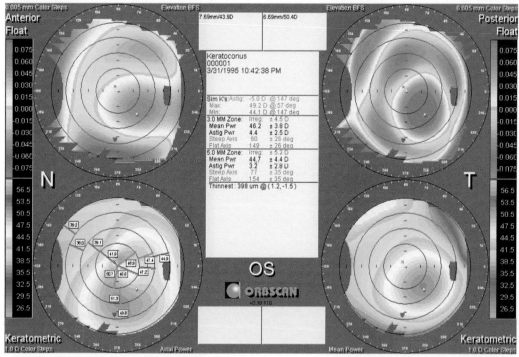

FIGURE 15.7: Lazy-C associated with central corneal asymmetry

2. *Bow-tie/broken bow-tie pattern:* The so-called "lazy-C" on the axial power map is very suspicious when the astigmatism shifts > 20° from a straight line (Figure 15.7).

3. *Central corneal asymmetry:* A change within the central 3 mm optical zone of the cornea of more than 3 diopters from superior to inferior (yellow flag) can be correlated with the present of vertical coma (Figure 15.7). However, this may be merely a sign of asymmetric astigmatism, and is not necessarily indicative of pathology.

COMPOSITE/INTEGRATED INFORMATION

1. **Correlation of signs with the highest point on the posterior elevation**. This is probably the *strongest topographic sign* indicative of early keratoconus.[7] If the highest point on the posterior elevation coincides with the highest point on the anterior elevation, the thinnest point on pachymetry, and the point of steepest curvature on the power map, never perform laser refractive surgery. This implies that the thinnest point represents a structural weakness, which causes a forward bending on the cornea (Figure 15.4).

2. **Efkarpides criteria**. The ratio of the radius in mm of the anterior BFS divided by the radius in mm of the posterior BFS. Surprisingly in normal corneas this ratio will be around 1.21. Between 1.23 and 1.27 we should be suspicious and look for other abnormalities. But when this ratio is 1.27 or higher this cornea should never be treated with laser (Figure 15.8).

3. **Bent/warped cornea.** Similarity between the anterior and posterior profiles implies a forward bending of those areas shown above BFS. If this bending is in association with the thinnest point on the

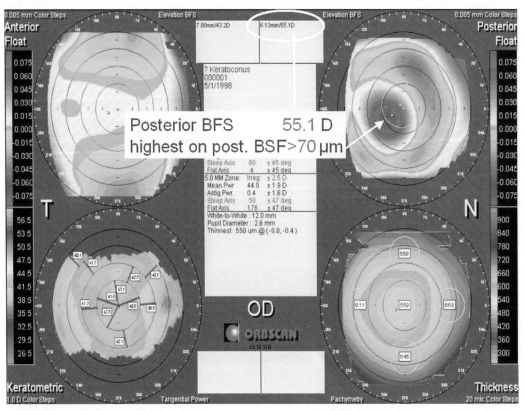

FIGURE 15.8: Efkarpides: 7.8 mm/6.13 mm = 1,273. In this obvious case also other red flags appear

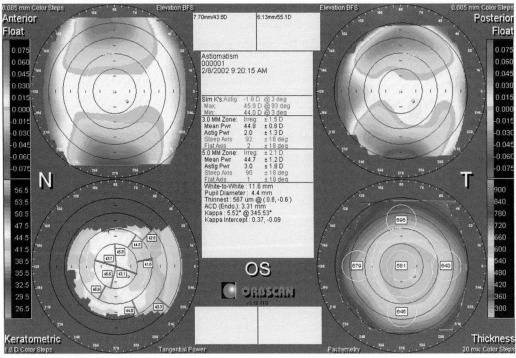

FIGURE 15.9: Bent/warped cornea: asymmetry of anterior and posterior elevation

cornea, it could relate to a structural weakness in the cornea. This sign needs to be evaluated within the context of the other parameters[8] (Figure 15.9).

4. **Inferotemporal displacement of the highest point** on the anterior as well as the posterior elevation profile can be indicative of early keratoconus (Figure 15.10).

5. Nature is surprisingly often very symmetrical, also our corneas. When a difference of more than 1D of astigmatism between two eyes is detected, there exists a higher risk of ectasia postoperatively.

6. Never forget to look at the information in the center of the quad maps. An **irregularity** of >1.5 D in the 3 mm central zone and of > 2.0 D in the 5 mm central zone should alert us (R Lindstrom, MD). This sign is probably the weakest of all, but should not be ignored (Figure 15.11).

7. **Normal band scale.** For the anterior and posterior elevation maps a normal band means an elevation within +/– 0.25 microns of the best fit sphere (BFS). The normal band for the total corneal power map is 40 to 48 diopters and for corneal thickness is between 500 and 600 microns. One pop-up means caution, two means concern and three pop-ups means a no-go situation (Figure 15.12 to 15.14).

8. If one eye fails on the indices but the other eye does not: NEVER TREAT EITHER EYE.

The above-mentioned indices can become useful in the armamentarium of preoperative evaluations for potential LASIK candidates towards safe and effective outcomes.

With newer technology integration using wavefront guidance (Zywave-B and L) we can detect higher order aberrations in the form of coma and increased RMS values (Gulani AC: Wavefront principles:

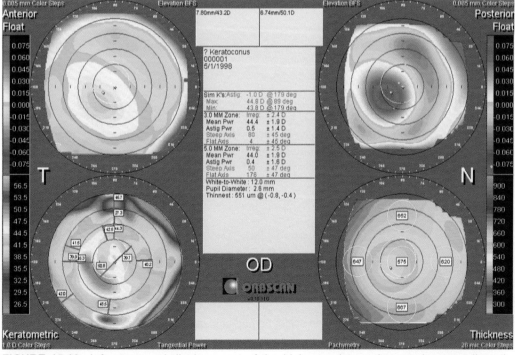

FIGURE 15.10: Inferotemporal displacement of the highest point on the anterior as well as the posterior elevation profile can be indicative of early keratoconus

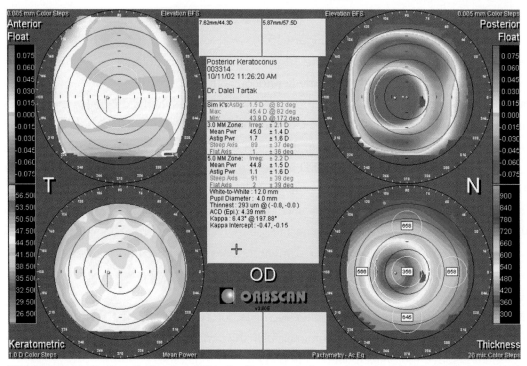

FIGURE 15.11: An irregularity of >1.5 D in the 3 mm central zone and of > 2.0 D in the 5 mm central zone should alert us. This sign is probably the weakest of all, but should not be ignored

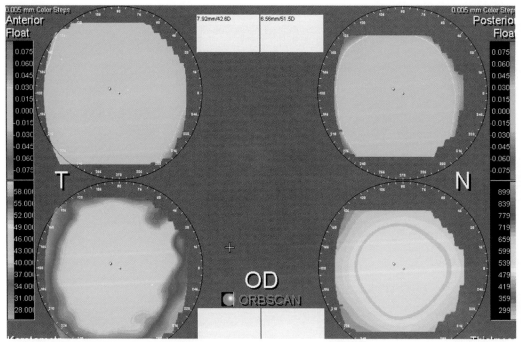

FIGURE 15.12: Normal band scale: no pop-ups: cornea within normal band

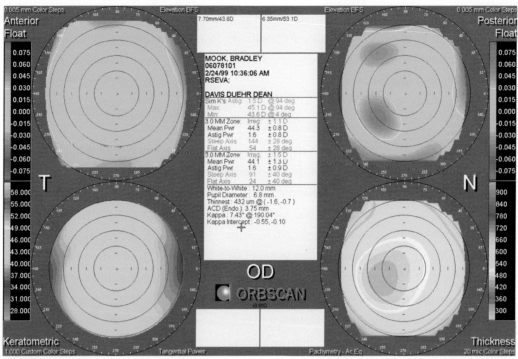

FIGURE 15.13: Normal band scale with two pop-ups: one in the pachymetry map and one in the posterior elevation map: there is great concern about this corneas ability to undergo lamellar refractive surgery

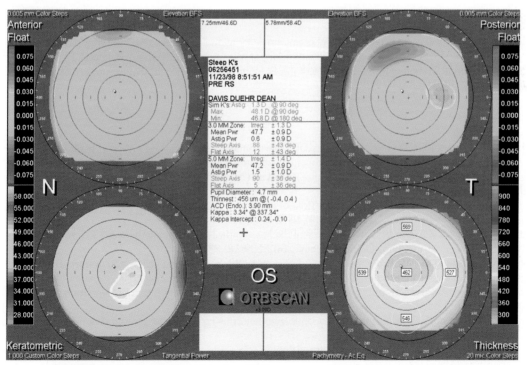

FIGURE 15.14: Normal band scale with three pop-ups: definitely a no-go situation

dimplified and applied. Instructional course. ESCRS, Paris, Sept 2004) aiding earlier detection of keratoconus and other potential ectatic corneal conditions. Pellucid marginal degeneration is mostly the cause of corneal topographic changes when correlated with higher levels of trefoil. Keratoconus will induce most likely higher levels of coma.

FUTURE THOUGHTS

I (Gulani AC, MD) would suggest moving in a direction that will incorporate a dynamic corneal imaging system (Dynamic corneal imaging: Prof Gunther Grabner et al: University Eye Clinic, Paracelsus Private Medical University, Salzburg, Austria), videotopography for measurement of the tear film and its contour (Janos Nemeth et al from the First Department of Ophthalmology, Semmelweis University, Budapest, Hungary; the Computer and Automation Research Institute, Hungarian Academy of Sciences, Budapest, Hungary; and the Department of Statistics, National Health Insurance Fund Administration, Budapest, Hungary). Wavefront incorporation[9] to rule out other internal optical elements keeping corneal measurement precise and non-contaminated. We could even consider confocal visiualization along with posterior corneal analysis to give clinical relevance to our findings besides artifactual assumptions.

Thus a technology that would combine, biomechanical forces, elasticity modules, wavefront analysis, confocal imaging, high-speed videography and dynamic testing even during the refractive surgery in real time would be my Gold Standard in corneal refractive surgery. I am privileged to be involved presently in this direction and shall look forward to sharing my insights in the next generation of this textbook.

ACKNOWLEDGMENTS

The work presented above was not the achievement of any single individual, but is the result of support and encouragement by many colleagues and friends. Those who played an important role, include Dr. Frederik Potgieter, Dr John Vukich, and our good friend, Philippe Dumarey from Bausch & Lomb), Belgium. Without their input and support, this work would not be possible.

REFERENCES

1. Charles N, Charles M, Croxatto JO, Charles DE, Wertheimer D. Surface and Orbscan II slit-scanning elevation topography in circumscribed posterior keratoconus, J Cataract Refract Surg 2005;31(3):636-9.
2. Seiler T, Quurke AW. Iatrogenic keratectasia after LASIK in a case of forme fruste keratoconus. J Cataract Refract Surg 1998;24(7):1007-9.
3. Rao SN, Raviv T, Majmudar PA, Epstein RJ. Role of Orbscan II in screening keratoconus suspects before refractive corneal surgery. Ophthalmology 2002;109(9):1642-6.
4. Pflugfelder SC, Liu Z, Feuer W, Verm A. Corneal thickness indices discriminate between keratoconus and contact lens-induced corneal thinning. Ophthalmology 2002;109(12):2336-41.
5. Ghergel D, Hosking SL, Mantry S, Banerjee S, Naroo SA, Sha S. Corneal pachymetry in normal and keratoconic eyes: Orbscan II versus ultrasound. J Cataract Refract Surg 2004;30(6):1272-7.
6. Arntz A, Duran JA, Pijoan JI. Subclinical keratoconus diagnosis by elevation topography. Arch Soc Esp Oftalmol 2003;78(12):659-64.
7. Auffarth GU, Wang L, Volcker HE. Keratoconus evaluation using the Orbscan Topography System. J Cataract Refract Surg 2000;26(2):222-8.
8. Cairns G, McGhee CN. Orbscan computerized topography: attributes, applications and limitations. J Cataract Refract Surg 2005;31(1):205-20.
9. Gulani AC, Probst L, Cox I, Veith R. Wavefront in Lasik: The Zyoptix. Platform. Ophthalmol Clin N Am 2004;17: 173-81.

Chapter

16

Presbyopic LASIK

Amar Agarwal
Athiya Agarwal
Sunita Agarwal
Guillermo Avalos

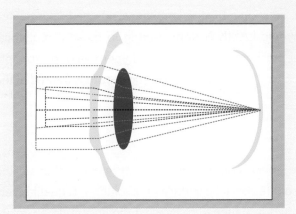

INTRODUCTION

Presbyopia, is the final frontier for an ophthalmologist. In the 21st century the latest developments, which are taking place, are in the field of presbyopia. In presbyopia, the nearest point that can be focused gradually recedes, leading to the need for optical prosthesis for close work such as reading and eventually even for focus in the middle distance.

PREVIOUS EXCIMER LASER TECHNIQUES

Presbyopic Photorefractive keratectomy (PRK) has been tried. In this using the excimer laser, a mask consisting of a mobile diaphragm formed by two blunt blades was used to ablate a 10-17 micron deep semilunar-shaped zone immediately below the papillary center, steepening the corneal curvature in that area.

Monofocal vision with LASIK has also been tried to solve the problem of presbyopia. The goal in such cases is to make the patient anisometropic. In this one eye is used for distance vision and the other for near vision. This is obviously not indicated in all subjects. The residual consequences are partial loss of stereopsis, asthenopia, headache, aniskonia and decreased binocularity.

HISTORY

Guillermo Avalos [1,2] started the idea of Presbyopic LASIK. This is called the PARM technique. He held a live surgical conference in Mexico where he had invited the Agarwals to perform Phakonit and the no-anesthesia cataract surgery technique. There he discussed with them the idea of Presbyopic Lasik and when they came back they started the technique.

PRINCIPLE

The objective is to allow the patient to focus on near objects while retaining his ability to focus on far objects, taking into account the refractive error of the eye when the treatment is performed. With this LASIK technique the corneal curvature is modified, creating a bilateral multifocal cornea in the treated optical zone. A combination of hyperopic and myopic LASIK is done aiming to make a multifocal cornea. We determine if the eye is presbyopic plano, presbyopic with spherical hyperopia or presbyopia with spherical myopia. These may also have astigmatism in which case the astigmatism is treated at the same time.

PROLATE AND OBLATE CORNEA

It is important for us to understand a prolate and oblate cornea before we progress further on the technique of Presbyopic LASIK. The shape of spheroid (a conoidal surface of revolution) is qualitatively prolate or oblate, depending on whether it is stretched or flattened in its axial dimension. In a prolate cornea the meridional curvature decreases from pole to equator and in an oblate cornea the meridional curvature continually increases. The optical surfaces of the normal human eye both cornea and lens is prolate. This shape has an optical advantage in that spherical aberration can be avoided. Following LASIK the prolateness of the anterior cornea reduces but is insufficient to eliminate its spherical aberration. Thus one should remember the normal cornea is prolate. When myopic LASIK is done the cornea becomes oblate. When hyperopic LASIK is done the cornea becomes prolate.

Every patient treated with an excimer laser is left with an oblate or prolate shaped cornea depending upon the myopia or hyperopia of the patient. The approach to improve visual quality after LASIK is to apply geometric optics and use the patient's refraction, precise preoperative corneal height data and optimal postoperative anterior corneal shape in order to have a customized prolate shape treatment.

TECHNIQUE

First of all a superficial corneal flap is created with the microkeratome. The corneal flap performed with the microkeratome must be between 8.5 to 9.5 mm in order to have an available corneal surface for treatment of at least 8 mm. In this way, the laser beam does not touch the hinge of the flap. In India the (Bausch & Lomb) Lasik machine is used and in Mexico the Apollo machine is used. Once the flap has been created a hyperopic ablation in an optical zone of 5 mm is done (Figure 16.1). The treated cornea now has a steepness section. The cornea is thus myopic, prolate. This allows the eye to focus in a range that includes near vision but excludes far vision.

With this myopic-shaped cornea, one now selects a smaller area of the central cornea that is concentric with the previous worked area. The size of the area is a 4 mm optical zone. A myopic LASIK is now done with the 4 mm optical zone (Figure 16.2). The resulting cornea now has a central area (oblate) that is

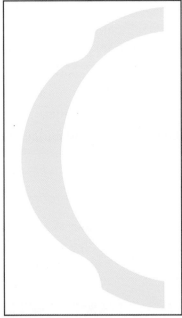

FIGURE 16.1: Hyperopic lasik done on the cornea. Myopic prolate cornea produced

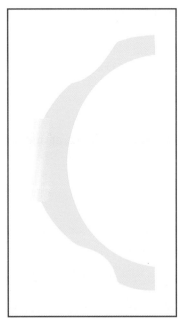

FIGURE 16.2: Myopic lasik done. Myopic ablation of 4 mm optical zone performed to create a central oblate cornea

223

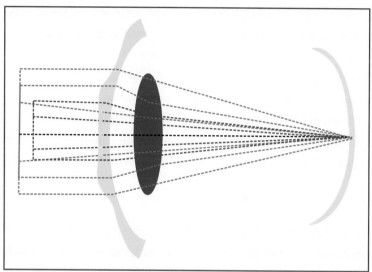

FIGURE 16.3: Schematic diagram of a presbyopic cornea in which hyperopic and myopic lasik has been done. The patient can thus focus for near and distance

configured for the eye to focus on far objects and a ring shaped area that allows the eye to focus on near objects (Figure 16.3). The flap is now cleaned and replaced back in position.

KERATOMETRY AND PACHYMETRY

Pachymetry is not important for this procedure. The preoperative keratometry reading is extremely important. The postoperative keratometer reading should not exceed 48 D. The keratometer reading should be taken from topography and not from a manual keratometer machine. For each hypermetropic diopter corrected, the corneal curvature increases in 0.89 keratometric diopters as an average. It is recommended to treat patients with keratometry in the range between 41 to 43 D to obtain postoperative curves under 48 D. If the cornea is more than 48 D, it produces undesired optical alterations like glare, halos, decreased visual acuity and decreased contrast sensitivity. The preoperative and postoperative keratometer readings should be nearly the same for the patient to be comfortable.

ASTIGMATISM

If astigmatism is present, it is recommended to use as a limit 2.5 D. One should also remember there is an induced astigmatism of 0.5 to 0.75 D created by the corneal shape after the surgery and this can decrease one or two lines of uncorrected visual acuity.

PLANO EXAMPLES

224

Now let us look at treating presbyopic patients who are basically plano for distance.

EXAMPLE 1

Let us take a patient who is plano for distance and is 20/20. For near on addition of + 2 D the patient is J1. The pre-operative keratometer let us say is 41 D.

There are three steps in the presbyopic LASIK treatment.

1 STEP: For distance—No treatment is required as the patient is plano 20/20

2 STEP: For near—Hyperopic LASIK is done of + 2 D. A 5 mm optical zone is taken. We have already mentioned that each dioptre of hyperopia corrected changes the corneal curvature by 0.89 D, which is approximately 1 D. So the keratometer changes from 41 to 43 D (approximately)

3. STEP: Myopic LASIK of minus 1 D with a 4 mm optical zone. So keratometer now becomes 42 D.

Regression occurs for hyperopia treatment to about 1 D, so we have done myopic ablation of minus 1 and not minus 2 D. The pre-op keratometer reading was 41 D and postoperative keratometer reading is 42 D, which is nearly the same.

HYPEROPIC EXAMPLES

Now let us look at presbyopic LASIK being performed in a hyperopic eye.

EXAMPLE 2

Let us take a patient who is hyperopic for distance and is 20/20 with + 1 D. For near on addition of + 3 D the patient is J1. The pre-operative keratometer let us say is 42 D.

There are three steps in the presbyopic LASIK treatment.

1. STEP: For distance—Hyperopic LASIK is done of + 1 D with a 5 mm optical zone. So keratometer changes from 42 D to 43 D.

2. STEP: For near—Hyperopic LASIK is done of + 3 D. A 5 mm optical zone is taken. We have already mentioned that each dioptre of hyperopia corrected changes the corneal curvature by 0.89 D, which is approximately 1 D. So the keratometer changes from 43 to 46 D (approximately)

3. STEP: Myopic LASIK of minus 2 D with a 4 mm optical zone. So keratometer now becomes 44 D.

Regression occurs for hyperopia treatment to about 1 D, so we have done myopic ablation of minus 2 and not minus 3 D. The pre-op keratometer reading was 42 D but after making the patient plano it is 43 D. The postoperative keratometer reading is 44 D, which is nearly the same.

Though we have to correct totally 4 D for hypermetropia we take it in two steps. One should not do it in one step as that much hyperopia corrected in one step makes the central cornea too steep to perform the myopic ablation.

EXAMPLE 3

Let us take a patient who is hyperopic for distance and is 20/20 with + 3 D. For near on addition of + 3 D the patient is J1. The pre-operative keratometer let us say is 44 D.

The preoperative keratometer reading is 44 D and we have to correct 3 D for distance and 3 d for near. So, if we do presbyopic Lasik we will make the keratometer reading 50 D. So, one should not treat such patients with presbyopia LASIK.

MYOPIC EXAMPLE

Now let us look at myopic patients.

EXAMPLE 4

Let us take a patient who is myopic for distance and is 20/20 with minus 2 D. For near on addition of + 2 D the patient is J1. This means the patient is plano for near. The preoperative keratometer let us say is 43 D.

There are three steps in the presbyopic LASIK treatment.

1. STEP: For distance—Patient is myopic so no treatment is required.
2. STEP: For near—Hyperopic LASIK is done of + 2 D. A 5 mm optical zone is taken. We have already mentioned that each diopter of hyperopia corrected changes the corneal curvature by 0.89 D, which is approximately 1 D. So the keratometer changes from 43 to 45 D (approximately)
3. STEP: Myopic LASIK of minus 3 D with a 4 mm optical zone. So keratometer now becomes 42 D.

Regression occurs for hyperopia treatment to about 1 D, so we have done myopic ablation of minus 3 and not minus 4 D. The pre-op keratometer reading was 43 D but patient was myopic by 2 D, so actually the keratometer reading should be 41 D. D. The postoperative keratometer reading is 42 D, which is nearly the same.

We did myopic ablation of 3 D, as patient is myopic of 2 D and presbyopic of 2 D. Regression factor taken is 1 D.

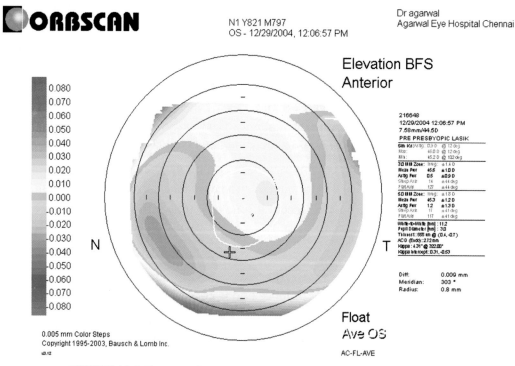

FIGURE 16.4: Preoperative topography of a patient before presbyopic lasik

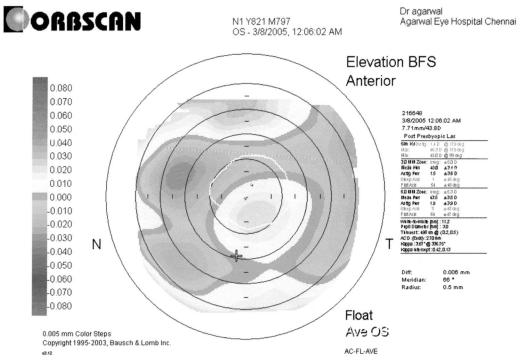

FIGURE 16.5: Postoperative topography of a patient after presbyopic lasik

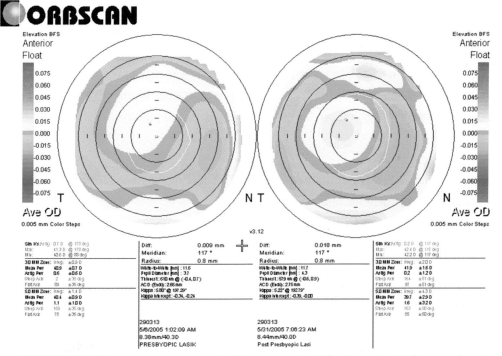

FIGURE 16.6: Preoperative topography (picture on the left) of a patient before presbyopic lasik and picture on the right shows the postoperative topography of the patient after presbyopic lasik

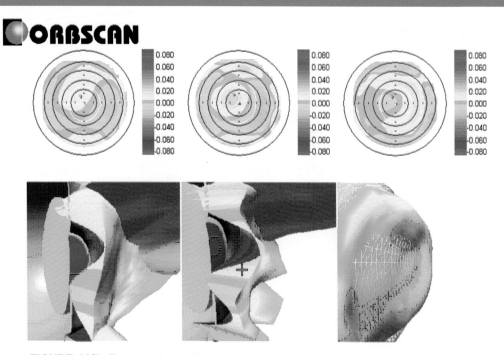

FIGURE 16.7: Preoperative and postoperative topography of a patient after presbyopic lasik shown in a 3 D pattern

TOPOGRAPHY

Figure 16.4 and 16.5 show the pre- and postoperative corneal topography in a patient in whom presbyopic lasik has been done. This patient was 20/20 and J1 postoperatively without glasses.

Figure 16.6 shows another case in whom presbyopic lasik was done. The figure on the left is the preoperative picture and the one on the right is the postoperative figure. Figure 16.7 is the same patients topographic photos showing pre and post surgery in a 3 D pattern.

SUMMARY

This idea of presbyopic LASIK is not the end of it all. This technique needs further improvizations to become the technique of choice for one and all.

REFERENCES

1. Guillermo Avalos. Presbyopic LASIK—The PARM Technique in Amar Agarwal's Presbyopia: A Surgical Textbook. Slack Inc, USA, 2002.
2. Agarwal T et al. Presbyopic LASIK—The Agarwal Technique in Amar Agarwal's Presbyopia: A Surgical Textbook. Slack Inc, USA, 2002.

Aberrometry and Topography in the Vector Analysis of Refractive Laser Surgery

Noel A Alpins
Gemma Walsh

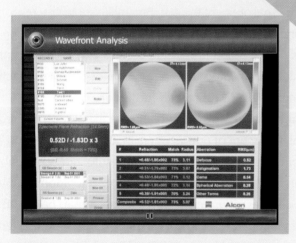

INTRODUCTION

Refractive laser surgery techniques such as laser in situ keratomileusis (LASIK) and photorefractive keratectomy (PRK) are effective methods of treating spherical myopic errors up to 12 D and hyperopic errors up to 6 D, with good visual outcomes. However, generally more than half of the people who are suitable candidates for refractive surgery have enough astigmatism to warrant its inclusion in the surgical correction. As astigmatism has both direction and magnitude, its incorporation into the treatment makes planning more complex. It has been shown that vector analysis could likely improve the visual outcome of spherocylindrical treatments by combining the topographic and refractive astigmatic components to target a reduced level of corneal astigmatism compared to using refractive parameters alone. [1][2][5]

MEASUREMENT OF ASTIGMATISM

There are three differing categories of astigmatism; naturally occurring regular astigmatism, naturally occurring irregular astigmatism and secondary irregular astigmatism associated with ocular trauma, disease, infection or previous ocular surgery.[1] There are many different ways to measure astigmatism, some assessing corneal astigmatism only, and the others measuring refractive astigmatism including the internal optics of the eye. It is important in routine clinical practice to utilize more than one method in the pre-operative examination.

The manifest subjective refraction is a measure of the spherocylindrical correction required for the patient's perception of their best vision. The principal contribution to the cylindrical error is the corneal astigmatism, but also includes astigmatism from the internal optics of the eye (such as the crystalline lens) as well as the interpretation of the image by the cerebral cortex. The measured result depends on many variables such as chart illumination and contrast, test distance and room lighting. The newer technology of wavefront analysis provides a spatially oriented refractive map of the pathway of light through the eye, which provides a greater amount of information on the refractive system than the manifest refraction data alone. It too includes the internal optics of the eye, but unlike subjective responses does not include the conscious percept of the cerebral cortex, thus giving no information regarding the non-optical interpretation of astigmatism images on the retina and visual cortex. This subjective value conventionally forms part of the ablative treatment and is an important component for patient satisfaction. The application of wavefront analysis in the treatment plan is discussed further on.

Keratometry is a useful objective test to measure average corneal curvature at the paracentral region of the cornea. However, as it requires the manual alignment of optical mires to identify the steepest and flattest corneal axes, there is a potential problem with reproducing reliable results due to variability between different observers. Corneal topography, or computer assisted videokeratography (CAVK), provides a more detailed quantified view of the corneal astigmatism displayed as a map based on the measurement of refractive power of thousands of separate points over the entire cornea. Average topographical astigmatism can be represented by a simulated keratometry value, which is a mean value derived from a number of constant reference points. It is a best fit compromise, and determined in various ways by the different types of topographers.

SURGICAL PLANNING—REFRACTION, TOPOGRAPHY, OR BOTH?

In an ideal world the goal of astigmatic refractive surgery is to completely eliminate astigmatism from the eye and its optical correction. However, it has since been recognized that this is not possible in the majority of cases due to the inherent differences between corneal astigmatism (represented by the simulated keratometry value from topography) and refractive astigmatism (represented by lower [second] order aberrations from aberrometry) correcting the eye.[4,5] Most surgeons traditionally treat the refractive value alone based on the principle that treating what the patient perceives to give their best corrected vision will provide a superior visual outcome.

However, this is not necessarily the case. Disregarding the shape of the cornea while changing it flies in the face of the fundamental principles of corneal surgery. In fact, simple arithmetic analysis shows that an excessive amount of corneal astigmatism may be left if treatment is applied exclusively based on the parameters derived from the refractive cylinder magnitude and axis.[2,3] This occurs because failing to align the maximum ablation closer to the flattest corneal meridia results in off-axis loss of effect when reducing corneal astigmatism. Consequently, lower (second) order astigmatic aberrations and (third order) coma would not be minimized, with more remaining than otherwise necessary.[1] This may result in post-surgical symptoms such as reduced visual acuity and contrast sensitivity, creating difficulty with night driving and thus actually diminishing satisfaction in a proportion of patients.

As it becomes more widely recognized that a zero overall astigmatism is mostly unattainable, effective contemporary methods target astigmatism outcomes that combine both the refractive and topographic measurements in the analytical planning process. This should ensure the distribution of the remaining astigmatism to achieve the optimal outcome. That is, choosing a maximal treatment that leaves the minimum amount of astigmatism and in the most favorable orientation. With-the-rule astigmatism is more prevalent in the younger population undergoing laser vision correction, and is thought to be more visually tolerable to refractive perception than against-the-rule astigmatism (Javals rule).[3,5,8]

VECTOR ANALYSIS BY THE ALPINS METHOD

The surgical planning and analysis process is expedited by the implementation of computer and software technology. Calculations performed for the publication of this chapter utilized the ASSORT program developed by the first author (the Alpins Statistical System for Ophthalmic Refractive surgery Techniques). It employs the principles of vector planning and analysis[1-6] and can utilize a paradigm that favors with-the-rule astigmatism that minimizes measurable postoperative refractive astigmatism quantified as second order aberrations.

The amount and axis of astigmatic change that the surgeon intends to induce is called the target induced astigmatism vector (TIA). This is determined by using an optimal combination of refractive and topographic data, as seen in the example later on. The surgically induced astigmatism vector (SIA) is the astigmatic change actually induced by the surgery. It is possible to determine whether the treatment was on-axis or off-axis, and also whether too much or too little treatment was applied by examining the various relationships between the SIA and TIA. The correction index (CI) is the ratio of the SIA to TIA and ideally is 1.0. An overcorrection occurs if the CI is greater than 1.0 and less than 1.0 for an undercorrection. The magnitude of error (ME) is the arithmetic difference between the magnitudes of the SIA and TIA. This is positive for overcorrections and negative for undercorrections. The angle of error (AE) is the angle contained by the SIA and TIA vectors. If the achieved correction is orientated counterclockwise (CCW) to where it was intended then the AE is positive. If the achieved correction is clockwise (CW) to the intended axis then the AE is negative.

An absolute measure of success of the surgery is described by the difference vector (DV). This is the induced astigmatic change that would enable the initial surgery to achieve its initial intended target, and is ideally zero. The DV is a useful dioptric measure of uncorrected astigmatism. A relative measure of success is the index of success (IOS) which is calculated by dividing the DV by the intended change, the TIA. This is also preferably zero.

As previously mentioned, the corneal and refractive astigmatisms are rarely equivalent. This difference may be represented vectorially by the ocular residual astigmatism (ORA).[9] In other words, the ORA is the noncorneal component of total refractive astigmatism, and quantifies by magnitude and axis orientation the minimum intraocular second order astigmatism aberrations. It is also the amount of corneal astigmatism expected to remain after treatment guided by refractive values alone, to neutralize this intraocular astigmatism.

ABERROMETRY AND WAVEFRONT GUIDED TREATMENT

Wavefront technology has added new understanding of the eye's refractive characteristics. It offers theoretical guidance to reduce spherical aberrations by achieving the most effective prolate aspheric profile and appears to be successful in this endeavor in the initial treatment studies. However, wavefront-assisted Lasik does not address the amount of resultant corneal astigmatism, and therefore is similar to Lasik based on manifest refraction. In addition, as aberrometry includes the internal optics of the eye in its calculations, any changes over time to the crystalline lens may undermine any benefit gained from the wavefront ablation.[1,7]

Furthermore, if wavefront guided ablation corrects all ocular aberrations at the corneal surface, it would produce an uneven corneal treatment resulting in induced corneal irregularities. This might be an undesirable result when it is widely recognized that a regular cornea with orthogonal and symmetrical astigmatism gives a superior visual result.[1,6] Permanently changing regional corneal shape in this manner is also complicated by the fact that this form of treatment may in fact be neutralized by epithelial healing.[7]

While wavefront guided ablation may not be the path to "super vision" as it was first thought to be, it does provide useful refractive information. Rather than employing wavefront data exclusively, it can be combined with the vector planning method described in this chapter to produce an optimal treatment with reduced post surgical aberrations.

COMBINING WAVEFRONT ANALYSIS AND TOPOGRAPHY WITH VECTOR PLANNING

A typical wavefront analysis is depicted in Figure 17.1. The spherocylindrical refraction as measured by the wavefront device at the spectacle plane is +0.52/-1.83x3. The two dimensional illustration of the wavefront analysis on the left shows a moderate level of mixed astigmatism with a typical saddle appearance. The higher order spherical aberrations are quantified as root-mean-square values in the lower right hand corner of the display. The spherical component of the correction (+0.52) is shown as the defocus. The cylindrical component is displayed beneath this. Third order aberrations (coma and trefoil) are listed separately, with 4th order spherical aberrations. 'Other terms' indicates 5th order and higher order aberrations.

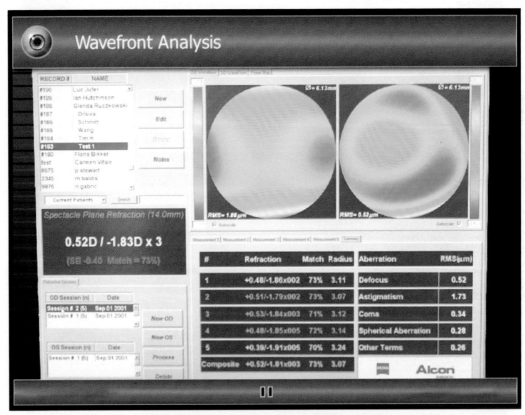

FIGURE 17.1: A typical wavefront analysis display

Figure 17.2 displays a topographical map of the matching astigmatic eye. The typical bow-tie appearance of the regular corneal astigmatism is evident. In this example the astigmatism measures 2.62 D at the steepest meridian of 96 degrees as quantified by the simulated keratometry values. These parameters can then be examined together with those from the wavefront analysis spherocylindrical (second order) values to produce an optimal treatment by using the Alpins method contained in the ASSORT program. This is shown in the treatment planning screen in Figure 17.3. In this diagram the treatment has been set to a base of 100% emphasis for correction of refractive astigmatism parameters.

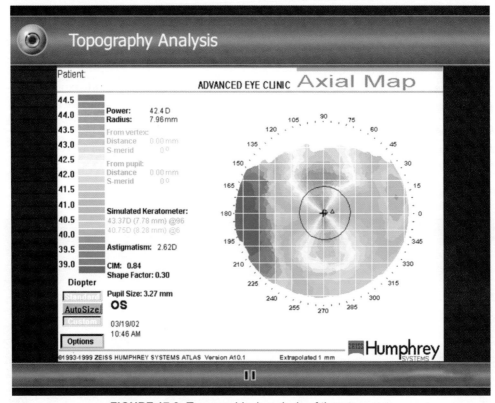

FIGURE 17.2: Topographical analysis of the same eye

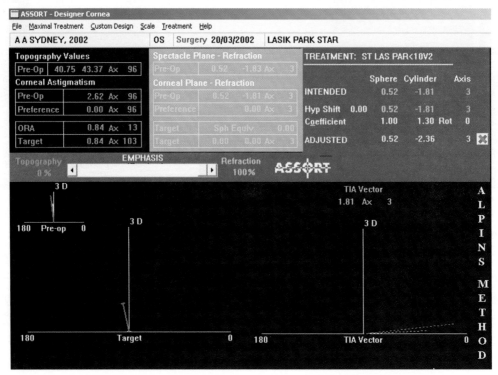

FIGURE 17.3: The ASSORT surgical planning module for this eye

Spectacle plane - refraction			
Pre-Op	0.52	−1.83 Ax	3

Corneal plane - refraction			
Pre-Op	0.52	−1.83 Ax	3
Prefrerence		0.00 Ax	3

Target	Sph equiv		0.00
Target	0.00 Ax	0.00 Ax	3

FIGURE 17.4: The top central section of the ASSORT screen displaying the preoperative refractive data obtained from the wavefront analysis (both spectacle and corneal plane values) and the chosen refractive spherocylindrical target

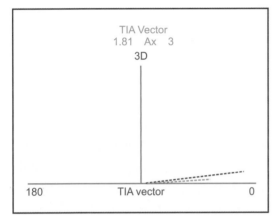

FIGURE 17.5: The lower right hand graph on the ASSORT screen with a polar display of the TIA vector

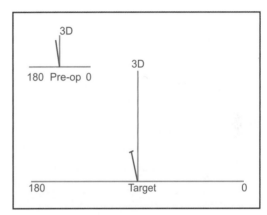

FIGURE 17.6: Pre-operative and post-operative target astigmatism vectors. The post-operative refractive target value is zero with the target corneal astigmatism vector displayed in green

This treatment screen in Figure 17.3 has been disassembled further for ease of understanding the various components. Figure 17.4 is the top central section on the ASSORT treatment screen, displaying the preoperative spherocylindrical refractive values taken from the wavefront analysis and also the corneal plane conversion. The cylindrical component here is 1.81 D of astigmatism at axis 3. This Figure 17.also displays the spherocylindrical target for the treatment, which in this case is zero.

The treatment vector being employed is shown in the polar diagram in Figure 17.5. Here the TIA is 1.81D at axis 3. The pre and post operative target astigmatism values are shown in Figure 17.6. The post-operative refractive target value is zero with the target corneal astigmatism value (obtained from Figure 17.7 below) displayed in blue.

The simulated keratometry values from the preoperative topographical map are shown in Figure 17.7. Also displayed here are the ORA and the target for the corneal postoperative astigmatism. A vectorial calculation is used to determine the ORA, which in this case is 0.84 D. That is, there is a calculated amount of 0.84 D of intraocular astigmatism that cannot be eliminated from this eye. As the spherocylindircal refractive target has already been guided to zero, this can only leave the whole of the remaining astigmatism on the cornea at a near vertical meridian of 103 degrees to neutralize the ORA 90 degrees away, as seen in the target value of Figure 17.7.

Topography Values				
Pre-Op	40.75	43.37	Ax	96

Corneal astigmatism

Pre-Op	2.62	Ax	96
Prefrerence	0.00	Ax	96

ORA	0.84	Ax	13
Target	0.84	Ax	103

FIGURE 17.7: The top left hand box of the ASSORT screen displaying the corneal topographical preoperative values and the targeted corneal postoperative value. The minimum amount of astigmatism is displayed as the ORA, which in this case matches the magnitude target for the corneal astigmatism and is 90 degrees away

However, as the emphasis is shifted towards the left, the treatment is more closely aligned to the principal corneal meridian. Figure 17.8 shows the optimal treatment for this eye, with the emphasis placed at 33% topography and 67% refraction. The ORA is still 0.84 D, but now it is apportioned between the refraction and the cornea. Here less corneal astigmatism is targeted and has been reduced to 0.56D at an unchanged meridian 103 (Figure 17.9). The remaining 0.28 D which is included in the spherocylindrical target of a spherical equivalent of zero, is not necessarily detected by the perceptive system at these levels, particularly as it is orientated favorably towards with-the-rule. Thus, with this method of vectorial planning, although the targeted sphero-cylindrical outcome is not zero, but 0.14/-

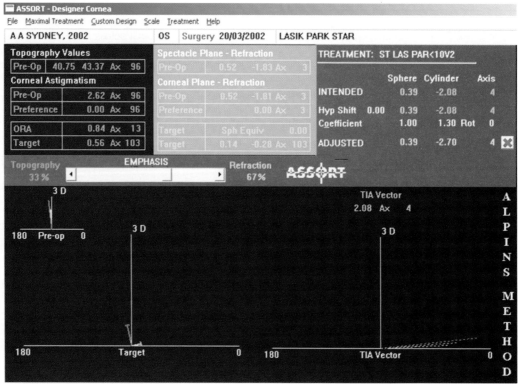

FIGURE 17.8: The ASSORT treatment screen displaying the optimal treatment for the same eye. Here the emphasis bar has been shifted 33% towards the left so that not all of the surgical emphasis is placed on complete refractive astigmatism correction

Topography Values				
Pre-Op	40.75	43.37	Ax	96

Corneal astigmatism			
Pre-Op	2.62	Ax	96
Prefrerence	0.00	Ax	96

ORA	0.84	Ax	13
Target	0.56	Ax	103

FIGURE 17.9: The optimal treatment for the same eye. Here the amount of corneal astigmatism remaining after treatment has been reduced by one third to 0.56D, though the total ORA remains unchanged at 0.84D

FIGURE 17.10: The new spherocylindrical target for this eye is not zero, but 0.14/-0.28 x 103. This distributes the ORA between the post-operative refractive and corneal modes to produce a more favorable corneal shape and therefore less second order aberrations following surgery. The favorably orientated and minimal refractive target is not likely to be perceived by the patient

Spectacle plane - refraction			
Pre-Op	0.52	−1.83 Ax	3

Corneal plane - refraction			
Pre-Op	0.52	−1.81 Ax	3
Prefrerence		0.00 Ax	3

Target	Sph equiv		0.00
Target	0.14 Ax	−0.28 Ax	103

0.28×103 as displayed in Figure 17.10, the measured postoperative refractive and wavefront astigmatism is likely to be negligible.

Despite not targeting a zero sphero-cylindrical outcome, by directing the remaining astigmatism away from the cornea the overall astigmatism is also less, and there are fewer aberrations remaining. This treatment results in an overall higher patient satisfaction.

TREATMENT OF IRREGULAR ASTIGMATISM

Differences in the two opposite superior and inferior hemidivisions of the corneal topographical contour map are widely prevalent. This is known as irregular astigmatism and occurs if the two sides of the bow-tie representation differ in magnitude (asymmetrical) or are not aligned at 180 degrees to each other (nonorthogonal), or most commonly a combination of the two.[1,6] Irregular astigmatism may also be identified optically using wavefront devices. Unlike other methods of astigmatism analysis, the method described in this chapter may theoretically also be applied independently to each hemidivision in a cornea displaying pre-existing idiopathic irregularity. This would theoretically allow analysis and treatment of this irregular astigmatism to produce an orthogonal, symmetrical cornea.

The target refractive and corneal astigmatism values must be considered separately for each hemimeridian, with individual treatment plans required for both the superior and inferior topographic magnitudes and meridian values with the common refractive astigmatism value. From this, minimum target astigmatism values may be calculated for each part of the cornea, and their orientations are used to guide the choice for the optimal TIA for that side.[6]

The vectorial difference between the two opposite semimeridian values for magnitude and axis in each corneal part is called the topographic disparity (TD). When displayed on a 720 degree double-angle vector diagram, the TD quantifies the irregular astigmatism of the cornea in dioptres, and the treatment required to reduce or eliminate the irregular astigmatism can be determined from this.[6]

The information gained from computerized topography regarding the corneal height (either directly such as the Z dimension on the Orbscan device, or indirectly inferred from slope measurement) may be translated into planned tissue ablation patterns using the Munnerlyn formula. This ablative pattern may then be applied at specific points on the corneal surface to reduce the irregularity.[1] There are various methods to link topographical information with tailored ablation, though a real time preoperative link is yet to be achieved.

In this way, the corneal shape may be manipulated by asymmetrical surgical treatment to the irregular hemidivisions of the cornea, allowing the achievement of any corneal shape (thus producing regular astigmatism where selected). In cases of irregular astigmatism a rearrangement rather than a reduction of the corneal astigmatism may be of benefit, as regularizing the cornea may improve best-corrected visual acuity to better approach the goal of supernormal vision.

SUMMARY

Due to natural differences in the vast majority of eyes between total astigmatism as measured by refraction and corneal astigmatism, it is impossible to completely eliminate astigmatism from the eye's optical system and its correction. It can therefore be beneficial to combine both these elements when considering the plan for refractive laser surgery to produce an optimal, individualized outcome. If the treatment plan utilizes manifest refraction data alone, it may actually increase the postoperative aberrations, thereby reducing the final visual result.

The Alpins method of vector planning utilizes information from both corneal topography and manifest refraction/wavefront data to target less postoperative corneal astigmatism and minimize postoperative aberrations. Though this often means that the postoperative refractive astigmatism target is not zero, this minor refractive error (with a spherical equivalent of zero) that remains postoperatively in a favorable orientation may not be significant enough for patient perception. In fact, overall the patient satisfaction is potentially higher due to the lesser amount of lower order aberrations.

This method of vector planning and analysis may also be used to optimize treatment for each separate hemimeridian of the cornea in cases of irregular astigmatism. This would enable the surgeon to rearrange the corneal astigmatism and regularize the cornea, thus producing a potential increase in the best corrected visual acuity. Though a real time preoperative link to the topographical and wavefront information for this specialized ablation is yet to be formed, this integration of these diagnostic modalities utilizing vector planning may be a reality in the future.

REFERENCES

1. Goggin M, Alpins N, Schmid L, Management of irregular astigmatism. Current Opinion in Ophthalmology 2000, 11:260-266.

2. Alpins NA. Astigmatism by the Alpins Method. J Cataract Refract Surg 2001; 27:31-49.
3. Croes KJ. The Alpins Method: A breakthrough in astigmatism analysis. Medical Electronics, September 1998.
4. Alpins NA. A new method of analyzing vectors for changes in astigmatism. J Cataract Refract Surg 1993; 19: 524-33.
5. Alpins NA. New method of targeting vectors to treat astigmatism. J Cataract Refract Surg 1997; 23:65-75.
6. Alpins NA. Treatment of irregular astigmatism. J Cataract Refract Surg 1998; 24:634-46.
7. Alpins NA. Wavefront technology: A new advance that fails to answer old questions on corneal vs refractive astigmatism correction. J of Refractive Surg; November/December 2002: 737-9.
   Discusses wavefront technology and the benefits of incorporating it into the refractive laser surgery plan.
8. Javal E. Memoirs d'Ophthalmometrie. 1890, G Masson, Paris.
9. Duke-Elder S (Ed). System of Ophthalmology. Vol 5: Ophthalmic optics and refraction. St Louis, Mosby, 1970: 275-78.

Chapter

18

NAV Wave:
Nidek
Technique for
Customized
Ablation

Masanao Fujieda
Mukesh Jain
Peter Keller

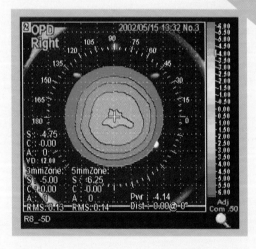

INTRODUCTION

NAV wave is a coupling of two brilliant technologies, to deliver customized ablation for the correction of refractive error. The OPD-Scan[R] system, combining wavefront analysis with corneal topography to map the aberrations of the entire optical system, is linked with Nidek's unique Final Fit Software to evaluate and convert the data to produce the precise ablation parameters for customized excimer laser ablation of the cornea.

OPD-SCAN

The OPD-Scan (Optical Path Difference Scanning System) is equipped with corneal topography, aberrometry, refractometry, keratometry and pupilometry functions within a single device overcoming the potential problems of inter-device misalignment. The OPD-Scan[R] measures both corneal topography using Placido disk reflection method as well as total ocular aberrations using dynamic skiascopy technology. Dynamic skiascopy currently provides the most direct measurement of any wavefront system without using a lenslet array or the projection of a grid target onto the retina. The technique of skiascopy has been successfully used in auto-refractometers but has now been modified to permit the additional measurement of higher order aberrations. The major difference between the dynamic skiascopy based OPD-Scan[R] and other skiascopy based auto-refractometers is that the OPD-Scan[R] can measure the distribution of refractive error in a wider corneal zone as it provides internally with a photo diode array at a conjugate position with the cornea.

A constant-speed single direction slit shaped infrared ray is projected towards the entrance pupil center as a thin beam and onwards to strike the retina. An aperture and a photo diode array that is conjugate with the retina for emmetropia collect the reflected light from the retina. There are four photodetectors above and four photodetectors below the optical axis. There are also two photodetectors, one of each side, which detect the center of the photodetector pairs. The basic principle is in many ways similar to confocal microscopy in that only the light reflected form the retina that passes through the aperture would reach the photodiode array. How the reflected light reaches the photo diode array depends on the positional relationship between the retina and aperture. We have just said only the reflected light that passes through the aperture will be collected. In the case of emmetropia eye, the aperture is positioned on the retina, and during the slit shape light goes across the aperture, the reflected light hits the all photo-diode cells simultaneously. Therefore, there is no time lag between different detection time and the time difference should be zero. In hyperopia, the aperture is positioned behind the retina and hence there is a time lag between different diodes detection time.

In the myopic eye, the aperture stop is located in front of the retina. The incoming slit-shaped light bundle bounces off the retina and the reflecting slit moves in an opposite direction compared to the incoming slit. This causes the some photodetectors cells to be stimulate earlier that the others. By correlating the time differences with refractive errors, a refractive error at each position on the cornea (photo diode position) with respect to the corneal center can be derived. By simple rotation of the measurement system through 180 degrees, the distribution of refractive errors can be obtained through 360-degree meridians.[1-2] The OPD scan also measures corneal topography using a Placido ring method and which has been widely utilized for almost two decades.

TOPOGRAPHY AND WAVEFRONT ANALYZER

The OPD-Scan is a combined corneal topography device and wavefront analyzer. The purpose of laser keratorefractive surgery is to photo ablate the cornea to alter its refracting power, and thereby improve unaided vision. The early systems were effective at reducing primary defocus and astigmatism but often led to increased higher order aberrations. Customized ablation now offers the potential to correct not just the lower order errors but also the majority of significant higher-order aberrations to achieve better vision. Generally, the Treatment Area consists of an Optical Zone and a Transition Zone. The optical zone plays the largest role in optical performance and should be larger than the pupil diameter whereas the Transition Zone blends the OZ with the untreated cornea to avoid abrupt changes in shape that are thought to trigger unwanted healing effects. The Transition Zone is also thought to play an important role in improving visual performance under Scotopic conditions as the pupil enlarges however, it is impossible to design the Transition Zone from Wavefront Analyzer information alone without thought to the cornea over relying areas outside the entrance pupil.

A major functional difference between Dynamic-Skiascopy and Hartmann-Shack type devices lies in the range of measurements capability:

OPD-Scan principle: Sphere: –20 to +22D, Cylinder: 0 to ±12D
Hartmann-Shack principle: Sphere: –15D to +7D, Cylinder: 0 to ±6D

OPD POWER MAP

The data generated by the OPD is typically displayed in map form showing the distribution of wavefront errors of the entire eye (D). Figure 18.1A illustrates the OPD map of a -4.75 D spherical model eye. In this map, the refractive error at a desired position on the cornea within a 6mm diameter is displayed. Since the map is of a spherical model eye uncorrected for spherical aberration, the measured errors vary with each concentric zone; the outermost concentric zone being more negative (reddish) than the central zone. In this figure, the terms, Sphere, Cylinder, and Axis have their conventional meaning and are displayed in the middle left for the central zone as: S: –4.75, C: –0.00, A: 0.0. This is repeated for 3mm and 5mm annulus zones immediately below the central data and show increasingly negative defocus errors in the periphery. Figure 18.1B illustrates the OPD map of a 3D cylindrical model eye. In this map of with-the-rule astigmatism the steeper meridian (in the 0 to 180° direction) and flatter meridian (in the 90 to 270° direction) are observed as a color-coded butterfly pattern. It is also clear from the map that even in this cylindrical model eye there is significant spherical aberration.

The OPD-Scan[R] also allows the mapping of various individual aberrations described in terms of Zernike coefficients from the wavefront data. The low-order components (up to 5) that can be corrected with spectacle lenses and some high-order components (6 and higher) can be displayed. Figure 18.2A illustrates an OPD map of an emmetropic human eye. This map is color-coded in three greenish colors

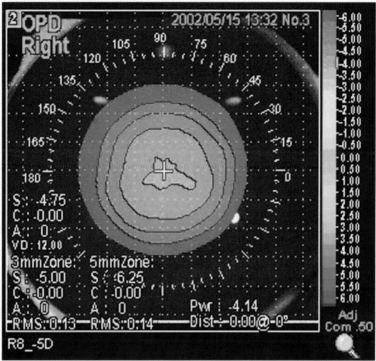

FIGURE 18.1A: OPD map of a –4.75D spherical model eye

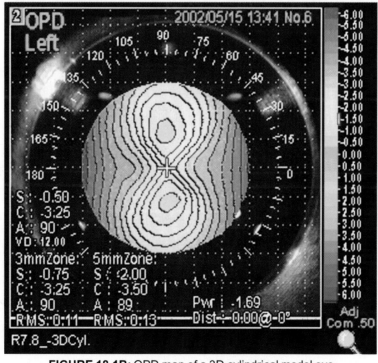

FIGURE 18.1B: OPD map of a 3D cylindrical model eye

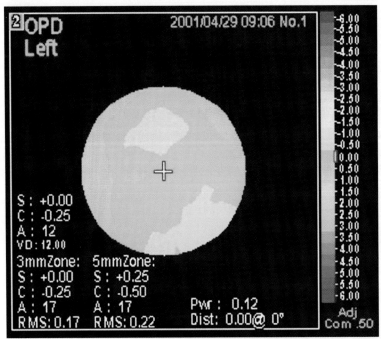

FIGURE 18.2A: OPD map of an emmetropic human eye

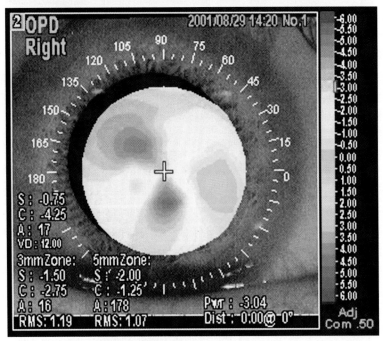

FIGURE 18.2B: OPD map of a myopic astigmatism eye

for simple pattern recognition. Figure 18.2B shows an eye with myopic astigmatism and Figure 18.2C shows a hyperopic astigmatism eye. The OPD-Scan[R] produces maps that are easily interpreted, using display techniques familiar to corneal topography maps. Just as computer assisted corneal topography devices raised the standard of keratometry, so too do wavefront devices provide us with a wealth of information over and above sphere, cylinder and axis.

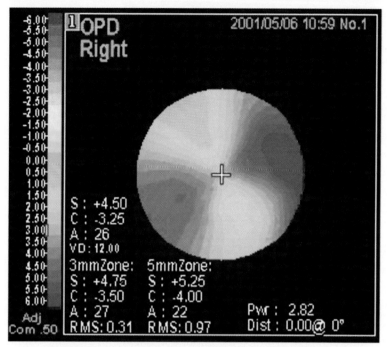

FIGURE 18.2C: OPD map of a hyperopic astigmatism eye

In addition, it is easily perceived whether the map has a butterfly pattern and illustrates symmetric or asymmetric astigmatism from the symmetry of the butterfly pattern. The OPD map provides us with more visual and multifactorial refractive information compared to a conventional auto refractometer that provides S, C and A data only.

OPD POWER MAP AND WAVEFRONT MAP

To explain how the OPD-Scan[R] measures optical aberrations begins with the duality of light, and that light can be thought to propagate in waves. The wavefront is defined as a plane perpendicular to the direction in which light travels and deviations from the ideal wavefront are termed wavefront errors and these errors tell us about the optical properties of the system. To illustrate this point consider the following diagram, Figure 18.3, of a simplified schematic eye with light reflected back out of the eye from a single point P on the retina. For a perfectly emmetropic eye the exiting wavefront will be a plane wave perpendicular to the Z-axis. However in this case the eye is myopic so the wavefront converges to a point P' where it intersects the reference axis. The difference in slope between the wavefront and the ideal wavefront allows the construction of the wavefront error map for multiple discrete points. The difference is often described using Zernike polynomials with each coefficient relating to a particular type of aberration such as Defocus, Astigmatism, Coma, Trefoil and so on.[4] Thus, one can tell the type and amount of aberrations that the eye produces. This information is useful for comparing preoperative and postoperative changes in ocular aberration quantitatively.

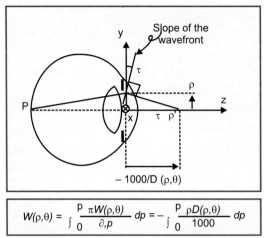

$$W(\rho,\theta) = \int_0^p \frac{\pi W(\rho,\theta)}{\partial,p} dp = - \int_0^p \frac{\rho D(\rho,\theta)}{1000} dp$$

FIGURE 18.3: Conversion between wavefront aberration and refractive errors

OPD MAP AND CORNEA TOPOGRAPHY MAP

This section describes one example in which a comparison between corneal topography and OPD map provides new information. Figure 18.4 illustrates the OPD map of total ocular refraction and the corneal refractive power map among corneal topographic maps for the same eye. The Corneal refractive map illustrates the distribution of corneal refractive powers calculated by Snell's law showing corneal astigmatism of about 2D. The OPD map on the left reveals total refractive astigmatism of 0.5 D at most with the difference being most likely due to crystalline lens astigmatism perpendicular to and therefore canceling the corneal astigmatism of 2D. Quite clearly the full corneal astigmatism of 2D should not be corrected whether it be by contact lenses or refractive surgery. To surgically correct refractive error demands an understanding of both the total ocular refractive status and the corneal surface ensuring a quick and correct diagnosis. The change in total refraction can be converted into an equivalent change in corneal surface shape and power. The Target Refractive map, method of calculating a shape of ablation, is obtained by adding the ocular refractive error map as measured by the OPD, to the corneal refractive power map. Either of them can be optically calculated from each other, but Axial and Instantaneous maps among topography maps cannot be calculated directly from the OPD map.

Relational expression: Refractive + OPD ≈ Target Refractive

ALIGNING TOPOGRAPHY DATA WITH OPD DATA

The abovementioned Target Refractive maps merge corneal information (Refractive) and total refractive information (OPD). It is important to avoid problems due to any change in eye alignment when moving from one device to another when collecting total ocular refraction data and corneal topography data. This potential problem is overcome with the OPD-scan by incorporating the two devices within the one instrument. The OPD-Scan[R] compensates for any positional shift between the Refractive map and OPD map by determining the location of the First Purkinje images its reference point.

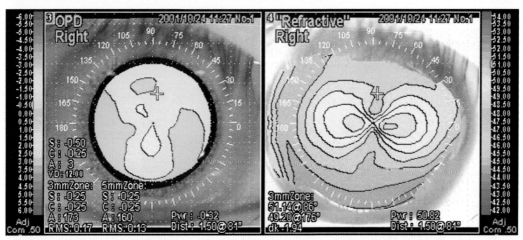

FIGURE 18.4: OPD map of total ocular refraction and corneal topography map for the same eye

MEASUREMENT OF PUPILLARY DIAMETER

The OPD-Scan[R] can measure the diameter and center position for both Photopic and Scotopic pupils as shown in Figure 18.5. To prevent halos and glare, the ablated area should be outside the nighttime dilated pupil. It would be ideal to compare a pupil image exposed to the laser with Photopic and Scotopic pupil diameters and respective pupil centers, and to align the laser axis with Scotopic pupil center. To avoid halo and glare due to poorly sized optical zones, the ablated area should be larger than the pupil under Scotopic conditions.

Scotopic   **Photopic**

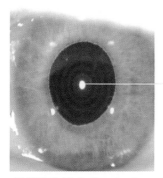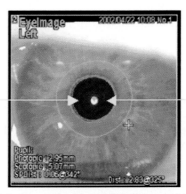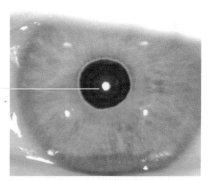

FIGURE 18.5: By aligning a bright corneal reflex of photopic pupil image with that of scotopic pupil image, it is possible to display the each pupil diameter, pupil center, and the distance between both pupil centers

FINAL FIT SOFTWARE: OUTLINE AND FEATURES

The Final Fit Software is designed to calculate ablation profile through analysis of both topography and OPD data obtained by the OPD-Scan[R] and generation of exact laser pulse shot data that controls the laser delivery system such as the movable apertures with the Nidek EC5000CX II refractive laser. With the Final Fit Software, the ablation profile data is divided into three components, as shown in Figure 18.6, so that they correspond to the ablation mechanism of the EC-5000CXII. Radially symmetric

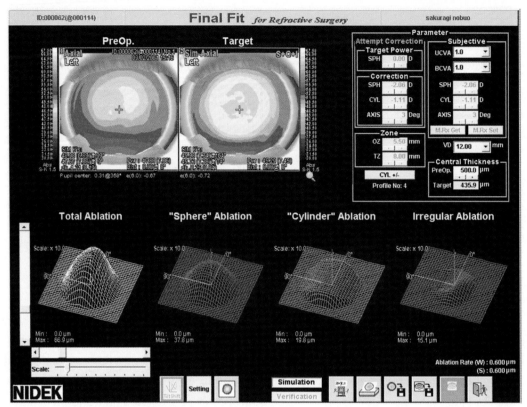

FIGURE 18.6: Final Fit software divides ablation profile data into three components; Sphere ablation, cylinder ablation and irregular ablation

components are ablated by scanning and rotating the rectangular laser beam controlled by the opening and closing of a diaphragm, linearly symmetric components are ablated by the laser beam controlled by the opening and closing of a slit mask, and irregular components are divided into small spots of 1 mm in diameter and ablated respectively, Multi Point Ablation.

The Final Fit software also displays preoperative and postoperative topography maps at the upper part of the screen, allowing the operator to optimize the conditions for operation such as the amount of correction, Optical Zone (OZ) and Transition Zone (TZ) for each eye (Figure 18.6).

CUSTOMIZED ABLATION

With the Final Fit software, the following ablation modes are available:

OZ	TZ
1. Spherical	OATZ * OATZ (Optimized Aspherical Transition Zone)
2. Topo-guided	OATZ
3. Wavefront-guided	OATZ

Spherical with OATZ Ablation

Spherical with OATZ ablation allows for customized ablation surgery in the periphery of the cornea to reduce nighttime halo, glare and the possible resultant decrease in contrast sensitivity. With the customized

Pre-op Profile a Profile b Profile c

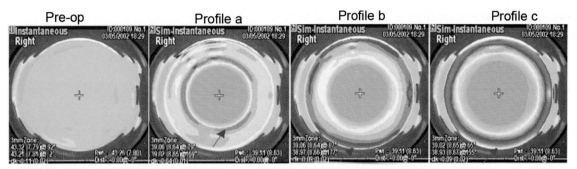

FIGURE 18.7: As the profile moves up from a to c, the red ring (indicated by "?") moves outward, the OZ and ablation depth increase. PMMA model eye; Hemisphere, 43.27D (7.8 mm), Parameter; Sph: –5 D, Cyl: 6 D, OZ: 5.0 mm, TZ: 9.0 mm, Ablation rate: 0.3 um/shot

ablation method, spherical lenses and cylindrical lenses are ablated in accordance with the amount of correction in the optical zone (OZ), and the ablated surface is smoothly connected with the non-ablated periphery of the cornea through the transition zone (TZ), This is to reduce nighttime halo, glare and a decrease in contrast sensitivity thought to be caused by abrupt changes in shape in the TZ.[5] The TZ shape can be determined by selecting the appropriate profile in Final Fit Software.

The Instantaneous corneal topography map is ideal for grasping subtle changes in corneal shape because the map better represents local corneal shape. Figure 18.7 shows that the position of the red ring representing the area with abrupt change in curvature changes with each power profile. As the profile moves up from a to c, the red ring moves to the periphery of the cornea, increasing the OZ and increasing the depth of ablation.

Topo-guided Customized Ablation

Topo-guided with OATZ ablation allows customized ablation for correcting pathological or postoperative corneal irregularities, such as decentered ablations. With the Topo-guided ablation method the larger irregularities are removed first. This ablation method allows the operator to ablate corneal irregularities with the minimum ablation depth. In these cases manifest refraction results can be unreliable but by removing much of the irregularities and then re-measuring and re-analyze the eye with the OPD-Scan superior results can be achieved.

Wavefront-guided Customized Ablation

Unlike some other wavefront analyzers, which calculate ablation depth directly from the amount of aberration, the OPD-Scan calculates ablation depth from what is required to change corneal surface power. As mentioned earlier, the preoperative refractive map and OPD map are used to generate the Target Refractive map, as well as corneal elevation data and the difference between the data used to determine the shape of ablation.

Wavefront-guided ablation allows for the display of an aberration-free area (OD) and to optimize the transition zone. The wavefront-guided ablation method is intended to reduce the amount of aberrations in the entire treatment zone (OZ + TZ). Although the above explanation presumes a target refractive endpoint of emmetropia this can be programed to achieve various levels of emmetropia as desired for example -1 D of myopia.

FEATURES OF THE FINAL FIT SOFTWARE

The features of the Final Fit are listed below:

- Preoperative and postoperative simulated Topography data allows an estimation of postoperative outcome—Safety
- The three ablation modes, normal (Spherical lens)/Topo-guided/Wavefront-guided ablation are selectable according to the eye to be operated on.—Quality of vision
- Vision quality can be enhanced by a smooth TZ with an OATZ (Optimized Aspherical Transition Zone)—Quality of vision
- The comparison function allows the operator to display preoperative, and postoperative topography map, the OPD map, and differential maps—Evaluation of postoperative outcome
- The topography data of the entire cornea and pupil contour displayed allows the operator to easily check the positional relationship between the treatment area and pupil, and distribution of powers. In addition, the OPD map allows the operator to check the distribution of refractive errors within a pupil (This is also available with the OPD-Scan)—Evaluation of postoperative outcome

CORRECTION OF CYCLO-TORSION

Little attention has been previously given to the possible shift of cylinder axis due to cyclotorsional rotation of the eye and many ophthalmic devices measure patients in the upright sitting position whereas

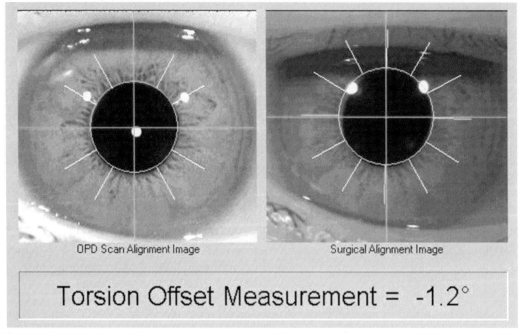

OPD Scan Alignment Image   Surgical Alignment Image

Torsion Offset Measurement = -1.2°

FIGURE 18.8: Torsion offset measurement calculated from eye images taken by OPD Scan and EC-5000CXII

during refractive surgery, the patient is in a recumbent position.[6] For this reason, when using the data obtained by the OPD-Scan in corneal refractive surgery, the eye rotation caused by this counter-rolling of the eyeball must be compensated. The OPD-Scan[R] analyzes iris pattern, pupil contour, pupil center and pupil size by capturing anterior eye images just after topography measurement. The pupil position information is then used for image registration and alignment as part of the Final Fit Calculations. The Final Fit Software generates ablation profiles and sends this together with the iris image registration data to the excimer laser system.

The iris image of the patient's eye lying on a bed will be captured by CCD camera installed in EC-5000 CXII laser system and then pupil center is calculated. Pupil center will also be determined against the iris image obtained by OPD Scan. Similar distinctive iris patterns will be detected from both iris images. The angle for some distinctive iris pattern will be measured from the baseline, which will go through each Pupil center and the angle difference between both images will be torsional angle error for as shown in Figure 18.8.

REFERENCES

1. MacRae S, Fujieda M. Customized Ablation using the NIDEK Laser, Customized Corneal Ablation. Slack 2001; 17:211-217.
2. Campbell C E, Benjamin WJ, Howland HC. Objective Refraction: Retinoscopy, Autorefraction and Photorefraction. In Benjamin WJ, Borlish IM (Ed): Borish's Clinical Refraction. Saunders 1998; 18: 594-600.
3. Thibos LN, Applegate RA. Assessment of Optical Quality in Customized Corneal Ablation: The Quest for SuperVision. Chapter 6, Slack Incorporated, New Jersey, USA, 2001.
4. Thibos LN, Applegate RA, Schwiegerling JT, Webb R, et al. Standards for Reporting the Optical Aberrations of Eyes, Vision Science and its Applications (OSA Trends in Optics and Photonics, Vol. 35), pp232-244, Optical Society of America, Washington, DC, 2000.
5. Wachler BS, Durrie DS, Assil KK, Krueger RR. Role of clearance and treatment zones in contrast sensitivity: significance in refractive surgery. J Cataract Refract Surg 1999; 25(1): 16-23.
6. Miller EF. Counter-rolling of the human eyes produced by head tilt with respect to gravity. Acta Otolaryngol 1962;54:479-501,
7. Wachler BS, Krueger RR. Agreement and repeatability of pupillometry using videokeratography and infrared devices. J Cataract Refract Surg 2000; 26(1): 35-40.

Section

III

Other Refractive Procedures

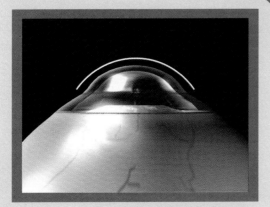

Chapter

19

Conductive Keratoplasty for Changing Corneal Curvature

Robeto Pinelli

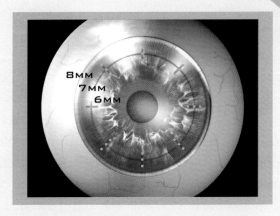

INTRODUCTION

Conductive Keratoplasty® (CK®) from Refractec, Inc. is a non-laser, radiofrequency-based procedure for treating presbyopia. The mechanism of action of CK is through the application of high frequency (radiofrequency) energy that the cornea converts to heat in a controlled fashion. Conductive keratoplasty requires no ablation or incisions and does not invade the central cornea.

In April, 2002, the United States Food and Drug Administration granted approval of the ViewPoint® CK System (Refractec, Inc., Irvine, CA) for the treatment of mild to moderate (0.75 D to 3.00 D) previously untreated, spherical hyperopia in persons 40-years-old or older.[1-3]

This was followed by the approval in March 2004 of CK to reduce the symptoms of presbyopia in presbyopic hyperopes (+1.00 to +2.25 D) or emmetropes through induction of a mild myopia in the non-dominant eye.[4] Other potential uses of the CK technique under investigation include treatment of over- or undercorrections following LASIK or other excimer laser procedures, enhancing outcomes of cataract surgery, and treating astigmatism (regular or irregular).

HISTORY OF CONDUCTIVE KERATOPLASTY

Early Thermokeratoplasty Procedures (second level section)

Thermokeratoplasty techniques aim to change corneal curvature through the application of heat, which shrinks corneal collagen. Although Lans attempted to shrink corneal collagen in rabbit eyes through thermal burns in the nineteenth century, it was not until the 1970s that various pathological conditions in humans, such as keratoconus and persistent corneal hydrops, were successfully treated with heated probes.[5,6] Although initially successful, corneal curvature returned to preoperative status and the complication rate was unacceptable.[7-9]

The Russian surgeon, Fyodorov, was the first to use thermokeratoplasty to change corneal refraction in 1981. Using a retractable probe tip, he and other investigators applied controlled thermal burns to treat spherical hyperopia and hyperopic astigmatism. The tip was heated to 600° C, and corneal penetration depth was reported to be 95%.[10-12] Although hyperopic corrections of up to 8.0 D were achieved, later studies showed lack of predictability and marked regression.[13,14]

Also in the early 1980s, Rowsey and colleagues developed the Los Alamos thermokeratoplasty probe. This instrument heated stromal collagen by means of radiofrequency waves, rather than by direct thermal conduction from a heated instrument. However, the topographical effect with this probe was short-lived, and testing was terminated.[15-17]

Following the report by Seiler and associates of stable corneal steepening achieved in blind eyes with a pulsed holmium:YAG laser used in the contact mode,[18] Sunrise Technologies of Fremont, California began to develop a non-contact method of holmium:YAG laser treatment for hyperopia. The clinical studies with two-year follow-up were published in 1996 and 1997.[19,20] The U.S. Food and Drug Administration approved the Hyperion LTK device in June 2000, based on a study cohort of 612 eyes, with 80% available for analysis at 12 months and only 12% at 24 months postoperatively.[21] The present Sunrise Hyperion LTK noncontact system provides three algorithms for pulse energy versus age of the patient. The physician must choose between an algorithm that substantially overcorrects initially but provides more long-term effect or one that overcorrects less but has less effect over time.

Laser Thermal Keratoplasty became unpopular because it lacked predictability and stability, and the device is no longer manufactured by Sunrise Technologies.

Conductive Keratoplasty Technology (second level section)

In the 1990s, Antonio Mendez, M.D. studied radiofrequency as an alternative to procedures that applied heat directly to the corneal surface.[22] His success in denaturing collagen and steepening of the cornea led to the development of the Conductive Keratoplasty® procedure (CK®), performed with the ViewPoint® CK System (Refractec, Inc., Irvine, California).

Unlike previous thermokeratoplasty methods that used a laser to generate heat intrastromally, conductive keratoplasty uses radiofrequency energy to shrink corneal collagen. The procedure is performed with the ViewPoint® CK System, and is based on the delivery of a precise amount of radiofrequency energy through a fine tip inserted into the peripheral corneal stroma. Treatment is applied in a ring pattern outside of the visual axis at a defined number of treatment spots, with a greater number of spots applied to achieve a greater effect (Figure 19.1). A full circle of treatment spots acts like a belt tightening the cornea in the periphery so that the central cornea steepens (Figure 19.2). During conductive keratoplasty treatment, corneal tissue is exposed to the same temperature at the bottom of the probe as at the top of the probe (corneal surface). This is in contrast to non-contact holmium LTK, which has a significant axial gradient and produces the highest temperatures at the corneal surface. The footprint

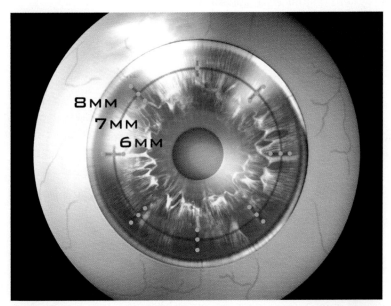

FIGURE 19.1: This shows the optical zone marks made by the marker to guide the surgeon in placement of the treatment spots. A circular mark is made on the 7 mm optical zone with the CK marker. An inner hatch mark lies on the 6 mm and an outer hatch mark on the 8 mm optical zone

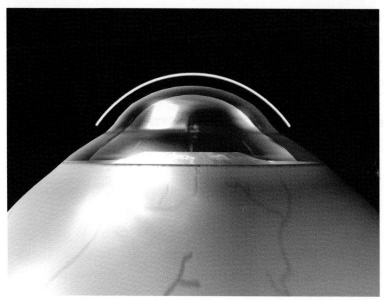

FIGURE 19.2: The conductive keratoplasty technique cinches the peripheral cornea which increases the curvature of the central cornea

after conductive keratoplasty is cylindrical and extends deep into the stroma to approximately 80% depth. This is in contrast to the conical stromal footprint made with the LTK technique.

THE CK SYSTEM

The ViewPoint® CK® system (Figure 19.3) consists of a portable console, corneal marker, lid speculum (choice of Lancaster, Barraquer, or Cook) that acts as the electrical return path for the radiofrequency

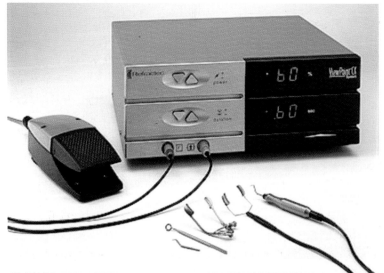

FIGURE 19.3: ViewPoint™ CK System. The ViewPointä CK system from Refractec, Inc. consists of a portable console, a corneal marker, choice of lid specula, a handpiece that holds the Keratoplast™ Tip, and a foot pedal

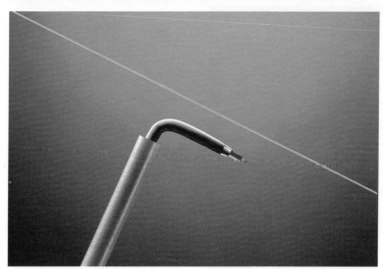

FIGURE 19.4: Keratoplast™ Tip. The Keratoplast™ Tip, (shown next to a 7-0 suture). The tip is 450 μm long and 90 μm wide and is used to deliver radiofrequency energy into the corneal stroma at the marked treatment points. A cuff on the probe assures correct depth of penetration

energy delivered by the tip, a handpiece (probe) that holds the 450 μm long and 90 μm wide stainless steel tip (Keratoplast™ Tip) (Figure 19.4), and a foot pedal. An insulated stop at the base of the probe controls the depth of penetration of the Keratoplast tip. Energy is delivered into the cornea by activation of the foot pedal.

Conductive keratoplasty uses the optimal combination of radiofrequency energy characteristics, including current, waveform, frequency, and duration of exposure, to raise the temperature of corneal collagen long enough to cause localized shrinkage of collagen fibers. Treatment application at the system default parameters causes the surrounding tissue to undergo a temperature increase. As the heated tissue dehydrates, its resistance to radiofrequency current increases. Since current seeks the path of least resistance, the current path moves up the shaft of the Keratoplast tip.

Tissue heating progresses from bottom (deep in the stroma) to top (corneal surface), and creates a thermal lesion that is uniformly cylindrical. The Keratoplast tip only *delivers* radiofrequency energy and heats up only in response to the increase in tissue temperature. The tip acts as a heat sink (takes heat away) rather than as a heat source (supplies heat). Histology studies on a pig cornea show that the cylindrical thermal lesion (footprint) formed as a result of CK treatment extends to approximately 80% of the depth of the stroma (Figure 19.5).

THE CK PROCEDURE

Patients suitable for the CK procedure should be 40 years of age or older, have visual acuity correctable to at least 20/40 in both eyes, and pachymetry readings of 560 mm or more at the 6 mm optical zone. Contact lens wearers should have a stable refraction. Patients undergoing CK for the treatment of presbyopia should have a history of monovision contact lens wear or success with a contact lens trial of

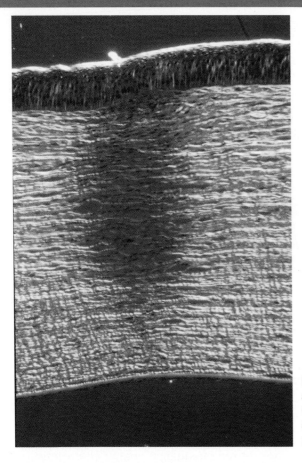

FIGURE 19.5: CK footprint. A polarized light micrograph of a histological section from a pig cornea, seven days after CK treatment. The footprint (dark region) is cylindrical and approximately 80% of corneal depth. Deep treatment penetration contributes to permanence of effect

monovision. Hard lens wearers should discontinue lens use three weeks and soft contact lens wearers two weeks before the procedure.

Patients should have no more than 0.75 D of refractive astigmatism, as determined by cycloplegic refraction. Assessment of preoperative topography is important to outcome. Avoid atypical or unusual corneas, such as those with keratoconus or pellucid marginal degeneration and be aware of potential sources of induced cylinder. These include corneas with a decentered apex or peripheral, asymmetric, or non-orthogonal astigmatism. Also avoid surgery on eyes with significant dryness or tear-function compromise. Preoperative testing includes slit lamp examination, keratometry, pachymetry, corneal topography and, for patients having treatment for presbyopia, dominance assessment, near and distance vision assessment, and monovision tolerance assessment.

Following screening, the surgeon can develop a treatment plan for each patient that considers patient age, accommodative amplitude, and desired distance or near correction. For the improvement of near vision in presbyopic emmetropes and hyperopes, the goal is to overcorrect the non-dominant eye by inducing slight to moderate myopia, –1.0 to –2.0 D (myopic endpoint) through the application of 16 to 24 CK treatment spots. If the dominant eye is significantly hyperopic, it can be targeted for +0.50 to -0.25 D. Most well selected patients treated for presbyopia will initially need only 16 spots in one eye. Treated patients display a reduction of symptoms of presbyopia without compromising binocular functional distance vision.

The procedure is performed with topical anesthesia. The surgeon places a lid speculum in the eye to be treated to obtain maximal exposure and provide the electrical return path. While the patient fixates on the microscope's light, cornea is then marked with a with a gentian-violet-dampened CK marker. Centration with the marker is very important, as is confirmation of satisfactory sphericity with the ring light. The surgeon then inserts the Keratoplast tip into the stroma at defined spots in a ring pattern around the peripheral cornea according to the supplied nomogram. Placement of the Keratoplast tip perpendicularly to the corneal surface at the treatment markings is also highly important. The cuff around the probe, which settles perpendicular to the cornea, helps to achieve perpendicular placement. Energy is applied by depressing the foot pedal. An increasing number of spots and rings are used for higher amounts of correction. The CK procedure takes only a few minutes to complete. Postoperative care includes instillation of a topical antibiotic solution, a topical nonsteroidal anti-inflammatory agent, and artificial tears, as needed.

Treatment of Presbyopia

The FDA clinical study for approval of CK for the correction of presbyopia (NearVision[SM] CK®) was conducted in 5 centers in the United States. The treatment goal was to improve near vision in non-dominant eye of hyperopic or emmetropic presbyopes and, if needed to improve distance vision in the dominant eye. A total of 150 patients (188 eyes) with symptoms of presbyopia were enrolled and treated with CK. One hundred twelve eyes were treated for near vision correction and 38 eyes for distance correction as well as near (bilateral correction). Patients were an average of 53 years old; 96% of all patients were Caucasian, and 61% were female. The mean intended correction for eyes treated for near was +2.03 D ± 0.63 D. The range of correction was +0.75 D to 3.00 D. Eyes treated for partial near correction (intermediate distance target) were excluded from analysis (N=14).

Of the eyes treated for near with an intended correction of +1.25 to 2.25 D (16 to 24 CK spots), 105/130 (81%) and 49/64 (77%) had J2 or better binocular UCVA-Near at 6 months and 12 months, respectively . For UCVA-Near of J3 or better, the percentage was 117/130 (90%) and 57/64 (89%), compared with 20/133 (15%) that had this uncorrected binocular near acuity preoperatively. Binocular UCVA-Distance results showed 95% and 97% with 20/20 or better acuity at 6 and 12 months, respectively, 100% and 98% for 20/25 or better at 6 and 12 months, respectively, and 100% with 20/32 or better at 6 and 12 months .

The combination of binocular UCVA-Distance of 20/20 or better with UCVA-Near of J2 or better was achieved by 100/130 (77%) at 6 months and 48/64 (75%) at 12 months. For combined binocular UCVA-Distance of 20/20 or better with UCVA-Near of J3 or better the percentages were 110/130 at 6 months and 56/64 (87%) at 12 months.

The 6-months cohort of patients showed no loss of contrast sensitivity under mesopic conditions. Best spectacles corrected visual acuity (BSCVA) before CK compared with BSCVA following CK was unchanged through postoperative month 12. Also, BSCVA before CK compared with UCVA-Near following CK was unchanged through postoperative month 12.

Treatment of Hyperopia

A two-year, multicenter, prospective clinical trial (FDA phase III hyperopia trial) was conducted to evaluate the safety, efficacy, and stability of conductive keratoplasty when performed on eyes with +0.75 to +3.00 D of hyperopia and 0.75 D of cylinder or less. Preliminary one-year results were previously published.[1-3] The treatment goal was a full correction of spherical hyperopia (emmetropia), and no retreatments were performed. A total of 400 eyes were treated. Follow-up at 1 year was 98% and, at 2 years, 94%.

The mean age of enrolled patients was 55.3 ± 6.4 years. The mean baseline cycloplegic spherical equivalent (SE) refraction was +1.86 ± 0.63 D. Uncorrected distance visual acuity (UCVA) preoperatively was 20/40 or better in 26% of the eyes. Twelve months postoperatively, UCVA was 20/20 or better in 174/320 (54%), 20/25 or better in 239/320 (75%), and 20/40 or better in 293/320 (92%) of the eyes. Results were similar at 24 months. Mean MRSE values showed 199/320 (62%) within 0.50 D of intended correction at 12 months.

The mean change in MRSE per month was 0.03 D, 0.05 D, and 0.03 D, between months six to nine, nine to 12, and 12 to 24, respectively. Expressed as change per interval, the MRSE changed a mean of +0.25 ± 0.50 D between three and six months, +0.11 ± 0.41 D between six and nine months, 0.13 ± 0.33 D between nine and 12 months, and 0.28 ± 0.41 D between 12 and 24 months. At 6 months the eyes were essentially emmetropic (mean MRSE = -0.03 D). Corneal topography (Orbscan) shows postoperative central corneal steepening surrounded by mid-peripheral flattening (Figure 19.6).

CK CASE HISTORIES

Conductive Keratoplasty can also be performed for conditions other than hyperopia and presbyopia. However, the surgeon must be highly experienced with conventional CK procedures before undertaking such procedures. Below are case histories I performed using the CK system to place spots in specific locations on the cornea that were not in the conventional ring pattern and did not follow the nomograms for hyperopia or presbyopia treatment.

Case 1: CK for Treating Keratoconus

The 34-year-old patient requested a surgical technique to enhance his vision and, if possible, reduce or eliminate dependence on spectacles. The corneal map revealed a bilateral pellucid marginal degeneration. In his right eye UCVA was 20/400, BCVA was 20/40, and cylinder was -2.5 D @ 65°. In the left eye, UCVA was 20/400, BCVA was 20/40, and cylinder was -2.5 D @ 65°. Conductive Keratoplasty was discussed with the patient. Theoretically, the possibility of placing asymmetrical spots following the corneal map could induce the cones to move to the center of the cornea, thereby obtaining better quality of vision and perhaps a gain of lines of UCVA.

The author decided to place 3 spots in the flat axis of the right eye and one spot on the opposite side to counterbalance the tension induced in the corneal tissue from treating the right eye. Figure 19.7 shows the patient's pre-CK topography and Figure 19.8 shows the location on the cornea at which the

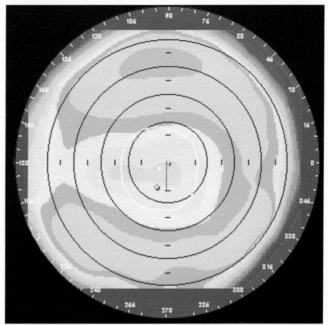

FIGURE 19.6A: 16- and 24-spot CK nomogram. Sixteen spots are applied at the 6 and 7 mm optical zones for correction of 1.00 to 1.625 D of correction and 24 spots are applied at the 6, 7, and 8 mm optical zones for 1.75 to 2.25D (ppt)

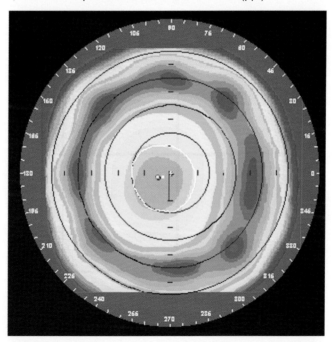

FIGURE 19.6B: Orbscan corneal topography pre- and post-CK. Corneal topography (Orbscan) shows postoperative central corneal steepening surrounded by mid-peripheral flattening

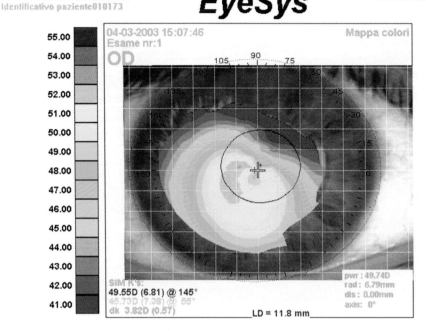

EyeSys

FIGURE 19.7: Preoperative corneal topography of patient with keratoconus

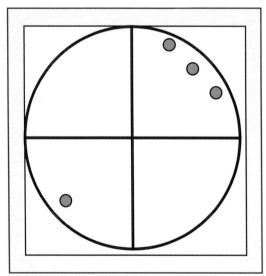

FIGURE 19.8: Location of CK spots placement of patient with keratoconus

CK spots were placed. The results six months postoperatively seem promising, with UCVA at 20/50 and BCVA at 20/40, cylinder -0.75 @ 90°. The post-CK corneal topography (Figure 19.9) shows the movement of the cones in the direction of the center of the cornea. Figure 19.10 shows post-CK slit lamp view of the patient with keratoconus.

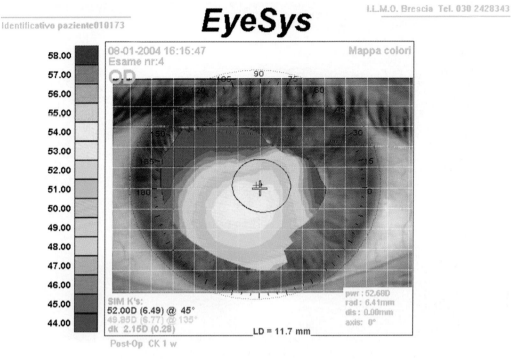

FIGURE 19.9: Post-CK corneal topography of patient with keratoconus

At this time the patient, happy and satisfied, asked to have surgery performed on the other eye. This case demonstrates that CK can be used to treat irregular astigmatism even though it requires additional follow up, as well as standardization of nomograms for such cases.

Case 2: CK for Post-cataract Surgery Astigmatism

A 71-year-old patient came to the Institute with a "visual problem" in the left eye. A phacoemulsification (sutureless) with the insertion of an Acrysof lens (Alcon) had been performed in another hospital. Uncorrected VA in the left eye was 20/50, BCVA was 20/30, and cylinder was + 1.5 D @ 70°. Corneal topography revealed regular post-cataract astigmatism (Figure 19.11). We did not know if the astigmatism had been induced by the incision, but it was not relevant to our treatment plan. After studying the topography map, I decided to place two spots, one in each flat axis, at the 7 mm optical zone (Figure 19.12). The post-CK corneal topography (Figure 19.13) shows no astigmatism, and the patient now has UCVA of 20/30 and a plano refraction, stable at the last examination (6 months). This case illustrates that Conductive Keratoplasty can be effective for treatment of post cataract surgery patients (hyperopic or astigmatic).

SUMMARY

Conductive keratoplasty is a non-laser procedure for changing corneal curvature to treat presbyopia, low to moderate spherical hyperopia, and other refractive conditions. The largest potential population

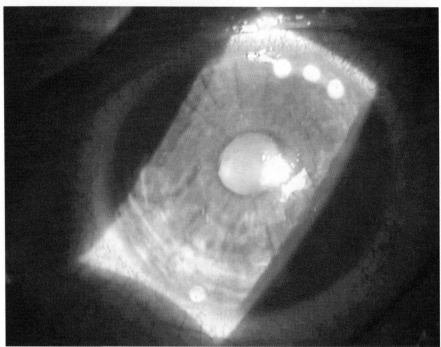

FIGURE 19.10: Post-CK slit lamp view of patient with keratoconus

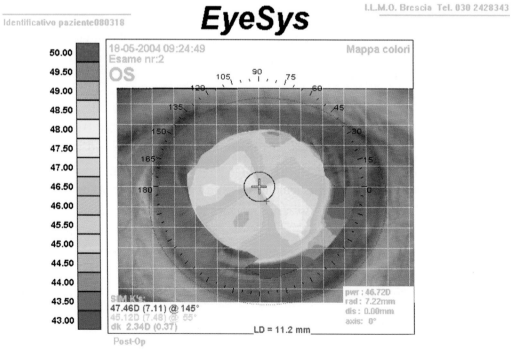

FIGURE 19.11: Preoperative corneal topography of patient with regular postcataract surgery astigmatism

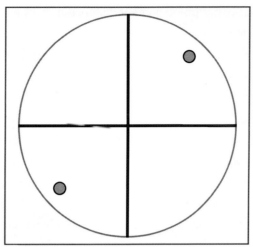

FIGURE 19.12: Location of CK spots placement
of patient with postcataract surgery astigmatism

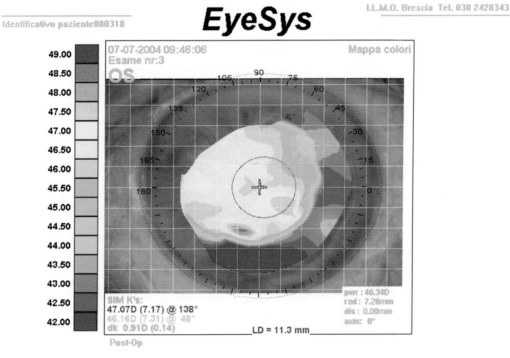

FIGURE 19.13: Post-CK corneal topography of patient with
post-cataract surgery astigmatism

for CK appears to be the presbyopes, many of whom are interested in a non-laser procedure that can extend the period of spectacle-free near vision.

Depth perception was maintained, binocular corrected distance acuity was better than preoperative level for 20/20, 20/32, and 20/40 acuities, and there was no loss of contrast sensitivity (quality of vision) from preoperative levels. Furthermore the presbyopia patient study showed that approximately 9/10 patients could see both 20/20 or better binocularly at distance and J3 or better at near without glasses. Patient satisfaction was high and 98% reported improvement in quality of vision. The procedure was remarkably safe with only 1% showing a transient loss of >2 lines of BSCVA.

Conductive Keratoplasty also has potential in the treatment of conditions other than hyperopia or presbyopia. The treatment plan for these must be designed by the surgeon for the patient's particular condition. At the Institute (Istituto Laser Microchirurgia Oculare, Brescia, Italy) we are treating keratoconus and astigmatism in post-cataract surgery patients by placing treatment spots on specifically chosen locations on the cornea. Other conditions we are studying and treating at the Institute are: 1) post-LASIK hyperopia performing CK spots on the flap (the effect seems to be more powerful compared to the CK applied to the virgin eye); 2) post-PRK hyperopia applying the CK spots only if we have enough pachimetry in 7/8 mm. optical zone; 3) post-PRK astigmatism (regular or irregular) and post-phakic IOL's hyperopia (here it is more easy being the cornea in a virgin condition). Conductive keratoplasty appears very promising for treating presbyopia and hyperopia, as well as a number of less common refractive conditions, easily, effectively, and safely.

Of course, a longer follow up is needed in order to evaluate the long term stability, effects and efficiency of this interesting technique in time.

REFERENCES

1. McDonald MB, Davidorf J, Maloney RK, Manche EE, Hersh P. Conductive keratoplasty for the correction of low to moderate hyperopia: 1-year results on the first 54 eyes. Ophthalmology 2002;109:637-49.
2. McDonald MB, Hersh PS, Manche EE, Maloney RK, Davidorf J, Sabry M. Conductive keratoplasty for the correction of low to moderate hyperopia: U.S. clinical trial 1-year results on 355 eyes. Ophthalmology. 2002; 109:1978-89.
3. Asbell PA, Maloney RK, Davidorf J, Hersh P, McDonald M, Manche E. Conductive Keratoplasty Study Group. Conductive keratoplasty for the correction of hyperopia. Trans Am Ophthalmol Soc. 2001;99:79-84.
4. McDonald, MB, Durrie DS, Asbell PA, Maloney R, Nichamin L. Treatment of presbyopia with conductive keratoplasty: six-month results of the 1-year United States FDA clinical trial. Cornea 2004;23:661-8.
5. Gassett AR, Kaufman HE. Thermokeratoplasty in the treatment of keratoconus. Am J Ophthalmol 1975;79:226-32.
6. Aquavella J, Buxton J, Shaw E. Thermokeratoplasty in the treatment of persistent corneal hydrops. Archives Ophthalmol 1977;95:81-84.
7. Aquavella JV, Smith RS, Shaw EL. Alterations in corneal morphology following thermokeratoplasty. Arch Ophthalmol 1976;94:2082-85.
8. Arentsen J, Rodriquez M, Laibson P. Histopathological changes after thermokeratoplasty for keratoconus. Invest Ophthalmol Vis Sci 1977;16:32-38.
9. Fogle JA, Kenyon KR, Stark WJ. Damage to the epithelial basement membrane by thermokeratoplasty. Am J Ophthalmol 1977;83:392-401.
10. Caster AI. The Fyodorov technique of hyperopia correction by thermal coagulation: A preliminary report. J Refract Surg 1988;4:105-08.
11. Neumann A, Sanders D, Salz J. Radial thermokeratoplasty for hyperopia. J Refract Corneal Surg 1989;5:50-54.
12. Neumann A, Fyodorov S, Sanders D. Radial thermokeratoplasty for the correction of hyperopia. J Refract Corneal Surg 1990;6:404-12.
13. Neumann A, Sanders D, Raanan M, DeLuca M. Hyperopic thermokeratoplasty: clinical evaluation. J Cataract Refract Surg 1991;17:830-38.
14. Feldman S, Ellis W, Frucht-Pery J, et al. Regression of effect following radial thermokeratoplasty in humans. J Refract Surg 1995;18:288-91.
15. Rowsey JJ, Doss JD. Preliminary report of Los Alamos keratoplasty techniques. Ophthalmology 1981;88:755-60.
16. Rowsey JJ, Gaylor JR, Dahlstrom R, et al. Contact Intraocul Lens Med J 1980;6:1-12.
17. Rowsey JJ. Electrosurgical keratoplasty: Update and retraction. Invest Ophthalmol Vis Sci 1987;28 (suppl):224.

18. Seiler T, Matallana M, Bende T. Laser thermokeratoplasty by means of a pulsed holmium:YAG laser for hyperopic correction. Refract Corneal Surg1990;6:355-59.

19. Koch DD, Abarca A, Villareal R, et al. Hyperopia correction by non-contact holmium:YAG laser thermokeratoplasty; clinical study with two-year follow-up.

20. Koch D, Kohnen T, McDonnell P, et al. Hyperopia correction by noncontact holmium:YAG laser thermal keratoplasty. U.S. Phase IIA Clinical Study with 2-year follow-up. Ophthalmology 1997; 104:1938-47.

21. United States FDA PMA P990078. Hyperion LTK System Device Labeling, Sunrise Technologies, Fremont, California, May 2000.

22. Mendez A, Mendez Noble A. Conductive keratoplasty for the correction of hyperopia. In Sher N (Ed): Surgery for Hyperopia and Presbyopia. Philadelphia: Williams and Wilkins: 1997;163-71.

Chapter

20

Intacs™: Refractive Correction with an Intracorneal Device

Terry E Burris
Debby Holmes-higgin

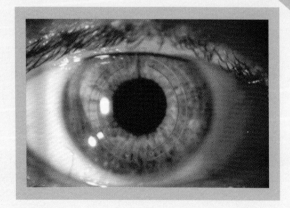

INTRODUCTION

Intracorneal ring technology has shown rapid development in the past twelve years, and clinical results are confirming outstanding results for the correction of low to moderate refractive myopias. The Intrastromal Corneal Ring Segments (ICRS® or Intacs®) are currently undergoing rigorous investigation in FDA regulated clinical trials in the US Results to date indicate the surgical procedure is safe and easily performed, visual results are excellent, and the device provides stable and predictable correction postoperatively. Enhancements can be easily performed by device exchange, and Intacs can be removed, reversing the refractive effect. Intacs are available in Europe and Canada for clinical use, and are anticipated to be FDA approved in the near future in the US.

HISTORY

The intrastromal ring concept was proposed by AE Reynolds in 1978. The device was to be placed in the corneal periphery through a single, peripheral radial incision. Central corneal curvature could be either flattened or steepened, respectively, by constricting or expanding the ring. As a refractive surgical device, the proposed benefits included surgical preservation of the central cornea, elimination of wound healing as a determinant of surgical outcome, rapid vision improvement, and capability to adjust or even reverse the procedure to expand patient options.

Later theoretical and animal study work on this device continued with funding from KeraVision, Inc. (Fremont, CA)[1] to confirm its feasibility. Human eye bank eye studies by Burris and associates[2] showed that ring thickness produced corneal flattening, which eliminated the need to constrict or expand the device. The current product, the intrastromal corneal ring segments (ICRS®), or Intacs™ corneal ring segments, is designed to correct low to moderate myopia by modulation of device thickness. Intacs have been approved for clinical use in Europe and Canada and FDA regulated clinical trials are currently being completed in the U.S.

Initial Clinical Studies

Non functional human eye studies of a full circle ring implant, the ICR® (Intrastromal Corneal Ring), were conducted in 1991 in Brazil and the US.[3,4] This 360° implant was made of polymethyl methacrylate (PMMA) and had an inner diameter of 6.8 mm, and outer diameter of 8.1 mm. The ICR was placed into a 360° intrastromal channel fashioned at two-thirds corneal depth, via a two millimeter radial incision. These studies demonstrated that the ICR could be easily implanted and safely tolerated by the cornea, achieve consistent corneal flattening, and with removal result in return of original corneal curvature.

The ICR was placed in the first ten human sighted eyes in 1991.[5] The most recently reported results (4 year) indicated that uncorrected visual acuity was 20/40 or better in nine eyes, eight eyes were within ±1.00 D of their intended correction as determined by manifest spherical equivalent refraction, and refractive effect was stable over time. One patient had the ICR removed at postoperative Month 6.

Phase II ICR clinical trials in the US were begun in 1993 under the direction of David Schanzlin, MD. These studies, conducted with either a radial or circumferential incision, further confirmed that the ICR was well tolerated in the cornea with predictable, stable optical correction of myopic eyes. Recently reported results indicated that, of sixty-six patients who had reached postoperative Month 12 at the reporting period, 85% had uncorrected visual acuity of 20/40 or better.[6]

Current US Clinical Studies

The original 360° ICR was modified to consist of two 150° PMMA arc segments (ICRS) in order to facilitate the surgical procedure and avoid potential incision related complications. Each device segment is inserted into its respective semi-circular shaped intrastromal channel made through a single 1.8 mm radial incision located in the superior cornea near the limbus. An Intacs in situ is presented in Figure 20.1. Original thicknesses of the Intacs for the US. Phase II and III clinical studies were 0.25, 0.30, 0.35, 0.40 and 0.45 mm; an additional thickness of 0.21 mm was added for the Phase III trial. The US clinical trials are currently ongoing and nearing completion.

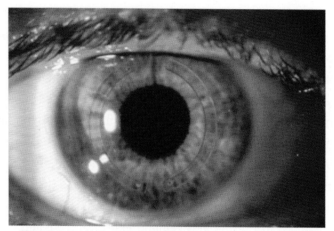

FIGURE 20.1: The Intacs refractive device placed in situ.

Surgical Procedure

The surgical procedure is illustrated in stepwise fashion by Figure 20.2 (A to G).[6] Patient preparation and Intacs placement are performed under topical anesthesia using techniques similar to LASIK.

The corneal geometric center is marked and peripheral corneal thickness is measured by ultrasonic pachymetry over the planned incision site, typically at the 12:00 meridian. A diamond knife is set to 68% of the peripheral corneal thickness and is used to create a 1.8 mm incision allowing introduction of the lamellar dissecting instruments (KeraVision, Inc., Fremont, CA). A pocket spreader (modified Suarez spreader) is used to initiate the lamellar dissection in both a clockwise and counterclockwise direction. A vacuum centering guide is applied to the globe, and the clockwise or counterclockwise stromal separator is introduced through the incision and rotated 180 to 190° to create a midperipheral semi-circular channel. The separator is rotated out of the channel, and the other separator is used to fashion the opposing half channel. The vacuum centering guide is removed. One of two Intacs is irrigated with BSS, inserted and rotated into either the clockwise or counterclockwise channel, and finely placed with a Sinskey hook. Its mate is similarly rotated into its respective portion of the channel. A single 10-0 or 11-0 nylon suture (optional)

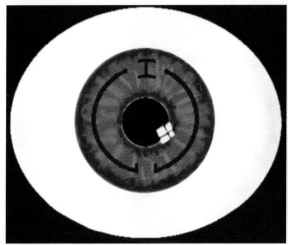

FIGURE 20.2A: Incision and placement for Intacs marked

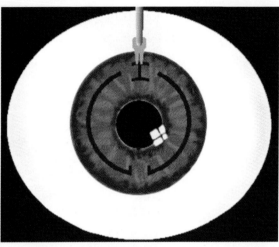

FIGURE 20.2B: Radial incision (~1.8 mm) made

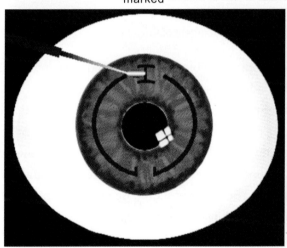

FIGURE 20.2C: Pocket created as a requisite for stromal separation and Intacs placement

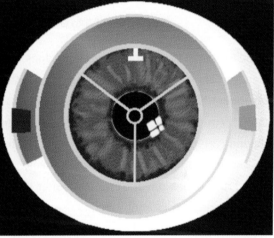

FIGURE 20.2D: Vacuum centering guide used to facilitate stromal separation

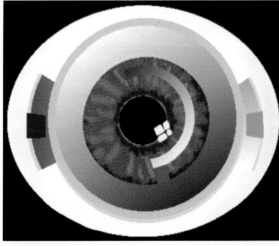

FIGURE 20.2E: Stromal separation in the clockwise direction

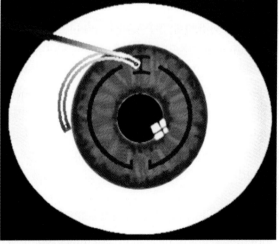

FIGURE 20.2F: Intacs segment inserted.

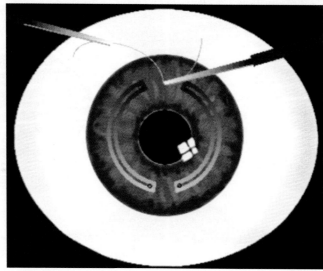

FIGURE 20.2G: Incision closed

FIGURES 20.2A to G: Surgical procedure for placement of the Intacs

is placed to ensure closure of the incision edges, drops of topical antibiotic/corticosteroid combination are applied and an eye shield taped into place for the immediate postoperative period.

Postoperative discomfort is managed with a topical non-steroidal anti-inflammatory agent such as Voltaren®. An antibiotic steroid combination drop, such Tobradex®, is used four times a day for one week, and can then be tapered rapidly over the following week. The nylon suture, if placed, is removed when loose, or by two weeks postoperatively. Any suture removal should be covered with antibiotic three to four times a day for four days after the removal. The patients should be examined about one week after cessation of antibiotic to ensure no late infections have occurred.

Clinical Outcomes

Visual Results

Month 12 postoperative results for the Phase II and III the US Intacs clinical trial cohort surveyed for the FDA pre-market approval (PMA) application were recently reported for three Intacs thickness.[7,8] Nominal predicted correction was –1.30 diopters for the 0.25 mm Intacs, –2.00 diopters for the 0.30 mm Intacs and –2.70 diopters for the 0.35 mm Intacs. Uncorrected visual acuity in 97% of patients (total n=410) was 20/40 or better (Figure 20.3). Ninety-nine percent of patients (409/410) had preserved best spectacles corrected visual acuity at postoperative Month 12 (Figure 20.4). One eye lost eleven ETDRS letters (about two lines) at postoperative Month 12, but had visual acuity (both uncorrected and best spectacles corrected) of 20/20.

Perioperative Observations and Complications

Perioperative observations with the Intacs are most representative of current surgical techniques reported for the FDA PMA cohort of 410 eyes.[7,8] Mild subconjunctival hemorrhages are seen at surgery from

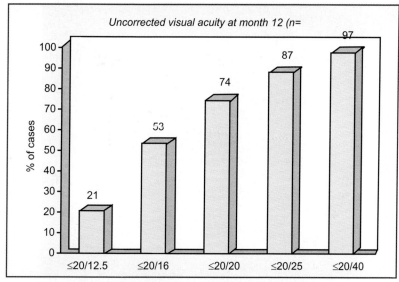

FIGURE 20.3: Uncorrected visual acuity at postoperative Month 12 with the Intacs

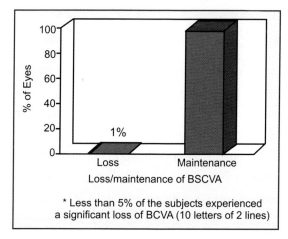

* Less than 5% of the subjects experienced a significant loss of BCVA (10 letters of 2 lines)

FIGURE 20.4: Best spectacles corrected visual acuity at postoperative Month 12 with the Intacs

manipulating the conjunctiva with surgical instruments. Adverse intraoperative complications for this clinical study cohort included one posterior corneal perforation into the anterior chamber, due to a deviation in surgical procedure, three anterior corneal surface perforations, due to superficial dissection of the intrastromal channel, and one case of subconjunctival chemosis, resulting from an allergic response to the surgical scrub. In all five cases the Intacs were not placed at the time the event occurred, although two of these patients subsequently had Intacs successfully placed in contralateral eyes. Best spectacles corrected visual acuity for patients experiencing intraoperative complications have returned to baseline, or improved, compared to preoperative values.

Postoperative Observations

Epithelial wound closure over the incision occurred for 96% of patients by Day 7 after receiving Intacs. All eyes had completely healed by Day 14. Small epithelial inclusion cysts were noted in 37.6% of

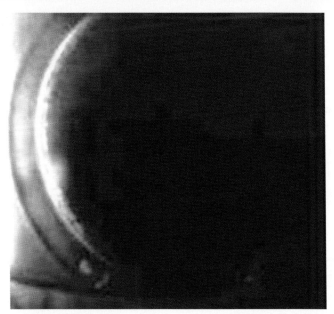

FIGURE 20.5: Mild channel haze and tiny refractile deposits in the lamellar channel are normal postoperative findings with the Intacs device.

patients at some point postoperatively, and appeared well embedded in the stroma with no fluorescein staining; these remained in only 7% of eyes at postoperative one year.

At Month 3, other clinically insignificant findings included mild channel haze, as well as tiny refractile deposits in the lamellar channel, and hazy cloudy deposits in the segment positioning holes, and / or at the ends of the segments in most patients (Figure 20.5). The location of the haze correlates with the zone of blunt lamellar stromal dissection, which is slightly larger than the width of the Intacs. Small amorphous chalky deposits develop adjacent to the ICRS in many patients. These increase for several months in many patients and tend to disappear by two years postoperatively. Haze and deposits have never been observed to extend outside the channel either peripherally or toward the visual axis for any patient.

Eight patients (8%) had corneal sensation losses of 20 mm or greater (Cochet-Bonnet aesthesiometry) at Month 3, and no patient had total loss of corneal sensation. This effect appears to be transient and principally limited to the central three millimeters of the cornea. No patient demonstrated signs of neurotrophic keratitis, such as punctate keratitis, filaments, epithelial breakdown or trophic ulceration. Subsequent study shows corneal sensation to be returning in all patients.

Postoperative adverse event occurred in 5/454 (1%) of the enrolled patient eyes in the PMA cohort. These included one incident of infectious keratitis, one incident of shallow segment placement, and two incidents of anterior chamber perforation during surgery. All adverse event patient eyes had a best spectacles corrected visual acuity of 20/20 or better at their last reported exam and none of them has experienced a permanent loss.

Twenty patients experienced induced astigmatism of greater than or equal to 1.0 D based on manifest refraction (Month 3). This is believed to be related to incisional healing effects and possibly due to suture tightness at surgery. Corneal topography in these cases confirm a typical with-the-rule induced cylinder effect originating from the area of the incision site at 12:00. In spite of the induced cylinder, nineteen of the twenty patients maintained uncorrected visual acuity of 20/40 or better. By Month 12, 15/410 patients (3.7%) had greater than one diopter of induced refractive astigmatism. Three patients (0.7%) experienced greater than one and a half diopters of induced astigmatism. All three of these patients had uncorrected visual acuity of 20/25 and best spectacles corrected visual acuity of 20/16 or better.

Corneal Topography

Corneal topography observations confirm that central corneal flattening increases incrementally with greater thickness Intacs.[2] In addition, postoperative corneal shape remains prolately aspheric, a potentially unique optical characteristic of the Intacs compared to other refractive correction procedures.[2,9-12] Color axial maps representing typical anterior corneal surface topography, preoperatively and with a 0.35 mm Intacs, are presented in Figure 20.6. These maps qualitatively illustrate the topographic flattening which occurs with Intacs. Preoperative prolate asphericity is accentuated with Intacs, but does not appear to be related to standard clinical visual performance measures including best spectacles corrected visual acuity and contrast sensitivity.[10-12]

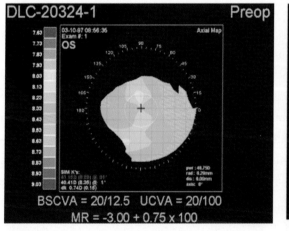 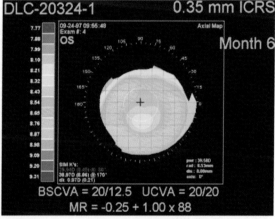

FIGURE 20.6: Color axial topography maps representing normal corneal topography before and after the Intacs refractive procedure.

Radius of curvature flattening profiles, adapted from methodology reported for previous corneal topography investigation,[13] were used to quantify induced topographic corneal flattening with each Intacs thickness. Flattening across the zero to six millimeter diameter optical zones was determined by subtracting the average postoperative axial radius of curvature values for each zone from respective preoperative values. Profiles have been designed to visually simulate mean axisymmetrical corneal curvature change; the zero millimeter zone mean value is placed at the center of each profile and each successive mean zone value is shown redundantly to each side. These profiles graphically illustrate average central and pericentral corneal flattening, in addition to showing trends of topographic change between the corneal diameter millimeter zones. Radius of curvature difference profiles indicated that

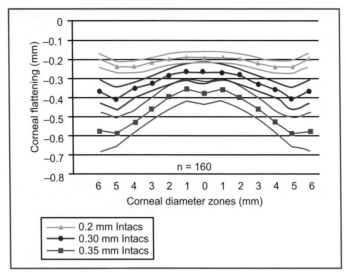

FIGURE 20.7: Mean (with 95% confidence intervals) radius of curvature flattening profiles for three different thickness Intacs.

flattening with Intacs was prolately aspheric; relatively more flattening occurred pericentrally than centrally (Figure 20.7). Confidence intervals (95%) suggested that the average radius of curvature change was significantly different between Intacs thicknesses for most millimeter diameter optical zones.

Anterior corneal surface topography with the Intacs has been typified. Color axial topography maps from eyes in the Phase III FDA clinical trial were classified by predominant qualitative pattern by two masked observers according to pre-specified topography classifications and guidelines.[14] The classification scheme was developed primarily from previously published works[15-21] and included the following prolate patterns: spherical (SPH), non-toric prolate asphere (PAS), symmetrically toric (STO), asymmetrically toric (ATO), multizonal (MZA), or non-central prolate asphere and unclassifiable (UNC). Preoperative and postoperative Month 6 corneas with the Intacs approximated patterns published for normal eyes, with a few exceptions.[15]

Reversibility of Refractive Effect after Intacs Removal

A unique characteristic of the Intacs refractive surgical procedure is its potential reversibility. Recently reported results for 449 eyes indicated that Intacs have been removed from 31 eyes (6.9%) with no apparent residual refractive effect.[8,22] Reasons for Intacs removal included dissatisfaction with correction achieved (12 eyes), dissatisfaction relating to glare and/or halos (16 eyes), bacterial infection (1 eye), and personal reasons (2 eyes). Manifest refraction spherical equivalent at Month 3 after Intacs removal returned to within one diopter of preoperative value for most eyes (Figure 20.8). Corneal topography analyses supported these refractive results.[23] Color axial trend maps for a sample eye clearly demonstrate the return of corneal curvature to approximate baseline levels after removal of the Intacs (Figure 20.9).

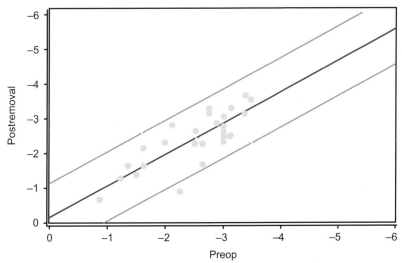

FIGURE 20.8: Manifest refraction spherical equivalent preoperatively and after removal (Month 3) of the Intacs for individual eyes.

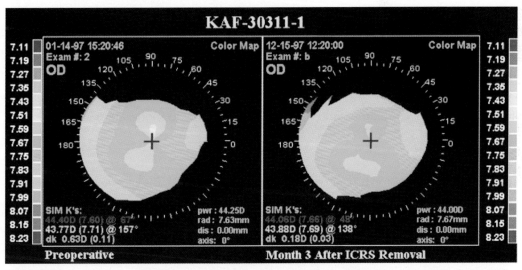

FIGURE 20.9: Color axial corneal topography trend map for a case eye preoperatively and after removal of the Intacs

Refinement of Refractive Effect with Intacs Exchange

Several patients have undergone Intacs exchange to treat over-or undercorrection. These brief procedures were easy to perform and preliminary reports indicate a good response.[8]

Safety Assurance and Further Indications

All the US FDA safety and efficacy endpoints have been reached for the 0.25, 0.30 and 0.35 mm Intacs and FDA market approval is expected soon in the United States. Intracorneal ring technology demonstrates a promising new technique for rapid, predictable vision correction with no removal of corneal tissue or surgical violation of the central cornea. At postoperative Month 12, uncorrected visual acuity is stable and best spectacles corrected visual acuity is maintained. Preliminary Intacs exchange data show enhancements to be easily performed and efficacious. Finally, Intacs are removable and the optical effect is reversible, making this technique uniquely appealing to patients who want to preserve future corrective options.

The effective range of treatment with the current Intacs design will likely apply to myopias up to five diopters, although newer permutations may have other refractive applications (i.e. astigmatism concurrent with myopia, hyperopia,). Astigmatism is not currently being corrected with the Intacs in the US clinical trials, although prototype device designs[24,25] and early patient results from Brazil have been reported.[26]

Complications of the US Intacs procedure to date have been few and easily managed. Importantly, there have been no complications resulting in permanent loss of uncorrected or best spectacles corrected visual acuity. Transient loss of corneal sensation is consistent with that seen in cataract surgery, incisional keratotomy and ablation procedures.[29-32] In all cases where the Intacs were removed, the refractive effect has been shown to be reversible.

The unique topography of the Intacs, showing maintenance of prolate corneal asphericity, has theoretical optical advantages that may be further exploited in the future.[9] One of our surgical refractive goals should be to minimize induced optical anomalies such as spherical aberration, which can degrade contrast sensitivity and image quality. Further studies of intracorneal implant technology and correlation with clinical outcomes will help refine our understanding of ocular optical principles as they apply to refractive surgery. Intacs have been approved for commercial use in the European Union, and may soon join the US refractive armamentarium for correction of low to moderate myopia.

REFERENCES

1. Fleming JR, Reynolds AI, Kilmer L, Burris TE, Abbott RL and Schanzlin DJ. The intrastromal corneal ring: Two cases in rabbits. J Refract Surg 1987; 3:227-32.
2. Burris TE, Baker PC, Ayer CT, Loomas BE, Mathis ML, Silvestrini TA. Flattening of central corneal curvature with intrastromal corneal rings of increasing thickness: an eye-bank eye study. J Cataract Refract Surg 1993;19(suppl):182-187.
3. Nosé W, Neves RA, Schanzlin DJ, Belfort R. Intrastromal corneal ring — one-year results of first implants in humans: a preliminary nonfunctional eye study. Refract and Corneal Surg 1993;9:452-8.
4. Assil KK, Barrett AM Fouraker BD, Schanzlin DJ. For the Intrastromal Corneal Ring Study Group. One-year result of the intrastromal corneal ring in nonfunctional human eyes. Arch Ophthalmol 1995;113:159-167.
5. Nosé W, Neves RA, Burris TE, Schanzlin DJ, Belfort R, Jr. Intrastromal corneal ring: 12-month sighted myopic eyes. J Refract Surg 1996; 12(1):20-28.
6. Schanzlin DJ, Asbell, PA, Burris TE and Durrie DS. The ICRS: Phase II results for the correction of myopia. Ophthalmology 1997; 104(7):1067-78.
7. Waring GO III, Abbott RL, Asbell PA, Assil KK, Burris TE, Durrie DS, Fouraker BD, et al. One-year outcomes of Intrastromal Corneal Ring Segments for the correction of -1.0 to -3.5 diopters of myopia. In American Academy of Ophthalmology Meeting, New Orleans, LA, 1998.
8. Waring GO III, Abbott RL, Asbell PA, Assil KK, Burris TE, Durrie DS, Fouraker BD, et al. One-year outcomes of Intrastromal Corneal Ring Segments for the correction of -1.0 to -3.5 diopters of myopia. Submitted for publication, Ophthalmology, 1998.
9. Burris TE, Holmes-Higgin DK, Silvestrini TA, Scholl JA, Proudfoot RA, Baker PC. Corneal asphericity in eye bank eye implanted with the intrastromal corneal ring. J Refract Surg 1997;13(6):556-567.
10. Holmes-Higgin, DK, Baker, PC, Burris, TE, Silvestrini, TA. Characterization of the aspheric corneal surface in ICRS® (Intrastromal Corneal Ring Segments) Patients. IOVS 1998;39(4):S74.

11. Holmes-Higgin, DK, Baker, PC, Burris, TE, Silvestrini, TA. Characterization of the aspheric corneal surface with the ICRS® (Intrastromal Corneal Ring Segments). Accepted for publication, J Refract Surg 1999.
12. Holmes-Higgin, DK, Burris, TE, Silvestrini, TA, Baker, PC, Torres, AR and the Phase III ICRS Study Group. Topographic corneal asphericity and visual outcome with the ICRS® (Intrastromal Corneal Ring Segments). In Pre-AAO International Society of Refractive Surgery Meeting. New Orleans, LA, 1998.
13. Waring GO, Hannush SB, Bogan SJ, Maloney RK. Classification of corneal topography with videokeratography. In: Schanzlin DS, Rubins B (Eds). Corneal Topography. New York, NY:Springer Verlag; 1992:47-73.
14. Burris TE, Holmes-Higgin DK, Asbell PA, Durrie DS, Schanzlin DJ. Month 3 corneal topography analysis of patients with the ICRS (Intrastromal Corneal Ring Segments). In American Academy of Ophthalmology Meeting, Atlanta, GE, 1996.
15. Bogan SJ, Waring GO, Ibrahim O, Drews C, Curtis L. Classification of normal corneal topography based on computer assisted videokeratography. Arch Ophthalmol 1990; 108:945-949.
16. Lin DTC, Sutton HF, Berman M. Corneal topography following excimer photorefractive keratectomy for myopia. J Cataract Refract Surg 1993; 19(Suppl):149-154.
17. Lin DTC. Corneal topographic analysis after excimer photorefractive keratectomy. Ophthalmology 1994;101(8):1432-1439.
18. Young JA, Siegel IM. Three dimensional digital subtraction modeling of corneal topography. J Refract Surg 1995; 11:188-193.
19. Hersh PS, Schwartz-Goldstein BH, and the PRK study group. Corneal topography of Phase III excimer laser photorefractive keratectomy. Ophthalmology 1995; 102:963-978.
21. Levin S, Carson CA, Garrett SK, Taylor HR. Prevalence of central islands after excimer laser refractive surgery. J Cataract Refract Surg 1995; 21:21-26.
22. Burris TE, Holmes-Higgin DK, Abbot RL, Asbell PA, Durrie DS, Verity SM, Schanzlin DJ. Corneal topography after removal of the ICRS. IOVS 39(4):S74.
23. Burris TE, Abbott RL, Asbell PA, Assil KK, Durrie DS, Fouraker BD, Lindstrom RL, McDonald JE II, Schanzlin DJ, Verity SM, Waring GO III. Reversibility of refractive effect after removal of the ICRS. In Pre-AAO International Society of Refractive Surgery Meeting. New Orleans, LA, 1998.
24. Holmes-Higgin DK, Burris TE, Silvestrini TA, Scholl JA, Proudfoot RA. Evaluation of topographic corneal astigmatism change in eye bank eyes with variable thickness ICR® prototypes. IOVS 1996;37(3):S66.
25. Burris TE, Holmes-Higgin DK, Silvestrini TA, Scholl JA, Proudfoot, RA. Preliminary eye bank eye topography studies with toric ICR prototypes developed to reduce astigmatism. IOVS 1996;37(3):S66.
28. Belfort R Jr, Nose W, Neves R, Burris TE, Silvestrini TA, Schanzlin DJ. Intra Corneal Implants. In World Congress on the Cornea IV Meeting, Orlando, FL, 1996.
29. Shivitz IA, Arrowsmith PN. Corneal sensitivity after radial keratotomy. Ophthalmology 1988;95:827-832.
30. Campos M, Hertzog L, Garbus JJ, McDonnell PJ. Corneal sensitivity after photorefractive keratectomy. Am J Ophthalmol 1992;114:51-54.
31. John T. Corneal sensation after small incision, sutureless, one-handed phacoemulsification. J Cataract Refract Surg 1995;21:425-428.
32. Mathers WD, Jester JV, Lemp MA. Return of human corneal sensitivity after penetrating keratoplasty. Arch Ophthalmol 1988;106:210-211.

IV

Cataract

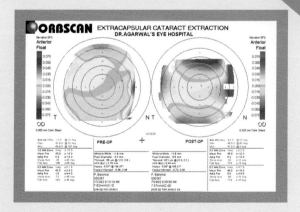

Chapter

21

Corneal Topography in Cataract Surgery

Sunita Agarwal
Athiya Agarwal
Amar Agarwal

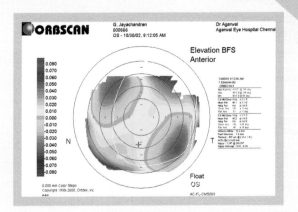

INTRODUCTION

Topography is defined as the science of describing or representing the features of a particular place in detail. In corneal topography, the place is the cornea, i.e. we describe the features of the cornea in detail.

The word Topography is derived[1,2] from two Greek words:

TOPOS- meaning place

and

GRAPHIEN- meaning to write

CORNEA

There are basically three refractive elements of the eye- namely; axial length, lens and cornea. The cornea is the most important plane or tissue for refraction. This is because it has the highest refractive power (which is about + 45 D) and it is easily accessible to the surgeon without going inside the eye.

To understand the cornea, one should realize that the cornea is a parabolic curve – its radius of curvature differs from center to periphery. It is steepest in the center and flatter in the periphery. For all practical purposes the central cornea, that is the optical zone is taken into consideration, when you are doing a refractive surgery. A flatter cornea has less refraction power and a steeper cornea has a higher refraction power. If we want to change the refraction we must make the steeper diameter flatter and the flatter diameter steeper.

KERATOMETRY

The keratometer was invented by Hermann Von Helmholtz and modified by Javal, Schiotz, etc. If we place an object in front of a convex mirror we get a virtual, erect and minified image (Figure 21.1). A keratometer in relation to the cornea is just like an object in front of a convex reflecting mirror. Like in a convex reflecting surface, the image is located posterior to the cornea. The cornea behaves as a convex reflecting mirror and the mires of the keratometer are the objects. The radius of curvature of the cornea's anterior surface determines the size of the image.

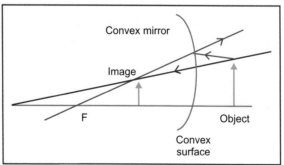

FIGURE 21.1: Physics of a convex mirror. Note the image is virtual, erect and minified. The cornea acts like the convex mirror and the mire of the keratometer is the object

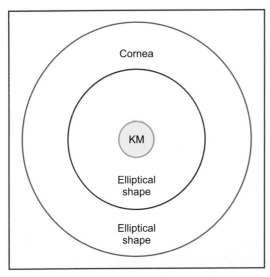

FIGURE 21.2: Keratometers measure the central 3 mm of the cornea, which generally behaves like a sphere or a spherocylinder. This is the reason why keratometers are generally accurate. But in complex situations like in keratoconus or refractive surgery they become inaccurate

The keratometer projects a single mire on the cornea and the separation of the two points on the mire is used to determine corneal curvature. The zone measured depends upon corneal curvature -–the steeper the cornea, the smaller the zone. For example, for a 36 D cornea, the keratometer measures a 4 mm zone and for a 50 D cornea, the size of the cone is 2.88 mm.

Keratometers are accurate only when the corneal surface is a sphere or a spherocylinder. Actually, the shape of the anterior surface of the cornea is more than a sphere or a spherocylinder. But keratometers measure the central 3 mm of the cornea, which behaves like a sphere or a spherocylinder. This is the reason why Helmholtz could manage with the keratometer (Figure 21.2). This is also the reason why most ophthalmologists can manage management of cataract surgery with the keratometer. But today, with refractive surgery, the ball game has changed. This is because when the cornea has complex central curves like in keratoconus or after refractive surgery, the keratometer cannot give good results and becomes inaccurate. Thus, the advantages of the keratometer like speed, ease of use, low cost and minimum maintenance is obscured.

The objects used in the keratometer are referred to as mires. Separation of two points on the mire are used to determine corneal curvature. The object in the keratometer can be rotated with respect to the axis. The disadvantages of the keratometer are that they measure only a small region of the cornea. The peripheral regions are ignored. They also lose accuracy when measuring very steep or flat corneas. As the keratometer assumes the cornea to be symmetrical it becomes at a disadvantage if the cornea is asymmetrical as after refractive surgery.

KERATOSCOPY

To solve the problem of keratometers, scientists worked on a system called Keratoscopy. In this, they projected a beam of concentric rings and observed them over a wide expanse of the corneal surface. But this was not enough and the next step was to move into computerized videokeratography.

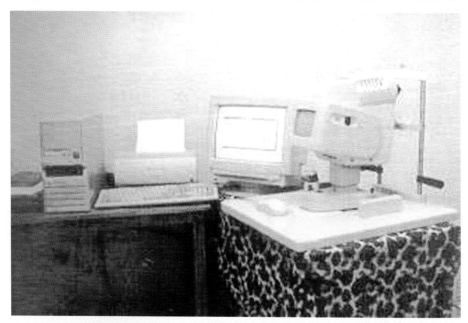

FIGURE 21.3: Placido type corneal topography machine

COMPUTERIZED VIDEOKERATOGRAPHY

In this some form of light like a placido disk is projected onto the cornea. The cornea modifies this light and this modification is captured by a video camera. This information is analyzed by computer software and the data is then displayed in a variety of formats. To simplify the results to an ophthalmologist, Klyce in 1988 started the corneal color maps. The corneal color maps display the estimate of corneal shape in a fashion that is understandable to the ophthalmologist. Each color on the map is assigned a defined range of measurement. The placido type topographic machines (Figure 21.3) do not assess the posterior surface of the cornea. The details of the corneal assessment can be done only with the Orbscan (Bausch & Lomb)) as both anterior and posterior surface of the cornea are assessed.

ORBSCAN

The ORBSCAN (Bausch & Lomb)) corneal topography system (Figure 21.4) uses a scanning optical slit scan that is fundamentally different than the corneal topography that analyses the reflected images from the anterior corneal surface. (Read Orbscan chapter) The high-resolution video camera captures 40 light slits at 45 degrees angle projected through the cornea similarly as seen during slit lamp examination. The slits are projected on to the anterior segment of the eye: the anterior cornea, the posterior cornea, the anterior iris and anterior lens. The data collected from these four surfaces are used to create a topographic map.

NORMAL CORNEA

In a normal cornea (Figure 21.5), the nasal cornea is flatter than the temporal cornea. This is similar to the curvature of the long end of an ellipse. If we see Figure 21.5 then we will notice the values written

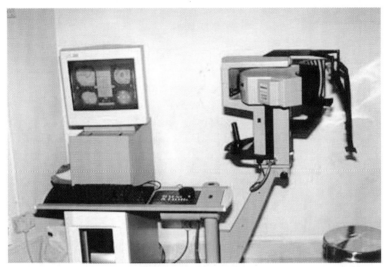

FIGURE 21.4: Orbscan

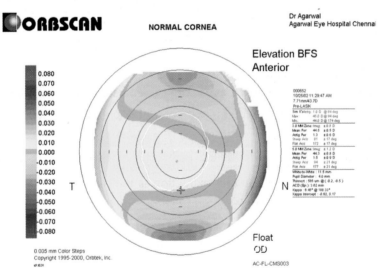

FIGURE 21.5: Topography of a normal cornea

on the right end of the pictures. These indicate the astigmatic values. In that is written Max K is 45 @ 84 degrees and Min K is 44 @ 174 degrees. This means the astigmatism is + 1.0 D at 84 degrees. This is with the rule astigmatism as the astigmatism is Plus at 90 degrees axis. If the astigmatism was Plus at 180 degrees then it is against the rule astigmatism. The normal corneal topography can be round, oval, irregular, symmetric bow tie or asymmetric bow tie in appearance. If we see Figure 21.6 we will see a case of astigmatism in which the astigmatism is + 4.9 D at 146 degrees. *These figures show the curvature of the anterior surface of the cornea. It is important to remember that these are not the keratometric maps. So the blue/green color denote steepening and the red colors denote flattening.* If we want the red to denote steepening then we can invert the colors.

289

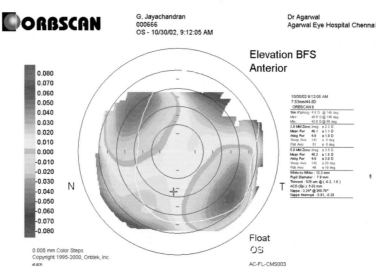

FIGURE 21.6: Topography showing an astigmatic cornea

CATARACT SURGERY

Corneal topography is extremely important in cataract surgery. *The smaller the size of the incision lesser the astigmatism and earlier stability of the astigmatism will occur.* One can reduce the astigmatism or increase the astigmatism of a patient after cataract surgery. The simple rule to follow is that- *wherever you make an incision that area will flatten and wherever you apply sutures that area will steepen.*

EXTRACAPSULAR CATARACT EXTRACTION

One of the problems in Extracapsular cataract extraction is the astigmatism which is created as the incision size is about 10-12 mm. In Figure 21.7, you can see the topographic picture of a patient after extracapsular cataract extraction (ECCE). You can see the picture on the left is the pre-op photo and the picture on the right is a post-op day 1 photo. Preoperatively one will notice the astigmatism is + 1.0 D at 12 degrees and postoperatively it is + 4.8 D at 93 degrees. This is the problem in ECCE. In the immediate postoperative period the astigmatism is high which would reduce with time. But the predictability of astigmatism is not there which is why smaller incision cataract surgery is more successful.

NON FOLDABLE IOL

Some surgeons perform phaco and implant a non-foldable IOL in which the incision is increased to 5.5 to 6 mm. In such cases the astigmatism is better than in an ECCE. In Figure 21.8, the pictures are of a patient who has had a non-foldable IOL. Notice in this the pre-operative astigmatism is + 0.8 D @ 166 degrees. This is the left eye of the patient. If we had done a phaco with a foldable IOL the astigmatism would have been nearly the same or reduced as our incision would have come in the area of the astigmatism. But in this case after a phaco a non-foldable IOL was implanted. The postoperative astigmatism one week post-op is + 1.8 D @ 115 degrees. You can notice from the two pictures the astigmatism has increased.

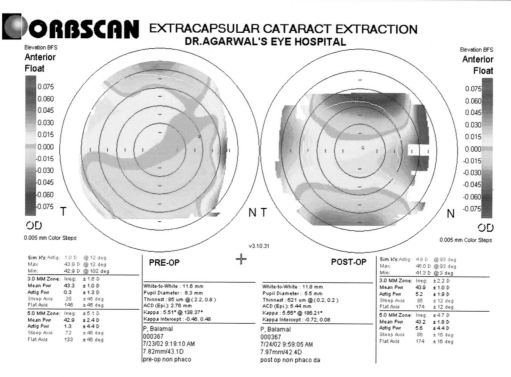

FIGURE 21.7: Topography after extracapsular cataract extraction (ECCE). The figure 21.on the left shows astigmatism of + 1.1 D at 12 degrees preoperatively. The astigmatism has increased to + 4.8 D as seen in the figure 21.on the right.

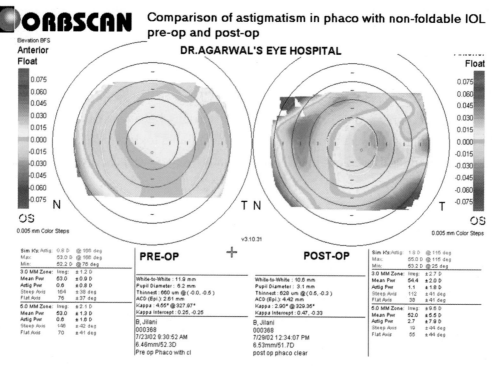

FIGURE 21.8: Topography of a non – foldable IOL implantation

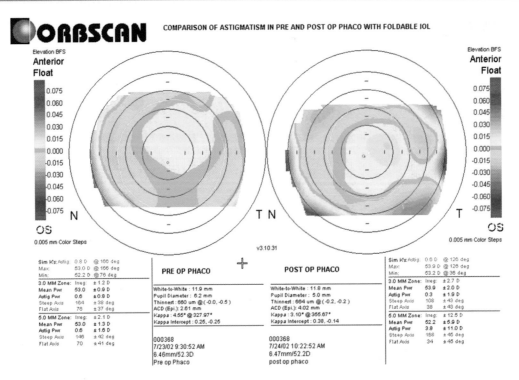

FIGURE 21.9: Topography of phaco cataract surgery with a foldable IOL implantation.

FOLDABLE IOL

In phaco with a foldable IOL the amount of astigmatism created is much less than in a non-foldable IOL. Let us look now at Figure 21.9. The patient as you can see has negligible astigmatism in the left eye. The picture on the left shows a pre-operative astigmatism of + 0.8 D at 166 degrees axis. Now, we operate generally with a temporal clear corneal approach, so in the left eye, the incision will be generally at the area of the steepend axis. This will reduce the astigmatism. If we see the post-op photo of day one we will see the astigmatism is only + 0.6 D @ 126 degrees. This means that after a day, the astigmatism has not changed much and this shows a good result. This patient had a foldable IOL implanted under the no anesthesia cataract surgical technique after a Phaco cataract surgery with the size of the incision being 2.8 mm.

ASTIGMATISM INCREASED

If we are not careful in selecting the incision depending upon the corneal topography we can burn our hands. Figure 21.10, illustrates a case in which astigmatism has increased due to the incision being made in the wrong meridian. The patient had a 2.8 mm incision with a foldable IOL implanted after a phaco cataract surgery under the no anesthesia cataract surgical technique. Both the pictures are of the right eye. In Figure 21.10, look at the picture on the left. In the picture on the left, you can see the patient has an astigmatism of + 1.1 D at axis 107 degrees. As this is the right eye with this astigmatism we should have made a superior incision to reduce the preoperative astigmatism. But by mistake we made a

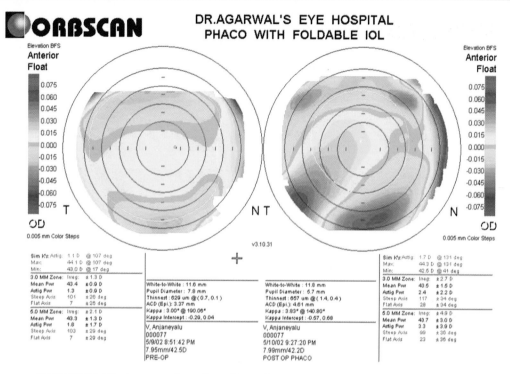

FIGURE 21.10: Increase in astigmatism after cataract surgery due to incision being made in the wrong meridian. Topography of a phaco with foldable IOL implantation.

temporal clear corneal incision. This has increased the astigmatism. Now if we wanted to flatten this case, we should have made the incision where the steeper meridian was. That was at the 105 degrees axis. But because we were doing routinely temporal clear corneal incisions, we made the incision in the opposite axis. Now look at the picture on the right. The astigmatism has increased from + 1.1 D to + 1.7 D. This shows a bad result. If we had made the incision superiorly at the 107 degrees axis, we would have flattened that axis and the astigmatism would have been reduced.

BASIC RULE

The basic rule to follow is to look at the number written in red. The red numbers indicate the plus axis. If the difference in astigmatism is say 3 D at 180 degrees, it means the patient has + 3 D astigmatism at axis 180 degrees. This is against the rule astigmatism. In such cases, make your clear corneal incision at 180 degrees so that you can flatten this steepness. This will reduce the astigmatism.

UNIQUE CASE

In Figure 21.11, the patient had a temporal clear corneal incision for Phaco cataract surgery under no anesthesia with a nonfoldable IOL. Both the pictures are of the left eye. The Figure 21.11 on the left shows the postoperative topographic picture. The postoperative astigmatism was + 1.8 D at axis 115 degrees. This patient had three sutures in the site of the incision. These sutures were put as a nonfoldable IOL had been implanted in the eye with a clear corneal incision. When this patient came for a follow up

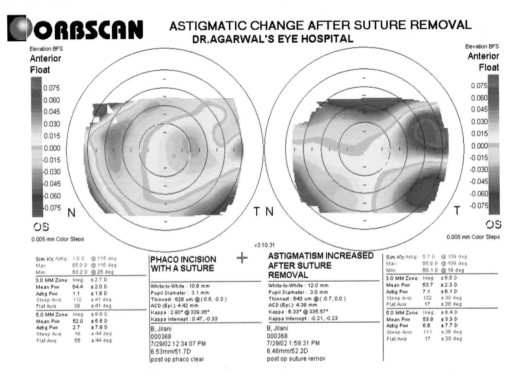

FIGURE 21.11: Unique case- topographic changes after suture removal

we removed the sutures. The next day the patient came to us with loss of vision. On examination, we found the astigmatism had increased. We then took another topography. The picture on the right is of the topography after removing the sutures. The astigmatism increased to + 5.7 D. So, one should be very careful in analyzing the corneal topography when one does suture removal also. To solve this problem one can do an astigmatic keratotomy.

PHAKONIT

Phakonit is a technique devised by Dr Amar Agarwal in which the cataract is removed through a 0.9-mm incision. The advantage of this is obvious. The astigmatism created by a 0.9-mm incision is very little compared to a 2.6 mm phaco incision. Today with the rollable IOL and the Acritec IOL's which are ultra-small incision IOL's one can pass IOL's through sub 1.4 mm incisions. This is seen clearly in Figure 21.12 and 13. Figure 21.12 shows the comparison aftert Phakonit with a Rollable IOL and Figure 21.13 with an Acritec IOL. If you will see the preoperative and the postoperative photographs in comparison you will see there is not much difference between the two. In this case a rollable IOL was implanted. The point which we will notice in this picture is that the difference between the preoperative photo and the one day post-op photo is not much.

SUMMARY

Corneal topography is an extremely important tool for the ophthalmologist. It is not only the refractive surgeon who should utilize this instrument but also the cataract surgeon. The most important refractive

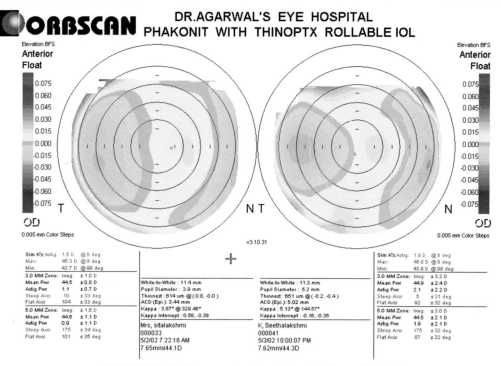

FIGURE 21.12: Topography of a phakonit with a rollable IOL

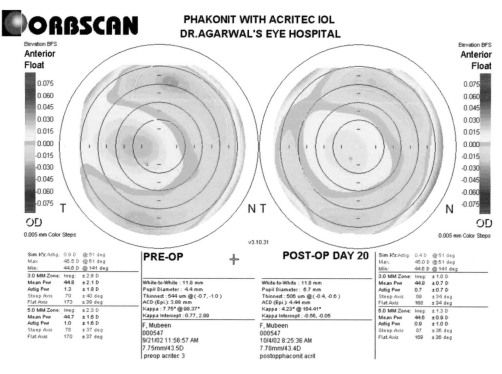

FIGURE 21.13: Topography of a phakonit with an acritec IOL

surgery done in the world is cataract surgery and not LASIK (Laser-in-situ keratomileusis) or PRK (Photorefractive keratectomy). With more advancements in corneal topography, Topographic- Assisted Lasik will become available to everyone with an Excimer Laser. One might also have the corneal topographic machine fixed onto the operating microscope so that one can easily reduce the astigmatism of the patient.

REFERENCES

1. Gills JP, et al. Corneal topography: The State–of-the Art; New Delhi; Jaypee Brothers, 1996.
2. Sunita Agarwal, Athiya Agarwal, Mahipal S Sachdev, Keiki R Mehta, I Howard Fine, Amar Agarwal. Phacoemulsification, Laser Cataract surgery and Foldable IOL's; New Delhi; Second edition; Jaypee Brothers Medical Publishers (P) Ltd., 2000.

Chapter 22

Corneal Topography in Phakonit with a 5 mm Optic Rollable IOL

Amar Agarwal
Soosan Jacob
Athiya Agarwal
Sunita Agarwal

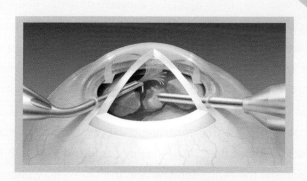

INTRODUCTION

Cataract surgery and intraocular lenses (IOLs) have evolved greatly since the time of intracapsular cataract extraction (ICCE) and the first IOL implantation by Sir Harold Ridley.[1] The size of the cataract incision has constantly been decreasing from the extremely large ones used for ICCE to the slightly smaller ones used in ECCE to the present day small incisions used in phacoemulsification. Phacoemulsification and foldable IOLs are a major milestone in the history of cataract surgery. Large post operative against-the-rule astigmatism were an invariable consequence of ICCE and ECCE. This was minimized to a great extent with the 3.2 mm clear corneal incision used for phacoemulsification but nevertheless some amount of residual postoperative astigmatism was a common outcome. The size of the corneal incision was further decreased by Phakonit [2-4] a technique introduced for the first time by one of us (Am. A), which separates the infusion from the aspiration ports by utilizing a sleeveless phaco probe and an irrigating chopper. The only limitation to thus realizing the goal of astigmatism neutral cataract surgery was the size of the foldable IOL as the wound nevertheless had to be extended for implantation of the conventional foldable IOLs.

ROLLABLE IOL

With the availability of the ThinOptX® rollable IOL (Abingdon, VA, USA), that can be inserted through sub-1.4 mm incision, the full potential of Phakonit could be realized. This lens was created and designed by Wayne Callahan from USA. Subsequently, one of the authors (Am. A) modified the lens by making the optic size 5 mm so that it could go through a smaller incision.

SURGICAL TECHNIQUE

Five eyes of 5 patients underwent Phakonit with implantation of an ultrathin 5 mm optic rollable IOL at Dr Agarwal's Eye Hospital and Eye Research Centre, Chennai. India.

The name PHAKONIT has been given because it shows phacoemulsification (PHAKO) being done with a needle (N) opening via an incision (I) and with the phaco tip (T). A specially designed keratome, an irrigating chopper, a straight blunt rod and a 15° standard phaco tip without an infusion sleeve form the main pre-requisites of the surgery. Viscoelastic is injected with a 26-G needle through the presumed site of side port entry This inflates the chamber and prevents its collapse when the chamber is entered with the keratome. A straight rod is passed through this site to achieve akinesia and a clear corneal temporal valve is made with the keratome (Figure 22.1A). A continuous curvilinear capsulorhexis (CCC) is performed followed by hydrodissection and rotation of the nucleus. After enlarging the side port a 20 Gauge irrigating chopper connected to the infusion line of the phaco machine is introduced with foot pedal on position 1. The phaco probe is connected to the aspiration line and the phaco tip without an infusion sleeve is introduced through the main port (Figure 22.1B). Using the phaco tip with moderate ultrasound power, the center of the nucleus is directly embedded starting from the superior edge of rhexis with the phaco probe directed obliquely downwards towards the vitreous. The settings at this stage are 50 percent phaco power, flow rate 24 ml/min and 110 mm Hg vacuum. When nearly half of

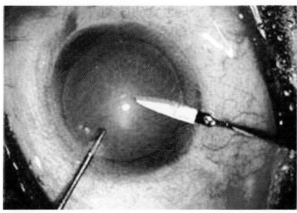

FIGURE 22.1A: Clear-corneal incision made with a specialized keratome. Note the left hand has a straight rod to stabilize the eye

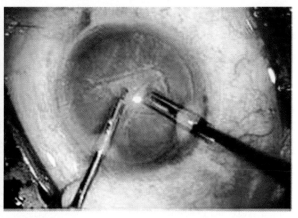

FIGURE 22.1B: Agarwal's phakonit irrigating chopper and sleeveless phako probe inside the eye

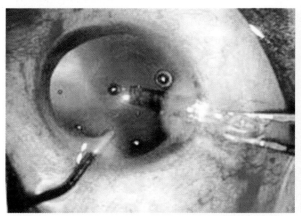

FIGURE 22.1C: The rollable IOL inserted through the incision

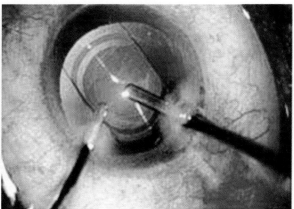

FIGURE 22.1D: Viscoelastic removed using bimanual irrigation aspiration probes

the center of nucleus is embedded, the foot pedal is moved to position 2 as it helps to hold the nucleus due to vacuum rise. To avoid undue pressure on the posterior capsule the nucleus is lifted slightly and with the irrigating chopper in the left hand the nucleus chopped. This is done with a straight downward motion from the inner edge of the rhexis to the center of the nucleus and then to the left in the form of an inverted L shape. Once the crack is created, the nucleus is split till the center. The nucleus is then rotated 180° and cracked again so that the nucleus is completely split into two halves. With the previously described technique, 3 pie-shaped quadrants are created in each half of the nucleus. With a short burst of energy at pulse mode, each pie shaped fragment is lifted and brought at the level of iris where it is further emulsified and aspirated sequentially in pulse mode. Thus, the whole nucleus is removed. Cortical wash-up is then done with the bimanual irrigation aspiration technique.

The lens is taken out from the bottle and placed in a bowl of BSS solution of approximately body temperature to make the lens pliable. It is then rolled with the gloved hand holding it between the index finger and the thumb. The lens is then inserted through the incision carefully (Figure 12.1C). The teardrop on the haptic should be pointing in a clockwise direction so that the smooth optic lenticular surface faces posteriorly. The natural warmth of the eye causes the lens to open gradually. Viscoelastic is then removed with the bimanual irrigation aspiration probes (Figure 12.1D). Figure 22.1 shows different steps of the surgery.

TOPOGRAPHIC ANALYSIS AND ASTIGMATISM

The preoperative best corrected visual acuity (BCVA) ranged from 20/60 to 20/200. The mean preoperative. astigmatism as detected by topographic analysis was 0.98 D ± 0.62 D (range 0.5 to 1.8 D).

The postoperative course was uneventful in all cases. The IOL was well centered in the capsular bag. There were no corneal burns in any of the cases.

Four eyes had a best-corrected visual acuity of 20/30 or better. One eye that had dry ARMD showed an improvement in BCVA from 20/200 to 20/60. Figure 22.2 shows a comparison of the pre and postoperative BCVA. The mean astigmatism on postoperative day 1 on topographic analysis was 1.1 ± 0.61 D (range 0.6 to 1.9 D) as compared to 0.98 D ± 0.62 D (range 0.5 to 1.8 D) preoperatively. The mean astigmatism was 1.02 ± 0.64 D (range 0.3 to 1.7 D) by 3 months postoperatively. Figures 22.3 and 22.4 shows mean astigmatism over time. Figures 22.5A and 22.5B show a comparison of the astigmatism over the pre- and postsurgical period.

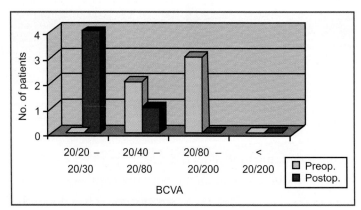

FIGURE 22.2: Comparison of pre- and postoperative BCVA

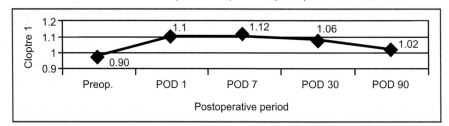

FIGURE 22.3: Mean astigmatism over time

MICROPHAKONIT (CATARACT SURGERY THROUGH A 0.7 MM TIP)

In 1998, Dr Amar Agarwal performed 1 mm cataract surgery by a technique called phakonit (Figure 22.7) (phako being done with a needle incision technology). This used the air pump or gas forced

Time	Eyes	Mean	Std. Dev.	Minimum	Maximum
Preop.	5	0.98	0.62	0.5	1.8
POD 1	5	1.1	0.61	0.6	1.9
POD 7	5	1.12	0.58	0.5	1.7
POD 30	5	1.08	0.62	0.5	1.8
POD 90	5	1.02	0.64	0.3	1.7

FIGURE 22.4: Table showing pre- and postoperative mean astigmatism

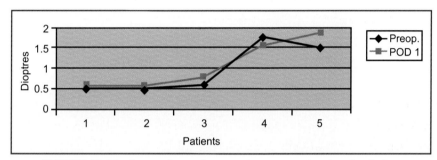

FIGURE 22.5A: Comparison of pre- and postoperative day 1 cylinder

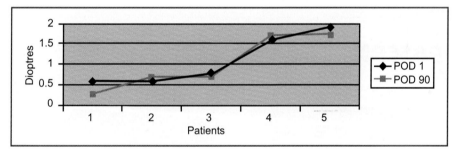

FIGURE 22.5B: Comparison of 1 day postoperative and
3 months postoperative astigmatism

infusion started by Sunita Agarwal to prevent any surge in the eye (Figure 22.8). Dr Jorge Alio coined the term *microincision cataract surgery* (MICS) for all surgeries including laser cataract surgery and phakonit. Dr Randall Olson first used a 0.8 mm phaco needle and a 21-gauge irrigating chopper and called it microphaco. On May 21st 2005, for the first time a 0.7 mm phaco needle tip with a 0.7 mm irrigating chopper was used by Dr. Agarwal to remove cataracts through the smallest incision possible as of now. This is called microphakonit (Figure 12.9). The 22-gauge(0.7 mm) irrigating chopper connected to the infusion line of with foot pedal on position. The phaco probe is connected to the aspiration line and the 0.7 mm phaco tip without an infusion sleeve is introduced through the clear corneal incision. Using the phaco tip with moderate ultrasound power, the center of the nucleus is directly embedded starting from the superior edge of rhexis with the phaco probe directed obliquely downwards toward the vitreous. The settings at this stage are 50% phaco power, flow rate 24 ml/min, and 110 mm Hg vacuum. Using the karate chop technique, the nucleus is chopped. Thus, the whole nucleus is removed.

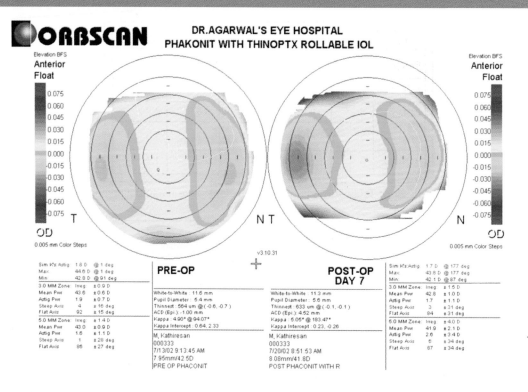

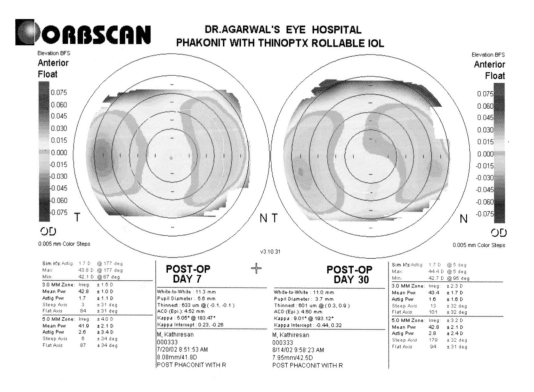

FIGURES 22.6A and B: Topographical comparison during different surgical periods

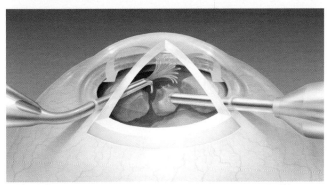

FIGURE 22.7: Phakonit done. Notice the irrigating chopper with an end opening. (Courtesy Larry Laks, MST, USA)

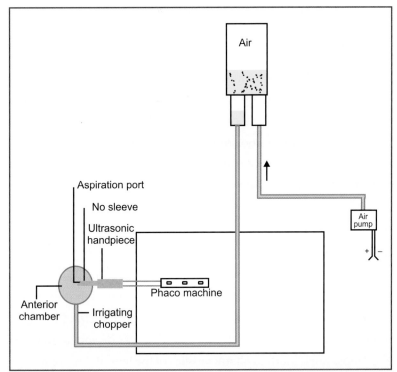

FIGURE 22.8: Air pump used to prevent surge in phaco and phakonit. In the air pump system, a locally manufactured automated device used in fish tanks (aquariums) to supply oxygen is utilized to forcefully pump air into the irrigation bottle. It has an electromagnetic motor that moves a lever attached to a collapsible rubber cap. There is an inlet with a valve that sucks in atmospheric air as the cap expands. On collapsing, the valve closes and the air is pushed into an intravenous (IV) line connected to the infusion bottle. The lever vibrates at a frequency of approximately 10 oscillations per second. The electromagnetic motor is weak enough to stop once the pressure in the closed system (i.e. the AC) reaches about 50 mm Hg. The rubber cap ceases to expand at this pressure level. A micropore air filter is used between the air pump and the infusion bottle so that the air pumped into the bottle is clean of particulate matter

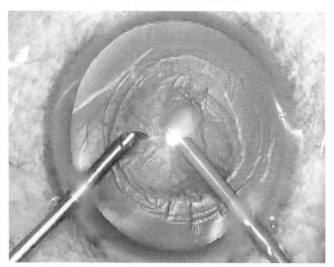

FIGURE 22.9: Microphakonit being performed with a 0.7 mm irrigating chopper and a 0.7 mm sleeveless phaco needle

Cortical washup is then done with the bimanual irrigation aspiration (0.7 mm set) technique. During the microphakonit procedure, gas forced infusion is used. The instruments are made by Larry Laks from Microsurgical Technology, USA. At the time of this writing, this is the smallest one can use for cataract surgery. With time, one would be able to go smaller with better instruments and devices. The problem at present is the IOL. We have to get good quality IOLs going through sub-1 mm cataract surgical incisions so that the real benefit of microphakonit can be given to the patient.

DISCUSSION

Cataract surgery has witnessed great advancements in surgical technique, foldable IOLs and phaco technology. This has made possible easier and safer cataract extraction utilizing smaller incision. With the advent of the latest IOL technology which enables implantation through ultrasmall incisions, it is clear that this will soon replace routine phacoemulsification through the standard 3.2 mm incisions. The ThinOptX® IOL design is based on the Fresnel principle. This was designed by Wayne Callahan (USA). Flexibility and good memory are important characteristics of the lens. It is manufactured from hydrophilic acrylic materials and is available in a range from –25 to +30 with the lens thickness ranging from 30 μm up to 350 μm. One of the authors (Am. A) has modified the lens further by reducing the optic size to 5 mm to go through a smaller incision. The lens is now undergoing clinical-trials in Europe and the USA.

In this study, no intraoperative complications were encountered during CCC, phacoemulsification, cortical aspiration or IOL lens insertion in any of the cases. The mean phacoemulsification time was 0.66 minutes. Previous series by the same authors showed more than 300 eyes where cataract surgery was successfully performed using the sub-1 mm incision.[3] Our experience and that of several other surgeons suggests that with existing phacoemulsification technology, it is possible to perform phacoemulsification through ultra-small incisions without significant complications.[2-6] In a recent study from Japan, Tsuneoka and associates[6] used a sleeveless phaco tip to perform bimanual phacoemulsification in 637 cataractous eyes. All cataracts were safely removed by these authors through an incision of 1.4 mm or smaller that was widened for IOL insertion, without a case of thermal burn and with few intraoperative complications. Furthermore, ongoing research for the development of laser probes[7,8] cold phaco, and microphaco confirms the interest of leading ophthalmologists and manufacturers in the direction of ultra-small incisional cataract surgery (Fine IN, Olson RJ, Osher RH, Steinert RF. Cataract technology makes strides. Ophthalmology Times, December 1, 2001, pp 12-15).

The postoperative course was uneventful in all the cases. The IOL was well centered in the capsular bag. There were no significant corneal burns in any of the cases. Final visual outcome was satisfactory with 4 of the eyes having a BCVA of 20/30 or better. One eye that had dry ARMD showed an improvement in BCVA from 20/200 to 20/60. Thus, the lens was found to have satisfactory optical performance within the eye. In our study, the mean astigmatism on topographical analysis was 0.98 ± 0.62 D (range 0.5 to 1.8 D) preoperatively, 1.1 ± 0.61 D (range 0.6 to 1.9 D) on postoperative day 1 and 1.02 ± 0.64 D (range 0.3 to 1.7 D) by 3 months post operatively. Figures 22.5A and B showing a comparison of the pre and postoperative astigmatism indicate clearly that Phakonit with an ultrathin 5 mm rollable IOL is virtually astigmatically neutral. Figures 22.6A and B depicting the topography comparison in different surgical periods show clearly the virtual astigmatic neutrality of the procedure and stability throughout the postoperative course.

There is an active ongoing attempt to develop newer IOLs that can go through smaller and smaller incisions. Phakonit ThinOptX® modified ultrathin rollable IOL is the first prototype IOL which can go through sub-1.4 mm incisions. Research is also in progress to manufacture this IOL using hydrophobic acrylic biomaterials combined with square-edged optics to minimize posterior capsule opacification.

CONCLUSION

Phakonit with an ultrathin 5 mm optic rollable IOL implantation is a safe and effective technique of cataract extraction, the greatest advantage of this technique being virtual astigmatic neutrality.

REFERENCES

1. Apple DJ, Auffarth GU, Peng Q, Visessook N. Foldable intraocular lenses: evolution, clinicopathologic correlations, complications. Thorofare: Slack , Inc., 2000.
2. Agarwal A, Agarwal A, Agarwal S, et al. Phakonit: phacoemulsification through a 0.9 mm corneal incision. J Cataract Refract Surg 2001; 27:1548-52.
3. Agarwal A, Agarwal A, Agarwal A, et al. Phakonit: lens removal through a 0.9 mm incision (Letter). J Cataract Refract Surg 2001; 27:1531-32.
4. Agarwal A, Agarwal S, Agarwal A. Phakonit and laser phaconit: lens removal through a 0.9 mm incision. In Agarwal S, Agarwal A, Sachdev MS, Fine IH, Agarwal A, (Eds): Phacoemulsification, laser cataract surgery and foldable IOLs. New Delhi: Jaypee Brothers Medical Publishers (P) Ltd., 2000; 204-16.
5. Tsuneoka H, Shiba T, Takahashi Y. Feasibility of ultrasound cataract surgery with a 1.4 mm incision. J Cataract Refract Surg 2001; 27:934-940.
6. Tsuneoka H, Shiba T, Takahashi Y. Ultrasonic phacoemulsification using a 1.4 mm incision: clinical results. J Cataract Refract Surg 2002;28:81-86.
7. Kanellpoupolos AJ. A prospective clinical evaluation of 100 consecutive laser cataract procedures using the Dodick photolysis neodymium: Yittrium-aluminum-garnet system. Ophthalmology 2001;108:1-6.
8. Dodick JM. Laser phacolysis of the human cataractous lens. Dev Ophthalmol 1991; 22:58-64.

Index